Modern Neuromuscular Techniques

For Churchill Livingstone:

Publishing Director, Health Professions: Mary Law
Project Development Manager: Katrina Mather
Project Manager: Wendy Gardiner
Designer: Judith Wright

Modern Neuromuscular Techniques

 with accompanying CD-ROM

Leon Chaitow ND DO

Osteopathic Practitioner and Senior Lecturer,
University of Westminster, London, UK

with contributions from

Judith DeLany LMT

(Chapter 10: American neuromuscular therapy)
Director of Neuromuscular Therapy Training Center,
St Petersburg, Florida, USA

Dennis J Dowling DO FAAO

(Chapter 11: PINS technique)
Professor and Chairman
The Stanley Schiowitz DO FAAO Department of Osteopathic Manipulative Medicine,
New York College of Osteopathic Medicine, New York Institute of Technology, Old Westbury,
New York, USA

Foreword by

David Peters MB ChB DO

Clinical Director, School of Integrated Health,
University of Westminster, London, UK

Illustrated by

Graeme Chambers BA (HONS)

Medical Artist

SECOND EDITION

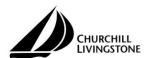

CHURCHILL LIVINGSTONE
An imprint of Elsevier Science Limited

First edition 1996
Second edition 2003

ISBN 0 443 07158 6

British Library Cataloguing in Publication Data
A catalogue record for this book is available from the British Library

Library of Congress Cataloging in Publication Data
A catalog record for this book is available from the Library of Congress

Every effort has been made by the author to contact holders of copyright to obtain permission to reproduce copyright material. However, if any have been inadvertantly overlooked, the publishers will be pleased to make the necessary arrangements at the first opportunity.

Note
Medical knowledge is constantly changing. As new information becomes available, changes in treatment, procedures, equipment and the use of drugs become necessary. The author, contributors and the publishers have taken care to ensure that the information given in this text is accurate and up to date. However, readers are strongly advised to confirm that the information, especially with regard to drug usage, complies with the latest legislation and standards of practice.

Neither the publishers nor the author will be liable for any loss or damage of any nature occasioned to or suffered by any person acting or refraining from acting as a result of reliance on the material contained in this publication.

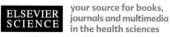

ELSEVIER SCIENCE — your source for books, journals and multimedia in the health sciences

www.elsevierhealth.com

Printed in China by RDC Group Limited

Contents

The CD-ROM accompanying this text includes video sequences of all the techniques indicated by the ⊙ icon. To look at the video for a given technique, click on the relevant icon on the CD-ROM. The CD-ROM is designed to be used in conjunction with the text and not as a stand-alone product.

Abbreviations

ACh	acetylcholine		**MI**	mechanical interface
ASIS	anterior superior iliac spine		**MPS**	myofascial pain syndrome
ATP	adenosine triphosphate		**MRT**	myofascial release technique
CFS	chronic fatigue syndrome		**NGF**	nerve growth factor
CNS	central nervous system		**NGP**	noxious generative point
CSF	cerebrospinal fluid		**NMT**	neuromuscular technique/therapy (USA)
CTM	connective tissue massage			
EAV	electroacupuncture according to Voll		**PINS**	progressive inhibition of neuromuscular structures
EMG	electromyography			
FMS	fibromyalgia syndrome		**PIR**	post-isometric relaxation
FPR	facilitated positional release		**PNF**	proprioceptive neuromuscular facilitation
GAS	general adaptation syndrome			
HIV	human immunodeficiency virus		**PRT**	positional release technique
HSZ	hyperalgesic skin zone		**PSIS**	posterior superior iliac spine
HVLA	high-velocity low-amplitude		**RI**	reciprocal inhibition
HVT	high-velocity thrust		**SCM**	sternocleidomastoid
INIT	integrated neuromuscular inhibition technique		**SCS**	strain/counterstrain
			STM	soft tissue manipulation
LAS	local adaptation syndrome		**TCM**	traditional Chinese medicine
MET	muscle energy technique		**TFL**	tensor fascia lata
			TMJ	temporomandibular joint

Foreword

This welcome new edition updates what was already a striking synthesis of theories and techniques. In it, clinicians will find diverse maps and explanations for the tantalising patterns of tender and trigger points they encounter every day. Having revealed a truly extraordinary overlapping of different systems of body mapping the author reviews and analyses them, making links to ways of evaluating each system and for using Neuro-Muscular Therapy (NMT) treatment.

This material alone would make the book essential reading, but in addition there are chapters explaining the origins of soft tissue distress and the generation of trigger and tender points.

The breadth of the book is impressive: while many of its sources are straight from the bodywork 'hall of fame' (F M Alexander, Barlow, Cyriax, Feldenkrais, Lewit, Janda, Stoddard) it also touches on less familiar territory: the emotional and even energetic anatomy of Rolf, Reich, Upledger and Boadella. In so many different ways this book made me aware of the wider horizons of therapeutic bodywork.

The second edition includes a great deal of new information expanding on the concept of NMT. Having found the first edition's section on fibromyalgia especially useful (and been particularly struck by the list differentiating it from myofascial pain syndrome) I was glad to find new sections on trigger point phenomena and myofascial release as well as the latest ideas on NMT in the treatment of fibromyalgia. In explaining the how and why of modern neuromuscular techniques, Leon Chaitow has been assisted by Judith (Walker) DeLany, who has presented details of American NMT. The section on associated techniques has grown too, with a chapter by Professor Dennis Dowling on progressive inhibition of neuromuscular structures (PINS) technique which incorporates up-to-date findings on ischaemic compression. Included too is a review of Dr Nimmo's original research (an American chiropractor who was a pioneer of trigger point therapy) which clearly adds to our understanding of NMT. A CD-ROM containing the complete text and video clips demonstrating techniques completes this rich offering.

I predict that almost every reader will find enlightening new avenues of knowledge and technique here, for the book outlines in effect a whole curriculum on soft tissue work. Perhaps the most important knowledge presented is on the diagnostic and therapeutic value of tender reflex points related to viscero-somatic and somatico-visceral reflexes. It seems more osteopaths have become interested in this area since the first edition – perhaps in part because of it – and I am sure the subject deserves more research to support NMT's potential role across many fields of healthcare. For those who want to explore further, the very extensive references given will enable them to do so.

Leon Chaitow has put the methods of European neuromuscular technique, originated by Stanley Lief DO and his cousin Boris Chaitow DC, into a broader context, and made NMT accessible and credible to a wider range of practitioners and therapists. NMT as Leon presents it, has already made a long-lasting impact on the ways many bodyworkers practice. The book's popularity and the need for a second edition surely confirm that this work will continue to be internationally influential.

2003

David Peters

Acknowledgements

Acknowledgements are divided between the heroes of the past, who developed NMT, and the clinicians and teachers of today, who have helped to widen the use of modern NMT. NMT has evolved over the past three quarters of a century to a position of international usage. It is now widely taught and practised in the USA and Europe, primarily in the UK. This would not have happened without the pioneering work of Stanley Lief ND DO DC, his son Peter Lief DO DC, and Stanley's cousin Boris Chaitow ND DC. As discussed in Chapter 2, Stanley Lief based his early version of NMT on the work of Ayurvedic physician Dewanchand Varma MD, who can therefore justifiably be regarded as the fountainhead of European NMT.

Boris Chaitow, with whom I was privileged to work in the early 1960s, died in 1995, during the editing of the first edition of this book. Boris happily contributed his thoughts and memories of the evolution of NMT in the days when he worked with Stanley Lief at Champneys, Tring, Hertfordshire in the mid-1930s (see some of Boris's quoted material in Chapters 2, 6 and 8 in particular). To Boris in particular I wish to express appreciation for the diligent instruction he provided in this apparently simple, yet fiendishly subtle approach to assessment and treatment of soft tissue dysfunction.

To Stanley and Peter Lief, Brian Youngs ND DO (extensively quoted in this text), Tom Moule ND DO, and his son Terry Moule ND DO (also quoted at length in Chapter 9) and the many others who helped to create NMT, my profound thanks.

NMT is now taught within the undergraduate bodywork scheme at the School of Integrated Health, University of Westminster, London, where its evolution can safely continue. My thanks to all those colleagues at the School who helped to create this safe environment for NMT to be taught, free of political/professional influences.

The American version of NMT, which has undoubtedly been influenced by the European version, but which owes much to the work of Raymond Nimmo DC, Janet Travell MD and David Simons MD, is now safely taught by a number of excellent tutors, including Judith (Walker) DeLany (see Chapter 10) and Paul St John. To all of these I need to express profound thanks for keeping NMT at the forefront of manual therapy. In particular my thanks go to Judith DeLany for her contribution to this book, and for her continuing time, effort and skill in conveying the NMT message to her profession, massage therapy, and to a wider audience of chiropractors, dentists and physical therapists.

To Dennis Dowling DO, who has contributed the chapter on his evolution of an NMT variation, PINS, my profound thanks.

This book, as was the first edition, is affectionately and gratefully dedicated to the memory of Stanley and Peter Lief, and Boris Chaitow.

2003   Leon Chaitow

1

Soft tissue distress

SOMATIC DYSFUNCTION

The musculoskeletal system is the means whereby we act out and express our human existence – 'The primary machinery of life' is what one of osteopathy's greatest researchers, Irwin Korr (1970), called it. While, medically speaking, the musculoskeletal system may lack the glamour and fascination of vital organs and systems, the fact is that the cardiovascular and neuroendocrine and digestive (and other) systems and organs exist only to service this great biomechanical structure through which we live and function. It is by means of our musculoskeletal system (not our kidneys or livers) that we perform tasks, play games, make love, impart treatment, perform on musical instruments, paint and, in these and a multitude of other ways, interact with one another and the planet.

The musculoskeletal system is also by far the greatest energy user in the body, as well as being one of our primary sources of pain, discomfort and disability, whether localised or general, referred or reflex, acute or chronic.

For the purpose of accuracy, a comprehensive term can be used to describe all lesions of the musculoskeletal system – osseous and soft tissue – and this term is 'somatic dysfunction'.

Somatic dysfunction can be defined as any impairment, or altered function, of related components of the somatic system (body framework), i.e. skeletal, arthrodial and myofascial structures, as well as related vascular, lymphatic and neural elements. This general expression

1

(somatic dysfunction) obviously requires specific definition in any given situation, which should include identification of the particular structure, tissue or area involved.

The objectives, if not the methods we are discussing, are not new. Carl McConnell, a major force in early 20th century osteopathy, discussed the soft tissues as follows (McConnell 1962):

A pathological point of prime importance, for example, is that osseous malalignment is sustained by ligamentous rigidity. This rigidity is incepted by way of muscular fascial and tendinous tensions and stresses. Every case portrays a uniqueness in accordance with location, architectural plan and laws, tissue texture, regional and strength ratios, resident properties, environmental settings, resolution of forces etc. Remember I am speaking of the solid biological background of individual pathogenesis, the veritable soil of prediseased conditions. The lack of either sufficient, or efficient, soft-tissue work, is one reason for mediocre technique and recurrence of lesions. The same is evident in the correction of postural defects.

The causes and the results of local and general somatic dysfunction, whether traumatic, functional, postural, pathological or psychological in origin, require a brief overview as we explore different aspects of the issues and the tissues involved, so that some of their possible solutions might become apparent.

Coherent and incoherent patterns

In Chapter 3 we will examine one of the major causes of somatic pain and dysfunction, myofascial trigger points, and the causes of this widespread phenomenon. At that time it will become clear that, while many forms of (referred) pain follow predictable and neurologically coherent pathways, there also exist patterns of pain and dysfunction that do not.

In this chapter our task is to evaluate a variety of influences on the evolution of soft tissue dysfunction, which follow a chronological sequence – the ways in which what is happening in an acute setting differs from what is taking place in a chronic situation, where an initial alarm state progressively gives way to a degree of organisation, adaptation, compensation and (if not

prevented) decompensation and dysfunction. It will also become clear that not all muscles respond to stressors in quite the same way.

Reporting stations

The reporting mechanisms in the soft tissues and joints (Travell & Simons 1983, 1992, Wall & Melzack, 1991) may be thought of as providing answers to a number of basic questions that the central nervous system (CNS) requires answering.

These questions are posed by Keith Buzzell (1970) as follows: 'What is happening in the peripheral machinery with respect to three questions? What is the present position? If there is motion, where is it taking us? And, third, how fast is it taking us there?'

The various neural reporting organs provide a constant information feedback to the CNS and higher centres as to the current state of tone, tension, movement, etc. of the tissues housing them. Such sensory information can be modulated and modified both by the influence of the mind and by changes in blood chemistry, to which the sympathetic nervous system is sensitive. A variety of inputs of information will give the answers to these important questions which allow the body to provide appropriate responses to the demands and adaptations constantly called for by varying situations. Some important structures involved in this internal information highway are summarised in Box 1.1.

There are various ways of 'manipulating' the neural reporting stations to produce physiological modifications in soft tissues – notably of the Golgi tendon organ in muscle energy techniques (METs) and of the spindle in various positional release (PR) techniques, such as strain/counterstrain (SCS) (Jones 1980, Stiles 1984).

Effect of contradictory information

Korr's words regarding the nature of the information that these, and other, reporting stations are providing to the CNS are worth recording (Korr 1976). He reminds us:

Box 1.1 Reporting stations

Ruffini end-organs
These are found within the joint capsule, around the joint, so that each is responsible for describing what is happening over an angle of approximately 15°, with a degree of overlap between it and the adjacent end-organ. These organs are not easily fatigued, and are recruited progressively as the joint moves, so that movement is smooth and not jerky. The prime concern of Ruffini end-organs is to maintain a steady position. They are also, to some extent, concerned with reporting the direction of movement.

Golgi end-organs
These, too, adapt slowly, and continue to discharge over a lengthy period. They are found in the ligaments associated with the joint. Unlike the Ruffini end-organs, which respond to muscular contraction that alters tension in the joint capsule, Golgi end-organs are not thus affected, and can deliver information independently of the state of muscular contraction. This helps the body to know just where the joint is at any given moment, irrespective of muscular activity.

Pacinian corpuscle
This is found in periarticular connective tissue, and adapts rapidly. It triggers discharges, and then ceases reporting in a very short space of time. These messages occur successively, during motion, and the CNS can therefore be aware of the rate of acceleration of movement taking place in the area. It is sometimes called an acceleration receptor.

There are other end-organs, but these three can be seen to provide information regarding the present position, direction and rate of movement of any joint.

Muscle spindle
This receptor is sensitive and complex. It detects, evaluates, reports and adjusts the length of the muscle in which it lies, setting its tone. Acting with the Golgi tendon organ, most of the information as to muscle tone and movement is reported. The spindles lie parallel to the muscle fibres, and are attached either to skeletal muscle or to the tendinous portion of the muscle. Inside the spindle are fibres that may be one of two types. One is described as a 'nuclear bag' fibre, and the other as a chain fibre. In different muscles the ratios of these internal spindle fibres differ. In the centre of the spindle is a receptor called the annulospiral receptor (or primary ending), and on each side of this lies a 'flower spray receptor' (secondary ending). The primary ending discharges rapidly, and this occurs in response to even

small changes in muscle length. The secondary ending compensates for this, because it fires messages only when larger changes in muscle length have occurred.

The spindle is a 'length comparator', and may discharge for long periods at a time. Within the spindle there are fine, intrafusal fibres that alter the sensitivity of the spindle. These can be altered without any actual change taking place in the length of the muscle itself, via an independent γ-efferent supply to the intrafusal fibres. This has implications in a variety of acute and chronic problems.

The proprioceptive role of muscles of the suboccipital region is directly related to the number of spindles per gram of muscle. There are an average of 36 spindles per gram in some of the suboccipital muscles, such as rectus capitis posterior minor, and 30.5 spindles per gram in rectus capitis posterior major, compared, for example, with 7.6 spindles per gram in splenius capitis and just 0.8 spindles per gram in gluteus maximus (Peck et al 1984). McPartland & Brodeur (1999) suggest that 'The high density of muscle spindles found in the RCPM muscles suggests a value . . . [which] lies not in their motor function, but in their role as "proprioceptive monitors" of the cervical spine and head.'

Buzzell (1970) describes the neural connections with the CNS thus:

The central connections of the spindle receptors are important. The annulospiral fibre has the only known monosynaptic relationship in the body. As the fibre passes to the cord, and through the dorsal horn, it goes without synapse, directly to the anterior horn cells that serve the muscle fibres in the vicinity of the spindle. This is the basis of the so called 'tendon reflex', which actually is not a tendon reflex, but simply a spindle response to a sudden elongation of the muscle.

In contrast, the secondary fibres have various synapses in their central connection which can be traced to higher cortical centres. Conscious activity may, therefore, provide a modifying influence, via these structures, on muscle tone. The activities of the spindle appear to provide information regarding length, velocity of contraction and changes in velocity. How long is the muscle? How quickly is it changing length? And what is happening to this rate of change of length? (Gray 1977).

Golgi tendon receptors
These structures indicate how hard the muscle is working, they reflect the tension of the muscle, rather than its length, as does the spindle. If the tendon organ detects excessive overload it may cause cessation of function of the muscle, to prevent damage. This produces relaxation.

The spinal cord is the keyboard on which the brain plays when it calls for activity or for change in activity. But each 'key' in the console sounds, not an individual 'tone', such as the contraction of a particular group of muscle fibres, but a whole

'melody' of activity, even a 'symphony' of motion. In other words, built into the cord is a large repertoire of patterns of activity, each involving the complex, harmonious, delicately balanced orchestration of the contractions and relaxations of many muscles. The brain 'thinks' in terms of whole motions, not individual muscles. It calls selectively, for the preprogrammed patterns in the cord and brain stem, modifying them in countless ways and combining them in an infinite variety of still more complex patterns. Each activity is also subject to further modulation, refinement, and adjustment by the afferent feedback continually streaming in from the participating muscles, tendons, and joints.

This means that the pattern of information fed back to the CNS and brain from neural reporting stations (proprioceptors, mechanoreceptors, nociceptors, etc.) reflects, at any given time, the steady state of joints, the direction as well as speed of alteration in position of joints, together with data on the length of muscle fibres, the degree of load that is being borne, along with the tension this involves. This total input is what occurs, rather than individual pieces of information, as outlined above, from particular reporting stations. But what if any of the mass of information being constantly received should be contradictory, and actually conflict with the other information being received?

Buzzell puts it this way:

It is possible, for example, for the excessive force exerted by external trauma to induce such hyperactivity of the joint and muscle receptors that the reports from that area become gibberish.

Should conflicting reports reach the cord from a variety of sources simultaneously, no discernible pattern may be recognised by the CNS. In such a case no adequate response would be forthcoming, and it is probable that activity would be stopped. Spasm, or splinting, could therefore result.

When somatosensory, vestibular or visual afferent systems provide conflicting information, a variety of symptoms may result. Somatosensory afferent systems depend on input from the soles of the feet, the neck and lumbar spine (Gagey 1986).

Neural 'cross-talk'

Korr (1976) discusses a variety of insults that may result in increased neural excitability: the triggering of a barrage of supernumerary impulses, to and from the cord, and also what he terms 'cross-talk', in which axons may overload and pass impulses to one another directly; muscle contraction disturbances, vasomotion, pain impulses, reflex mechanisms, disturbances in sympathetic activity, all may result from such activity, due to what might be relatively slight tissue changes, for example in the intervertebral foramina.

In addition, Korr states that when any tissue is disturbed, whether bone, joint, ligament or muscle, the local stresses feed constant information to the cord, and effectively jam normal patterned transmission from the periphery. These factors, combined with any mechanical alterations in the tissues, are the background to much somatic dysfunction.

He summarises thus (Korr 1976):

These are the somatic insults, the sources of incoherent, and meaningless feedback, that causes the spinal cord to halt normal operations and to freeze the status quo in the offending and offended tissues. It is these phenomena that are detectable at the body surface, and are reflected in disorders of muscle tension, tissue texture, visceral and circulatory function, and even secretory function; the elements that are so much a part of osteopathic diagnosis.

Mechanisms that alter proprioception
(Lederman 1997)

- Ischaemic or inflammatory events at the receptor site may produce diminished proprioceptive sensitivity due to metabolic byproduct build-up stimulating groups III and IV, mainly pain afferents (this also occurs in muscle fatigue).
- Physical trauma can directly affect receptor axons (articular receptors, muscle spindles and their innervations).
- In direct trauma to muscle, spindle damage can lead to denervation and atrophy (e.g. following whiplash) (Hallgren et al 1993).
- Structural changes in parent tissue leads to atrophy and loss of sensitivity in detecting movement, plus altered firing rate (e.g. during stretching).
- Loss of muscle force (and possibly wasting) may result when a reduced afferent pattern

leads to central reflexogenic inhibition of motor neurons supplying affected muscle.
- Psychomotor influences (e.g. feeling of insecurity) can alter patterns of muscle recruitment at the local level, and may result in disuse muscle weakness.

Trophic neural influences

Setting aside for the moment the obviously important feature of nerves, and their message-carrying functions, we need to consider the less understood role they play in transporting substances – proteins, phospholipids, glycoproteins, neurotransmitters, enzymes, mitochondria and more. Transportation takes place, at a rate of anything from 1 mm/24 h to several hundred millimetres per 24 h, depending on what is being transported and the presence, or absence, of interfering factors. Movement occurs in both directions along nerves, with retrograde (returning from the target tissues towards the CNS) transportation seemingly 'a fundamental means of communication between neurons and between neurons and non-neuronal cells' which strongly influences the 'plasticity of the nervous system', according to Korr's research (Korr 1981).

Patterson & Wurster (1997) note that substances known as nerve growth factors (NGFs) are supplied to the neural structures by the target (end) organ to which neurotrophic substances are being transported. 'If the end organ does not supply the NGF, the synaptic contact is lost.' They continue: 'Complete withdrawal of NGF or of the material delivered by the nerve to its end organ may result in loss of function ... The occurrence of the tissue tensions and fluid flow disturbances often associated with somatic dysfunctions can be factors in altering axoplasmic flows.'

Butler (1991) reports that there are two speeds of delivery of trophic substances via the nerves:

The fast transport moves at approximately 400 mm per day and the substances carried, such as neurotransmitters and transmitter vesicles, are for use in transmission of impulses at the synapse. This transport depends on an uninterrupted supply of

energy from the blood. Various toxic substances and deprivation of blood will slow or block the transport.

In the slow antegrade (delivery) transport (1–6 mm per day), cytoskeletal material is carried.

The return transportation (retrograde) along the nerve carries recycled transmitter vesicles and extracellular material. Butler suggests that 'It also seems likely that the retrograde flow carries "trophic messages" about the status of the axon, the synapse and the general environment around the synapse including the target tissues.'

Very significantly, Butler states: 'If the retrograde flow is altered by physical constriction, or from loss of blood flow, nerve cell body reactions are induced.'

Korr (1981) demonstrated that red (postural) and white (phasic) muscle fibres, which differ morphologically, functionally, chemically and, as we will discover later in this chapter, in their response to stress, can have all of their characteristic differences reversed if their innervation is 'crossed', so that red muscles receive white muscle innervation and vice versa. 'This means, in effect, that the nerve instructs the muscle what kind of muscle to be, and is an expression of a neurally mediated genetic influence', according to Korr (1981).

Neural influences on gene expression

Korr's research (1981) therefore suggests that it is the nervous system that largely determines which genes in a muscle will be suppressed, and which expressed, and this information is carried in the material being transported along the axons. (See Box 1.2 for additional influences on gene expression.)

When a muscle loses contact with its nerve (as in anterior poliomyelitis, for example) atrophy occurs, not as a result of disuse but because of loss of the integrity of the connection between nerve cells and muscle cells at the myoneural junction, where nutrient exchange occurs irrespective of whether or not impulses are being transmitted.

Box 1.2 Gene expression

As noted, Korr (1981) has demonstrated that obstruction of axonal transport modifies gene expression. Additional modulation of gene expression is now known to derive from biomechanical influences, specifically the status of minute structures – integrins – that penetrate the cell surface, acting as a communicating mechanism between the extracellular and intracellular environment.

'Integrin molecules carry tension from the extracellular matrix, across the cell surface to the cytoskeleton which behaves as a tensegrity matrix' (Wang et al 1993).

'Of particular interest are the roles of the integrins in the migration of cells that defend the body against disease and repair injuries' (Horwitz 1997, Hynes 1992).

The precise effects of tense, distorted, contracted, fibrosed or otherwise dysfunctional tissues on the integrins of the cells in these tissues, and subsequent gene expression, are topics for research, as are the potentially beneficial influences of appropriate bodywork designed to normalise such tissues (Oschman 2000).

Moving beyond neural and mechanical influences on gene expression, Martin (2001) interviewed functional medicine expert Jeffrey Bland, who observed:

Functional genomics derived out of the human genome project, in which it was thought that by dissecting the code of life in our 23 pairs of chromosomes, people would be able to understand how they were going to die. They would see locked in their genes heart disease, cancer, diabetes, arthritis,

whatever it might be, and they would tell from these genetic imperfections what day, and what disease, they would finally fall prey to . . . Mendelian determinism . . . said that locked into our genes, when the sperm met the egg, were these strengths and weaknesses that we call the recessive and dominant characteristics of inheritance, . . . [and that] basically if we had the genes for cancer we would die of cancer, [and] if we had the genes for heart disease we would die of heart disease. It turns out that the human genome project has discovered that the genes that we thought were hard-wired to produce these diseases, are not hard-wired at all. Within our genes are multiple messages, and the message that is expressed at any moment – that's in our phenotype – is a consequence of the environmental messages including diet, lifestyle, environment, that wash over our genes to give rise to different expression paths of the genes . . . some may be healthy, some may be unhealthy . . . what we're really seeing is that the major determinants for the expression of genetic patterns, over decades of living, are the decisions that we make, either consciously or subconsciously, every day. How we exercise, how we work, what our stress patterns are.

A picture emerges that suggests structural features, neural function, stress and emotion, as well as environmental factors including diet, all determine the way in which genetic predispositions are either modified, modulated, contained or expressed.

Korr (1981) also describes just how vulnerable these highways of nutrition are:

Any factor which causes derangement of transport mechanisms in the axon, or that chronically alters the quality or quantity of the axonally transported substances, could cause the trophic influences to become detrimental. This alteration in turn would produce aberrations of structure, function and metabolism, thereby contributing to dysfunction and disease.

What could cause such neurotrophic interference? Korr specifies 'Deformations of nerves and roots, such as compression, stretching, angulation and torsion', especially, he tells us, 'in their passage over highly mobile joints, through bony canals, intervertebral foramina, fascial layers and tonically contracted muscles'.

Mention by Korr, Butler and others of the changes that can have a negative influence on neurotrophic flow include altered circulatory status as well as hypertonicity. Trigger point

activity, as we will see in later chapters, should be capable of directly producing just such changes. Normalisation of trigger point activity, and the aetiological factors that produced them, utilising NMT for example, should therefore be at least one way of assisting more normal neurotrophic function.

More general normalisation of somatic dysfunctions, which include not just trigger points but the entire range of shortened, fibrotic, hypertonic, oedematous, inflamed, restricted or otherwise compromised soft and osseous structures, can therefore be seen to offer benefit in restoration of neurotrophic function, and therefore of body functions generally.

Maitland and Butler: 'abnormal neural movement'

Butler & Gifford (1989), building on the original work of Maitland (1986), have shown how what they term 'adverse tension' in the nervous system can impair its mobility and elasticity, and how many painful problems can result from this. Butler and Gifford's detailed analysis of the diagnosis and treatment of such restrictions and tensions is highly recommended to manual therapists. The tissues that surround neural structures are known as the mechanical interface (MI). These adjacent tissues are those that can move independently of the nervous system; for example, supinator muscle is the MI to the radial nerve, as it passes through the radial tunnel.

There is no general agreement as to the terminology that should be used in describing such biomechanical changes in the neural environment. Maitland et al (2001), for example, suggest that 'abnormal neural movement' is a more accurate description than 'neural tension'. Whatever we term the dysfunctional pattern, Butler and Gifford's focus on those 'adverse mechanical' changes that negatively influence neural function, and that cause a multitude of symptoms, including pain, has been a singular contribution to our understanding of some aspects of pain and dysfunction.

Any pathology in the MI can produce abnormalities in nerve movement, resulting in tension on the neural structure with unpredictable ramifications. Examples of MI pathology include nerve impingement by disc protrusion, or osteophyte contact, and carpel tunnel constriction. These problems would be regarded as mechanical in origin as far as the nerve restriction is concerned. Any symptoms resulting from mechanical impingement on neural structures will be more readily provoked in tests that involve movement rather than pure (passive) tension.

Chemical or inflammatory causes of neural tension can also occur, resulting in 'interneural fibrosis', which leads to reduced elasticity and increased 'tension', and would become obvious with tension testing of these structures.

Pathophysiological changes resulting from inflammation, or from chemical damage (i.e. toxicity), are noted by Butler & Gifford (1989) as commonly leading on to internal mechanical restrictions of neural structures in a different manner to mechanical causes such as those, for example, imposed by a disc lesion.

Korr (1970) states:

To appreciate the vulnerability of the segmental nervous system to somatic insults it must be understood that much of the pathway taken by nerves as they emerge from the cord is actually through skeletal muscle. The great contractile forces of skeletal muscles with the accompanying chemical changes exert profound influences on the metabolism and excitability of neurons. In this environment the neurons are subject to quite considerable mechanical and chemical influences of various kinds, compression and torsion and many others . . . slight mechanical stresses may, over a period of time, produce adhesions, constrictions and angulations imposed by protective layers. [Perhaps involving friction protectors such as meningeal extensions including nerve sheaths or nerve sleeves.]

Adverse mechanical tension changes do not necessarily affect nerve conduction, according to Butler and Gifford; however, Korr's research indicates that axonal transport may be affected.

From the perspective of the manual therapist, this knowledge is extremely important. The dysfunctional tissues and patients being treated by massage therapists, neuromuscular therapists, physiotherapists, Rolfers, Heller Workers, osteopathic and chiropractic practitioners, and those using movement therapies (Pilates, Feldenkrais, etc.), all have the potential to involve the mechanically interfacing structures in which neural tissues lie, and where normal mobility should be present (and often is not).

THE ROLE OF NEUROMUSCULAR TECHNIQUES

This book has, as a primary focus, the use of neuromuscular techniques (NMTs) in assessing and treating somatic dysfunction. The objectives of neuromuscular technique (NMT as practised in Europe) and neuromuscular therapy (NMT as practised in the USA) are summarised in Box 1.3.

To understand the context for application of such approaches, we need to appreciate temporal influences on the evolution of dysfunction: how, over time, a progression occurs that alters

---

Box 1.3 NMT: European (Lief's) neuromuscular technique and American neuromuscular therapy (Chaitow & Delaney 2000)

Neuromuscular technique, as the term is used in this book, refers to the manual application of specialised (usually) digital pressure and strokes, most commonly applied by finger or thumb contact. These digital contacts can have either a diagnostic (assessment) or therapeutic objective, and the degree of pressure employed varies considerably between these two modes of application. There are subtle differences between the European and American versions of NMT. Detailed descriptions of Lief's NMT will be found in Chapter 6, while the American NMT version is outlined by Judith DeLany in Chapter 10.

Additional complementary manual methods to NMT (both versions) include massage, muscle energy technique (MET), positional release technique (PRT), myofascial release technique (MRT) and variations of these soft tissue manipulation approaches.

Aims of NMT
Therapeutically, NMT aims to produce modifications in dysfunctional tissue, encouraging a restoration of functional normality, with a particular focus of deactivating focal points of reflexogenic activity, such as myofascial trigger points.

An alternative objective of NMT application is toward normalising imbalances in hypertonic and/or fibrotic tissues, either as an end in itself or as a precursor to joint mobilisation or manipulation.
NMT attempts to:

- offer reflex benefits
- deactivate myofascial trigger points
- prepare for other therapeutic methods such as exercise or manipulation

- relax and normalise tense, fibrotic muscular tissue
- enhance lymphatic and general circulation and drainage
- simultaneously offer the practitioner diagnostic information.

Neuromuscular therapy (USA) utilises similar manual methods, as well as re-education, rehabilitation and home-care approaches, to those utilised in European methodology.

NMT attempts to address a number of features that are all commonly involved in causing or intensifying pain and dysfunction (Chaitow & DeLany 2000) including, among others:

- *biochemical features* – nutritional imbalances and deficiencies, toxicity (exogenous and endogenous), endocrine imbalances (e.g. thyroid deficiency), ischaemia, inflammation
- *pyschosocial factors* – stress, anxiety, depression, etc.
- *biomechanical factors* – posture, including patterns of use, hyperventilation tendencies, as well as locally dysfunctional states such as hypertonia, trigger points, neural compression or entrapment.

NMT sees its role as attempting to normalise or modulate whichever of these (or additional) influences on musculoskeletal pain and dysfunction can be identified in order to remove or modify as many aetiological and perpetuating influences as possible (Simons et al 1999), without creating further distress or requirement for excessive adaptation.

---

acute responses, as the tissues locally, or the body as a whole, modify, accommodate, compensate and adapt to the demands, stresses and insults of daily life.

 General adaptation syndrome (GAS) and local adaptation syndrome (LAS), and connective tissue

Selye (1976) called stress the non-specific element in disease production. In describing the relationship between the general adaptation syndrome (GAS) – i.e. alarm reaction, resistance (adaptation) phase followed by the exhaustion phase (when adaptation finally fails), which affects the organism as a whole – and the local

adaptation syndrome (LAS), which affects a specific stressed area of the body, Selye also emphasised the importance of connective tissue. He demonstrated that stress results in a pattern of adaptation, individual to each organism. He further showed that, when an individual is acutely alarmed, stressed or aroused, homeostatic (self-normalising) mechanisms are activated – this is the alarm reaction of Selye's general (and local) adaptation syndromes.

If the alarm status is prolonged or repetitive, defensive adaptation processes commence and produce long-term – chronic – changes. In assessing (palpating) the patient, these neuromusculoskeletal changes represent a record of the attempts on the part of the body to adapt and adjust to the stresses imposed upon it as time passes. The results of repeated postural and traumatic insults of a lifetime, combined with changes of emotional and psychological origin, will often present a confusing pattern of tense, contracted, bunched, fatigued and ultimately fibrous tissue (Chaitow 1989).

The minutiae of the process are not, for the moment, at issue. What is important is the realisation that, due to prolonged stress of a postural, psychic or mechanical type, discrete areas of the body become so altered by the efforts to compensate and adapt that structural and, eventually, pathological changes become apparent. Researchers have shown that the type of stress

---

Box 1.4 Selective motor unit involvement

The effect of psychological influences on muscles seems to be more complex than a simplistic 'whole' muscle or regional involvement. It has been demonstrated that a small number of motor units in particular muscles may display almost constant, or repeated, activity when influenced psychogenically (Waersted et al 1993). The reaction time taken to perform tasks was evaluated in normal individuals, so creating a 'time pressure' anxiety. Researchers were able to demonstrate low-amplitude levels of activity (using surface EMG in trapezius muscles) even when the muscle was not being employed. It seems that, in spite of low total activity level of the muscle, a small pool of low-threshold motor units may be under considerable load for prolonged periods of time.

Such a recruitment pattern would be in agreement with the 'size principle' first proposed by Henneman (1957), which states that motor units are recruited according to their size. Motor units with type I (postural) fibres are predominant among the small, low-threshold units. If tension-provoking factors (e.g. anxiety) are frequently present, and the subject repeatedly recruits the same motor units, overload may follow, possibly resulting in a metabolic crisis and the appearance of type I fibres with an abnormally large diameter, or 'ragged-red' fibres, which are interpreted as a sign of mitochondrial overload (Edwards 1988, Larsson et al 1990). The implications of this information are profound, because they suggest that emotional stress can selectively involve postural muscle fibres that have a tendency to shorten over time when stressed (Janda 1983).

The possible 'metabolic crisis' suggested by this research has strong parallels with the evolution of myofascial trigger points as suggested by Simons, a topic that is discussed in greater detail in later chapters (Wolfe & Simons 1992).

---

involved can be entirely physical in nature (Wall & Melzack 1991) (e.g. a single injury or repetitive postural strain) or purely psychic in nature (Latey 1983) (e.g. chronically repressed anger). An example of localised emotional stress influences on muscle tissue is given in Box 1.4. Wider biomechanical responses to emotional stress are discussed later in this chapter.

More often than not a combination of emotional and physical stresses will so alter neuromusculoskeletal structures as to create a series of identifiable physical changes, which will themselves generate further stress, such as pain, joint restriction, general discomfort and fatigue.

As described in this and later chapters, predictable chain reactions of compensating changes will evolve in the soft tissues in most instances of chronic adaptation to biomechanical and psychogenic stress (Lewit 1992). Such adaptation is almost always at the expense of optimal function, as well as being an ongoing source of further physiological embarrassment.

A biomechanical stress response sequence
(Basmajian 1974, Dvorak & Dvorak 1984, Janda 1982, 1983, Korr 1978, Lewit 1985, Travell & Simons 1983, 1992).

When the musculoskeletal system is 'stressed', a sequence of events occurs which can be summarised as follows:

- 'Something' (see Causes of soft tissue dysfunction below) occurs that leads to increased muscular tone.
- Increased tone, if anything but short-term, leads to a retention of metabolic wastes.
- Increased tone simultaneously leads to a degree of localised oxygen lack (relative to the efforts being demanded of the tissues) – resulting in ischaemia.
- Increased tone might also lead to a degree of oedema.
- These factors (retention of wastes, ischaemia, oedema) result in discomfort or pain.
- Discomfort or pain leads to increased or maintained hypertonicity.

- Inflammation, or at least chronic irritation, may be a result.
- Neurological reporting stations in hypertonic tissues will bombard the CNS with information regarding their status, leading to a degree of sensitisation of neural structures and the evolution of facilitation – hyperreactivity (see Ch. 2).
- Macrophages are activated, as is increased vascularity and fibroblastic activity.
- Connective tissue production increases with cross-linkage, leading to shortened fascia.
- As all fascia/connective tissue is continuous throughout the body, any distortions that develop in one region can potentially create distortions elsewhere, so having a negative influence on structures that are supported by, or attached to, the fascia, including nerves, muscles, lymph structures and blood vessels.
- Changes occur in the elastic (muscle) tissues, leading to chronic hypertonicity and, ultimately, to fibrotic changes.
- Hypertonicity in a muscle will produce inhibition of its antagonist muscles.
- Chain reactions evolve in which some muscles (postural – type I) shorten, while others (phasic – type II) weaken.
- Because of sustained increased muscle tension, ischaemia in tendinous structures occurs, as it does in localised areas of muscles, and periosteal pain areas develop.
- Abnormal biomechanics occur, involving malcoordination of movement (with antagonist muscle groups being hypertonic (e.g. erector spinae) and weak (e.g. the rectus abdominis group)).
- The firing sequences of antagonistic and synergistic muscles alter.
- Joint restrictions and/or imbalances as well as fascial shortenings develop.
- Progressive evolution of localised areas of hyperreactivity of neural structures occurs (facilitated areas) in paraspinal regions or within muscles (trigger points).
- The degree of energy wastage due to unnecessarily maintained hypertonicity leads to generalised fatigue.

- More widespread functional changes develop – for example affecting respiratory function – with repercussions on the total economy of the body.

In the presence of a constant neurological feedback of impulses to the CNS/brain from neural reporting stations indicating heightened arousal (a hypertonic muscle status is the alarm reaction of the flight/fight alarm response), there will be increased levels of psychological arousal and an inability to relax adequately with consequent increase in hypertonicity. Functional patterns of use of a biologically unsustainable nature will emerge, probably involving chronic musculoskeletal problems and pain.

At this stage, restoration of normal function requires therapeutic input which addresses the multiple changes that have occurred as well as the need to re-educate the individual as to how to use their body – to breathe, to carry and to use themselves – in less stressful ways.

The chronic adaptive changes that develop in such a scenario lead to the increased likelihood of future acute exacerbations as the progressively chronic, less supple and resilient, biomechanical structures attempt to cope with new stress factors resulting from the normal demands of modern living.

CAUSES OF SOFT TISSUE DYSFUNCTION

Causes of biomechanical (musculoskeletal) distress

The 'something' that can contribute to the 'stress' sequence described includes:

1. Congenital factors (short or long leg, small hemipelvis, fascial, cranial and other distortions, hypermobility tendencies)
2. Overuse, misuse and abuse (and disuse) factors (such as injury or inappropriate patterns of use involved in work, sport or regular activities)
3. Postural stresses
4. Chronic negative emotional states (anxiety, etc.) – see Box 1.4

5. Reflexive factors (trigger points, facilitated spinal regions)
6. Pathology (arthritis, etc.).

As a result of the processes described above – most of which affect each and every one of us to some degree – acute and painful problems, overlaid on chronic soft tissue changes, become the norm – the raw material on which bodywork therapies focus.

Stressing the soft tissues

Forms of stress affecting the body can be categorised as follows: physiological, emotional, behavioural and structural (Barlow 1959).

Physiological. This might involve an overall increase of muscle hypertonicity/tension or localised soft tissue changes due to habitual patterns of use or from patterns of overuse. Occupational, sporting, leisure and general activities are all potential producers of such repetitive or constant stress involving the soft tissues (Janda 1982, 1988).

Emotional. All emotional changes are mirrored in muscular changes. Emotional attitudes such as anger or fear, as well as moods such as excitement, anxiety or depression, are known to produce altered muscular postures and patterns. There is a close relationship between habitual tension patterns and posture, and psychological attitudes and conflicts. The use of the body as a metaphor for emotional feelings ('pain in the neck') is well documented (Boadella 1978).

Reich (1949) outlined his understanding of the postures and defensive armouring produced by neurotic patients. He believed that such individuals often behaved as though they were 'half-dead' and that their normal functioning, on all levels, was diminished and restricted. He described an all too frequently seen pattern: 'They were disturbed sexually, they were disturbed in their work function, their bodily processes lacked rhythm, their breathing was uncoordinated' (Boadella 1978). Reich and his followers demonstrated how emotions can 'mobilise' or 'paralyse' the body, with continued and repeated stress producing 'blockages' and restrictions which, if unreleased, become self-perpetuating and are themselves the source of pain and further stress. The ability to relax is lost, and the drain on nervous energy is profound in such situations. The bioenergetic answer to this problem is to aid in the release of these tensions by a complex set of exercises, including facial expressions and body positions, accompanied by breathing techniques. These methods are doubtless successful in many cases, but what is important is recognition that neuromuscular changes, as evidenced by stiffness, pain and restriction, may often be a manifestation of deep psychological and emotional stress.

Behavioural. All movement requires muscular activity. Certain patterns of use establish themselves. Often, individual awareness of the pattern of use is diminished, and habitually used, repetitive actions take place with resultant muscular hypertonicity developing (Feldenkrais 1977). Altering habitual use patterns is far more difficult than altering the resultant soft tissue changes in the short term. Breathing patterns that are habitual, such as hyperventilation, could be included in this category of stress factors impacting the musculoskeletal system (Chaitow et al 2002, Timmons 1994).

Structural. Over and above inborn features, such as a short leg, acquired structural changes make further demands on the adaptive capacity of the body. Depending upon the mechanical and structural loads it bears and responds to, muscle tissue will change in texture, chemistry, tone, etc., and will also modify and alter the framework of the body, warping and cramping its potential for normal use. The body will be bent and distorted to meet the stresses imposed from without and within. Barlow (1959), whose work follows that of Alexander (1957), suggested that there is a self-regulating tendency in the way muscles behave in response to stress. The term 'postural homeostasis' implies a return to a balanced resting state after activity. Such regulation is usually at an unconscious level, and Barlow gives the example of a patient with persistent low back pain who, in the resting position, demonstrated a particular set of muscular distortions such as tense erector spinae muscles on the left and a tense trapezius on the right, together with a pelvic twist to the right. On activity all these spasms would become accentuated. Barlow employed postural re-education (Alexander technique) to restore balanced use; however, it is suggested that more long-lasting benefits might be achieved by the use of soft tissue normalisation, using NMT, muscle energy and myofascial release methods, plus appropriate manipulation – combined with re-education (such as the Alexander technique) – rather than simply relying on re-education without attention to the structural modifications (e.g. fibrosis) produced by the adaptation process. Any attempt to normalise structural changes without due attention to patterns of use would be equally unsatisfactory.

Mobilisation before rehabilitation?

These thoughts are supported by Dommerholt (2000), who points out:

In general, assessment and treatment of individual muscles must precede restoration of normal posture and normal patterns of movement. Claims that muscle imbalances would dissolve, following lessons in the Alexander technique are not substantiated in the scientific literature (Rosenthal 1987). Instead muscle imbalances must be corrected through very specific strengthening and flexibility exercises, since generic exercise programs tend to perpetuate the compensatory muscle patterns. Myofascial trigger points must be inactivated using either invasive or non-invasive treatment techniques. Associated joint dysfunction, especially of the cervical and thoracic spine must be corrected with joint mobilizations. Once the musculoskeletal conditions for 'good posture' have been met, postural retraining [Alexander or other methods], can proceed.

Hypermobility

Clearly hypermobility tendencies may be inborn; however, acquired hypermobility may result from trauma or over-zealous manipulation of particular joints.

Kappler (1997) cautions: 'A normal physiological reaction to a painful hypermobile joint is for muscles surrounding the joint to splint the joint, and protect it from excess motion. Physical examination reveals restriction of motion. Underneath the protective muscle splinting is the unstable joint.'

It may be useful to reflect that one way in which the body might maintain excess tone in a muscle offering such protective support would be for it to evolve trigger point activity. These distressed supporting muscles (and their associated trigger points) might best be left untreated until underlying use patterns can be modified. Kappler (1997) suggests: 'Management [of hypermobile structures] involves modifying patient activity that contributes to instability, mobilizing adjacent hypomobile joints, and prescribing active rehabilitation exercises.'

Understanding pain

Research into the mechanisms involved in muscular pain have evolved rapidly over the past 50 years. In 1959, Barlow suggested that in the absence of other pathology muscular pain resulted from:

● The muscle itself, through some noxious metabolic product, such as 'factor P' (Lewis 1942), or an interference in blood circulation due to spasm, resulting in relative ischaemia.

● The muscular insertion into the periosteum, such as that caused by an actual lifting of the periosteal tissue following marked, or repetitive, muscular tension (e.g. 'tennis elbow' and periosteal pain points, which are described and listed in Chapter 3) (Lewit 1992).

● The joint, which can become restricted and over-approximated. In advanced cases, osteo-arthritic changes can result from the regular microtrauma of repeated muscular misuse. Over-approximation of joint surfaces due to soft tissue shortening can also lead to uneven wear and tear, as, for example, when the tensor fascia lata structure shortens and crowds both the hip and lateral knee joint structures.

● Neural irritation, which can be produced spinally or along the course of the nerve as a result of chronic muscular contractions. These can involve disc and general spinal mechanical faults (Korr 1976) as well as abnormal neural status (Butler & Gifford 1991, Maitland et al 2001).

● Variations in pain threshold, largely to do with perception, which will make all these factors more or less significant and obvious (Wall & Melzack 1991).

Other models of pain genesis

Medical acupuncture model

Baldry (1993) describes the progression from muscle in a normal state to muscle in painful chronic distress as commonly involving initial or repetitive trauma (strain or excessive use) resulting in the release of chemical substances such as bradykinin, prostaglandins, histamine, serotonin and potassium ions. Sensitisation of A-δ and C (group IV) sensory nerve fibres may follow, with involvement of the brain (limbic system and the frontal lobe).

Trigger points (see Ch. 3), which evolve from such a progression, themselves become the source of new problems in their own locality, as well as at distant sites, as their sarcoplasmic reticulum is damaged and free calcium ions are released, leading to the formation of localised taut bands of tissue (involving the actin–myosin contractile mechanisms in the muscle sarcomeres). If free calcium and energy-producing adenosine triphosphate (ATP) is present, this becomes a self-perpetuating feature compounded by the relative (compared with surrounding tissues) ischaemia that has been identified in such chronically contracted tissues (Simons 1987). Local myofascial changes are considered in Chapter 3.

Note: Where pain has been produced by repetitive habits, postural and otherwise, with emotional and psychological overtones, the task of the therapist is complex because hypertonicity can often be only partially released or relaxed without resolving the underlying pattern of use. If repeated recurrence of painful episodes is to be minimised, a state of relative equilibrium of body structure and function is needed, which calls for treatment of structural restrictions as well as re-education regarding posture and use.

Stoddard's osteopathic perspective

Stoddard (1969), in discussing contracted musculature, describes its 'stringy' feel, resulting from the continuous contraction of some muscle fibres, and ascribes the cause to the underlying joint dysfunction. The resulting ache and pain, he believes, is usually a result of circulatory embarrassment as metabolic wastes build-up due to sustained muscular contraction. Muscular guarding is always seen to indicate deeper pathological changes (e.g. tuberculosis of the spine, osteomyelitis, disc herniation).

Stoddard sees the metabolic wastes, which may result from a degree of stasis, as causing a vicious cycle in perpetuating muscular contraction, leading eventually to fibrous changes. There is no indication that Stoddard considers such changes to be of primary importance in his treatment programme. He does stress the importance of exercises (to strengthen muscle groups) and of correct posture, but does not indicate any great interest in treatment of the soft tissues themselves.

While release of muscular restrictions and shortening could be considered a desirable step in the restoration of normality, it is worth emphasising that once adaptive fibrotic changes have taken place in the soft tissues (whether in response to emotional stress or anything else) these changes are no longer under purely neurological control and therefore cannot simply be 'released' (by exercises or anything else): they require a physical input that alters, stretches and effectively breaks down concretions such as fibrotic tissue.

Modern pain concepts

The complexity of muscular pain mechanisms becomes clearer as the diligent research and reporting of Mense & Simons (2001) is examined. Interestingly, many of the ideas promoted half a century ago, by Barlow and others, are confirmed by modern research, although far more detail is now available with regard to pain mechanisms.

A brief summary of the key elements described by Mense and Simons is offered below; however, this captures no more than a superficial glimpse of the material in their book.

Common subgroups of muscular pain are identified: *myofascial pain* resulting from trigger points (often also used to describe regional pain syndromes); *fibromyalgia* (also used to describe myoglossis, muscular induration, non-articular rheumatism and tendomyopathy); and *muscular pain* related to articular dysfunction. Mense and Simons consider that most other terms used to describe muscular pain can be subsumed into these three terms.

Gender differences (fibromyalgia occurs in a female : male ratio of approximately 4 : 1) relate largely to 'a higher sensitivity of the pain system in females'.

Sensitisation of nociceptors by vasoneuro-reactive substances (such as bradykinin and prostaglandins) leads to long-lasting tenderness of trigger points (Fig. 1.1). This is discussed further in Chapter 3.

This process of sensitisation involves local oedema, release of neuropeptides such as substance P, subsequent compression of venous vessels, venous congestion (which reduces blood supply) and therefore local ischaemia. Ischaemic conditions lead to the release of more brady-kinin, ensuring a vicious cycle, which engenders sensitisation of pain receptors.

In skeletal muscle, ischaemia results in interference with normal energy (ATP) production, which leads to disturbance of normal calcium pump activity, preventing actin and myosin filaments from releasing their contractured state. This is the hypothesised cause of 'taut bands', which are a key feature of myofascial trigger points (see Ch. 3).

Mense & Simons (2001) suggest that when inflammation occurs in muscle for a period as short as 12 days, the concentration of thin nerve fibres containing neuropeptides increases markedly, leading to a greater reporting of pain sensations (Reinert & Mense 1993).

The widely held belief that a pain–spasm–pain cycle exists is questioned by Mense & Simons (2001). Their arguments are too complex to summarise without losing accuracy, but the following remarks offer a glimpse:

The [pain–spasm–pain] cycle is assumed to start with a muscle lesion that excites nociceptors. The small-diameter group III and IV muscle afferent fibers from the muscle nociceptors excite interneurons in the

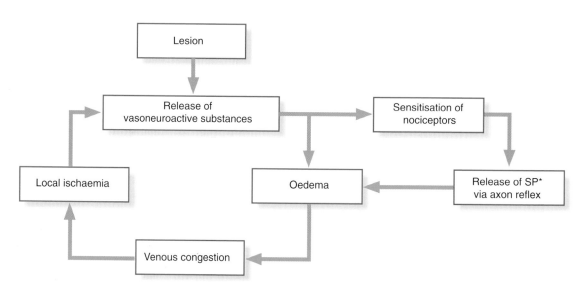

Figure 1.1 Schematic diagram showing hypothesised mechanism for sustained tenderness in trigger points. (SP = substance P) Redrawn from Mense S & Simons D, Muscle pain, Williams & Wilkins, 2001, with permission.

dorsal horn, which in turn activate α-motor neurons. Via their efferent fibers (α-motor axons) these motor neurons activate the neuromuscular endplate and cause spasm of the muscle. A longer-lasting spasm is painful and further activates muscle nociceptors.

Mense and Simons argue that although excitation of dorsal horn neurons by muscle nociceptors is established there is no proof that homonymous α-motor neurons are similarly activated: 'An acute noxious stimulus to a muscle is likely to inhibit rather than excite homonymous motor neurons if the muscle is an extensor.' They believe that because flexor muscle motor neurons display only short-lasting excitation (if any), and painful muscles frequently show little or no electrical activity when at rest, 'the postulated [pain–spasm–pain] reflex is not functional in every muscle and cannot explain long-lasting spasm.'

Apart from the idea that spasm results via reflex arcs, as outlined above, a variety of other working hypotheses exists to explain the phenomenon of spasm, none of which is proven. These include the possibility that joint nociceptors act as initiators resulting in reflex stabilisation via chronic muscle spasm. Mense and Simons reject this as being universally valid because 'in many cases of painful joint lesions . . . neighboring muscles are reflexly inhibited.'

Neuroplastic sensitisation involves a process in which nociceptive input to the cord or brainstem leads to synaptic sensitisation in the dorsal horn neurons. 'Following such an input, the neurons are thought to increase their excitability and exhibit enhanced responses to both pathologic and normal afferent inflow.' Central sensitisation is then thought to perpetuate nociceptive activity. This is a concept close to facilitation mechanisms, as hypothesised by osteopathic medicine, and discussed in Chapter 3.

There may be a malfunctioning of the descending antinociceptive system, in which central damping down of pain messages fails to be effective. Mense and Simons state: 'It is conceivable that a malfunction of the descending antinociceptive system, which might occur spontaneously, or following a central or peripheral lesion, leads to chronic pain sensations from deep tissues, even in the absence of a peripheral lesion.' Fibromyalgic pain may result from such a process.

Psychological factors modulate pain perception; however, controversially, Mense & Simons (2001) contend that whilst 'psychological stress can be a potent aggravating factor . . . as we learn more about the pathophysiology concerning the origin of muscle pain, the less psychogenic and more somatic it becomes.'

A variety of mechanical (e.g. poor posture, asymmetry) and systemic (e.g. anaemia, low thyroid function, vitamin B deficiency) factors may interact to aggravate and perpetuate painful conditions.

Mense and Simons insist that it is essential to be aware of, and able to distinguish between, pain and tenderness that is local, projected (caused by peripheral nerve irritation), referred and of central origin – and of overlaps between these.

Additional insights from Mense and Simons will be introduced in later chapters. At this stage it is useful to observe that pain is complex, confusing and demanding. The task of uncovering the mechanisms involved in any given patient's painful muscular condition calls for the ability to evaluate muscular and articular status, and neurological features, as well as identification of myofascial trigger points and fibromyalgia characteristics. One requirement for such a process is the ability to distinguish between different muscular responses to stress: overuse, misuse, disuse and abuse.

Different responses in postural and phasic muscles

It is not within the scope of this book to provide detailed physiological analysis; however, it is vital that the ways in which different muscle fibre types respond to stress are understood. To be sure there are several models in which different muscle groups are designated according to their main functions and characteristics, and an attempt is made in Box 1.5 to summarise these.

Box 1.5 Categorization of muscles

Postural and phasic muscles (sometimes called type I and type II)
Muscles have a mixture of fibre types, although there is usually a predominance of one type or another. There are those that contract slowly ('slow twitch fibres' or 'slow white fibres'), which are classified as type I. These have very low stores of energy-supplying glycogen but carry high concentrations of myoglobulin and mitochondria. These fibres fatigue slowly and are mainly involved in postural and stabilising tasks (Engel et al 1986, Woo et al 1987).

There are also several phasic/active type II fibre forms, notably:

- Type IIa fibres ('fast twitch' or 'fast red' fibres), which contract more speedily than type I and are moderately resistant to fatigue, with relatively high concentrations of mitochondria and myoglobulin.
- Type IIb fibres ('fast twitch/glycolytic fibres' or 'fast white fibres'), which are less fatigue-resistant and depend more on glycolytic sources of energy, with low levels of mitochondria and myoglobulin.
- Type IIm ('superfast' fibres), found mainly in the jaw muscles, which depend on a unique myosin structure which, along with a high glycogen content, differentiates this from the other type II fibres (Rowlerson 1981).

The implications of the effects of prolonged stress on these different muscle types cannot be emphasised too strongly, because long-term stress involving type I muscles indicates that they will shorten, whereas type II fibres undergoing similar stress will weaken without shortening over their whole length (they may, however, develop shortened areas within the muscle). It is important to emphasise that shortness or tightness of a postural muscle does not imply strength. Such muscles may test as strong or weak. However, a weak phasic muscle will not shorten overall and will always test as weak (Janda 1982).

Fibre type is not totally fixed, in that evidence exists as to the potential for adaptability of muscles, so that committed muscle fibres can be transformed from slow-twitch to fast-twitch and vice versa (Lin et al 1994).

An example of this potential, which is of profound clinical significance, involves the scalene muscles, which Lewit (1999) confirms can be classified as either postural or phasic. If the largely phasic scalene muscles, which are dedicated to movement, have postural functions thrust upon them (as in an asthmatic condition in which they will attempt to maintain the upper ribs in elevation to enhance lung capacity) and if, owing to the laboured breathing of such an individual, they are thoroughly and regularly stressed, their fibre type will alter and they will shorten, becoming postural muscles (Lin et al 1994). A list of postural and phasic muscles is given later in this chapter.

Stabilisers and mobilisers
Norris (1995a, b, c, d, e, 1998) designates muscles according to their major functions, i.e. as 'stabilisers' or 'mobilisers'. According to Norris, research has shown that muscles that are inhibited or weak may lengthen, adding to the instability of the region in which they operate. It is the 'stabiliser' muscles that have this tendency: if they are inhibited because of deconditioning they become unable adequately to perform the role of stabilising joints in their 'neutral posture'.

'Stabiliser' muscles, which are more deeply situated, slow twitch, and have a tendency to weaken and lengthen if deconditioned, include: transverse abdominis, multifidus, internal obliques, medial fibres of external oblique, quadratus lumborum, deep neck flexors, serratus anterior, lower trapezius, gluteus maximus and medius. These muscles can be correlated to a large extent (apart from quadratus lumborum) with muscles designated by Lewit (1999) and Janda (1982, 1983) as 'phasic'.

The more superficial, fast-twitch muscles which have a tendency to shortening (i.e. 'mobilisers' in Norris's terminology) include: suboccipital group, sternocleidomastoid, upper trapezius, levator scapulae, iliopsoas and hamstrings. These fall into the category of 'postural' muscles as described by Lewit (1992), Janda (1982) and Liebenson (1996).

Norris calls these 'mobilisers' because they cross more than one joint. This redefining of 'postural' as 'mobiliser' appears to be confusing, and many prefer to refer to these muscles simply as 'having a tendency to shortening' (Liebenson 1999).

Examples of patterns of imbalance that emerge as some muscles weaken and lengthen and their synergists become overworked, while their antagonists shorten, can be summarised as follows:

Underactive stabiliser	Overactive synergist	Shortened antagonist
Gluteus medius	Tensor fascia lata, quadratus lumborum, piriformis	Thigh adductors
Gluteus maximus	Iliocostalis lumborum, hamstrings	Iliopsoas, rectus femoris
Transversus abdominis	Rectus abdominis	Iliocostalis lumborum
Lower trapezius	Levator scapulae, upper trapezius	Pectoralis major
Deep neck flexors	Sternocleidomastoid	Suboccipitals
Serratus anterior	Pectoralis major/minor	Rhomboids
Diaphragm		Scalenes, pectoralis major

Box 1.5 *(cont'd)*

Multijoint or monoarticular muscles
Richardson et al (1999, 2000) have argued for the use of the terms multijoint muscles (also described as 'global' or 'deep' – slow twitch) and monoarticular muscles (also described as 'local' or 'superficial' – fast twitch). Richardson (2000) states:

For many years traditional exercise therapy was mainly focussed on building strength or endurance of whole muscle groups e.g. rotators of the trunk, extensors of the knee, internal rotators of the shoulder. Those involved in rehabilitative exercise gradually realized that people with injury not only needed general strength and endurance of whole muscle groups to perform an activity e.g. lifting a load, but also needed more specifically directed exercise.

More specifically exercise regimes were necessary to take into account that some individual muscles of a synergistic group:

(1) have distinct and different individual functions
(2) react in different ways to injury of the associated joint (reflex inhibition and excitation)
(3) react in different ways to lack of use or lack of gravitational load
(4) react in different ways to specific patterns of use (e.g. ballistic, repetitive activity)

In each of the above it can be easily predicted that individual muscles would fall consistently into basically two groups.

Group A
[Note: These are the 'phasic', stabiliser', multijoint (deep, global) muscles.]

(1) more linked with joint stabilisation
(2) more likely to undergo reflex inhibition with injury to associated joint
(3) more likely to atrophy quickly due to lack of use or lack of gravitational load
(4) more likely to decrease activity and change their function when exposed to ballistic repetitive exercise

Group B
[Note: These are the 'postural', 'mobiliser', monoarticular (superficial/local) muscles.]

(1) more linked with efficient movement of joints
(2) more likely to undergo reflex excitation with injury to associated joint
(3) not prone to atrophy quickly due to lack of use or lack of gravitational load
(4) more likely to become more active (and tighten) when exposed to ballistic repetitive exercise.

To minimise confusion, this book will follow the Janda/Lewit/Liebenson categorisations of postural and phasic muscles.

In this book the categorisation 'postural/phasic' (Janda 1982, 1996, Lewit 1992) is used, as this has been found by the principal author to be the most useful in clinical practice. What has been demonstrated is that, when stressed (overuse, misuse, abuse, disuse, etc.), postural muscles have a propensity to shorten, whereas phasic muscles undergoing similar 'stress' are inhibited, become weaker, and possibly lengthen (although localised contractures may be present).

Fetal position influences

Kolar (1999) reports that the muscles that tend to hypertonicity and shortening (i.e. 'postural' muscles) include most muscles shortened in the fetal position. These include finger, hand and wrist flexors; shoulder internal rotators and adductors; shoulder girdle elevators, as well as ankle plantar flexors and inverters; hip flexors, internal rotators and adductors.

The antagonists to these tend to become reciprocally inhibited (i.e. 'phasic' muscles). Janda (1996) suggests that these are the muscles whose neurodevelopment brings about the upright posture.

Role of the muscles in low back problems

If we examine the role of the muscular component of musculoskeletal structures, we find strong evidence for its involvement in many acute and chronic conditions. Jokl (1984) tells us that disuse muscular atrophy, following back injury, is a major factor in the progression from an acute back problem to a chronic one. Changes take place that are observable, histologically and biochemically, in the muscle fibres, and that are translated into functional changes. The effects of these changes involve decreased endurance and weakened muscles, as well as spasm. We should remind ourselves of the basic anatomy of the low back, which includes the division of the musculature into:

1. The *deep muscles*, connecting the adjacent spinous processes (interspinales), adjacent transverse processes (intertransversari) and the rotatores, connecting the transverse process below to the laminae above.

2. The *intermediate muscles* include multifidus, which connects the transverse processes to the spinous processes of the vertebra above.

3. The superficial group includes iliocostalis, longissimus and spinalis (erector spinae). The origin of this is on the ischium, and the insertion on the sixth and 12th ribs. Together with the psoas (major and minor) and the quadratus, these greatly influence spinal stability.

4. The prevertebral muscles, which further stabilise and support the spine, are those that encircle the abdomen, such as the internal and external oblique, and rectus abdominus muscles.

MUSCLE TYPES (see Box 1.5)

Any, or all, of these muscles can have a major influence on the onset of low back problems and pain. The division of muscles with regard to their different postural and phasic (volitional movement) types is worthy of re-emphasis. As mentioned above (p. 15), muscle fibres may be differentiated into types by virtue of their role, as well as their main energy source. For example, type I muscles require stamina, rather than speed of action, and derive their energy via oxidative phosphorylation. This is in contrast to type II muscles, which produce power and speed, and derive energy from carbohydrate sources via glycolytic breakdown.

The muscles that support the spine are mainly type I, endurance and stamina muscles. Their activities are in the main related to static, antigravity efforts, which require prolonged contraction, and these muscles are far more susceptible to disuse atrophy and shortening. The strength

of such muscles may not indicate much change, even after a period of disuse, but the endurance factor could be greatly affected. This necessitates a certain degree of caution when interpreting muscle strength tests involving the paravertebral musculature.

Jokl (1984) points out that electromyographic (EMG) studies indicate that paraspinal muscles show marked fatigue in individuals with low back pain. This fatigue factor may play a major part in worsening, or accentuating, an already demonstrable degree of dysfunction in this region. When such a situation exists (pain and easy fatigue of supporting musculature), it may be assumed that an increasing number of muscle fibres has been recruited in order to maintain spinal stability, which in turn results in increased muscular pressure. Jokl tells us that normal muscle can work for long periods without any EMG evidence of fatigue. As muscles become weaker, they work at an increased percentage of their maximum voluntary contraction. Ultimately this leads to muscle spasm, which allows ischaemia to develop, and pain to result.

The cycle of increased effort, local spasm and ischaemia, leading to pain, may ultimately result in paraspinal spasm and splinting.

The use of both neuromuscular and muscle energy techniques is indicated in such a situation, as a means of disrupting the cycle and, initially, relaxing the contracted muscles. NMT methods have a combined effect, both relaxing the tissues as well as increasing the vascularity and mobility of these structures. They become more 'extensible', to use Grieve's phrase (Grieve 1985). He enlarges on this aspect thus:

There is new evidence to support the view that suppleness and flexibility of muscle and connective tissue, are of prime importance. Long and continued occupational and postural stress, asymmetrically imposed upon the soft tissues, tends to cause fibroblasts to multiply more rapidly and produce more collagen. Besides occupying more space within the connective tissue element of the muscle, the extra fibres encroach on the space normally occupied by nerves and vessels. Because of this trespass, the tissue loses elasticity and may become painful when the muscle is required to do work in coordination with others. In the long term collagen would replace the active fibres of the muscle and since collagen is fairly resistant to enzyme breakdown these changes tend to be irreversible.

The explanations of Jokl, Korr, Patterson and Grieve, as discussed above, help us to gain a clearer picture of the structural changes that take place as stress factors operating over a period of time impact on the soft tissues.

Postural and phasic muscle lists

Type I postural muscles are prone to loss of endurance capabilities when disused or subject to pathological influences and become shortened or tighter, whereas type II phasic muscles, when abused or disused, become weak (Janda 1982, Lewit 1992).

Postural muscles that become hypertonic and shorten in response to dysfunction include (Fig. 1.2):

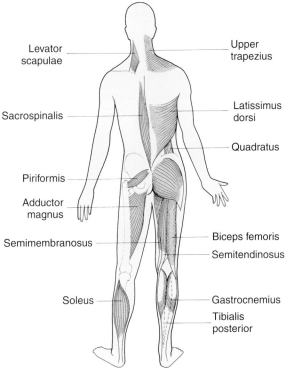

Figure 1.2B   Major postural muscles of the posterior aspects of the body.

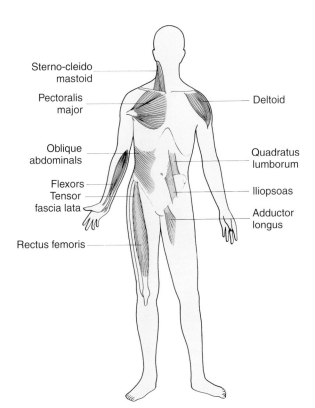

Figure 1.2A   Major postural muscles of the anterior aspects of the body.

- Trapezius (upper), sternocleidomastoid, levator scapulae and upper aspects of pectoralis major, in the upper trunk; and the flexors of the arms.
- Quadratus lumborum, erector spinae, oblique abdominals and iliopsoas, in the lower trunk.
- Tensor fascia lata, rectus femoris, biceps femoris, adductors (longus brevis and magnus) piriformis, hamstrings, semitendinosus.

Phasic muscles, which weaken (i.e. are inhibited), and may lengthen, in response to dysfunction, include:

- The paravertebral muscles (not erector spinae) and scaleni, the extensors of the upper extremity (flexors are primarily postural), the abdominal aspects of pectoralis major; middle and inferior aspects of trapezius; the rhomboids, serratus anterior, rectus abdominus; the internal and external obliques, gluteals, the peroneal muscles and the extensors of the arms.

- Muscle groups such as the scaleni are equivocal: they start out as phasic muscles but can end up as postural ones (see above).

Note: Lewit (1985) does not subscribe to the theory that phasic and postural muscles can be differentiated by virtue of their fibre type, as do Grieve and Jokl, but certainly subscribes to their differences in all other regards.

FIBROSITIS

Having evolved from 'muscular rheumatism', via fibrositis to the currently favoured term 'fibromyalgia', generalised muscular pain is a manifestation of multiple causative influences.

The great British orthopaedic physician and writer James Cyriax (1962) believed, like Stoddard, that all primary 'fibrositic' conditions were a result of articular lesions (dysfunctions). A secondary fibrositic change could result, he stated, from traumatic injury to soft tissues (e.g. capsular adhesion at the shoulder after injury) which he called fibrosis, not fibrositis. He saw fibrosis as scar tissue formation. Other secondary fibrositic conditions were said to result from rheumatoid disease, infection (such as epidemic myalgia) and parasitic infection (*Trichinella spiralis*). All other muscular and soft tissue dysfunctions, Cyriax regarded as one result of joint dysfunction, which then produced muscular protective spasm, muscular wasting, pain, etc., and which could be normalised only by correction of the joint lesion.

NMT theory and practice holds an almost precisely opposing view to that held by Cyriax – maintaining that appropriate normalisation of the soft tissues can, more often than not, achieve joint normalisation when restriction exists, without active manipulation of the joint, since most joint problems appear to be the direct result of myofascial dysfunction (Cantu & Grodin 1992, Janda 1988, Stiles 1984).

Cyriax did point out that fibrous tissue is capable of maintaining inflammation, originally traumatic, almost as a matter of habit. In such cases he opted for hydrocortisone injections as the appropriate measure to 'break' this habit. Such treatment can work, but such an approach all too often fails if underlying fibrotic changes have not been normalised or habits of use modified.

Fibrositis changes its name to fibromyalgia

In Chapter 3, in which the phenomenon of local soft tissue dysfunction, most notably myofascial trigger point activity, is analysed in detail, the evolution of thinking regarding 'fibrositis' is also examined. Fibromyalgia (the new incarnation of fibrositis), with its causes, associated conditions and diagnostic criteria, requires discussion in that context because of the confusion that currently exists regarding the overlap between fibromyalgia syndrome (FMS), myofascial pain syndrome (MPS) and chronic fatigue syndrome (CFS). The fascia of the body has profound influence, and it is to this focus that we now turn.

THE FASCIAL NETWORK
(DiGiovanna 1991, Frankel 1980, Warwick & Williams 1973)

Of major significance in understanding musculoskeletal function and dysfunction is the fact that the fascia comprises one connected network – from the fascia attached to the inner aspects of the skull to the fascia in the soles of the feet, there exists just one fascial structure. If any part of this is deformed or distorted, negative stresses may be imposed on distant aspects, and on the structures that it divides, envelops, enmeshes and supports, and with which it connects. There is ample evidence that Wolff's law applies, in that fascia accommodates to chronic stress patterns and deforms itself – something that often precedes deformity of osseous and cartilaginous structures in chronic diseases.

Note: Wolff's law states that biological systems (including soft and hard tissues) deform in relation to the lines of force imposed on them.

The musculoskeletal system, the mechanical component of the human machine, comprising as it does 60% of the mass of the body, exists in a state of structural and functional continuity between all of its hard and soft tissues, and fascia is the ubiquitous elastic–plastic, gluey, component that invests, supports and separates, connects and divides, wraps and gives cohesion to the rest of the body – the fascial, connective tissue network. It is the connective tissues/fascia that provide most of that continuity. Any tendency to think of a local 'lesion' as existing in isolation should be discouraged as we try to visualise a complex, interrelated, symbiotically functioning assortment of tissues comprising skin, muscles, ligaments, tendons and bones, as well as the neural structures, blood and lymph channels, and vessels that bisect and invest these tissues – all given shape, cohesion and functional ability by the fascia (connective tissue).

Apart from its immense role in the support, structural organisation and motion of the body, fascia is involved in numerous complex biochemical activities:

● Connective tissue provides a supporting matrix for more highly organised structures and attaches extensively to muscles. Individual muscle fibres are enveloped by endomysium, which is connected to the stronger perimysium which surrounds the fasciculi. The perimysium's fibres attach to the even stronger epimysium, which surrounds the muscle as a whole and attaches to fascial tissues nearby.

● Because it contains mesenchymal cells of an embryonic type, connective tissue provides a generalised tissue capable of giving rise, under certain circumstances, to more specialised elements.

● It provides, by its fascial planes, pathways for nerves, blood and lymphatic vessels, and structures.

● Many of the neural structures in fascia are sensory in nature.

● It supplies restraining mechanisms by the differentiation of retention bands, fibrous pulleys and check ligaments, as well as assisting in the harmonious production and control of movement.

● Where connective tissue is loose in texture, it allows movement between adjacent structures

and, by the formation of bursal sacs, reduces the effects of pressure and friction.

● Deep fascia ensheathes and preserves the characteristic contour of the limbs, and promotes the circulation in the veins and lymphatic vessels.

● The superficial fascia, which forms the panniculus adiposus, allows for the storage of fat and also provides a surface covering which aids in the conservation of body heat.

● By virtue of its fibroblastic activity, connective tissue aids in the repair of injuries by the deposition of collagenous fibres (scar tissue).

● The ensheathing layer of deep fascia, as well as intermuscular septa and interosseous membranes, provides vast surface areas for muscular attachment.

● The meshes of loose connective tissue contain the 'tissue fluid' and provide an essential medium through which the cellular elements of other tissues are brought into functional relation with blood and lymph. Connective tissue has a nutritive function and houses nearly a quarter of all body fluids (Dicke 1978).

● The histiocytes of connective tissue comprise part of an important defence mechanism against bacterial invasion by their phagocytic activity. They also play a part as scavengers in removing cell debris and foreign material.

● Connective tissue represents an important 'neutraliser' or detoxicator to both endogenous toxins (those produced under physiological conditions) and exogenous toxins (those introduced from outside the organism). The mechanical barrier presented by connective tissue has important defensive functions in cases of infection and toxaemia.

Fascia, then, is not just a background structure with little function apart from its obvious supporting role, but is a ubiquitous, tenacious, connective tissue that is involved deeply in almost all of the fundamental processes of the body's structure, function and metabolism.

In therapeutic terms there can be little logic in trying to consider muscle as a separate structure from fascia, because they are so intimately related. Remove connective tissue from the

---

Box 1.6 Biomechanical terms relating to fascia

Creep
Continued deformation (increasing strain) of a viscoelastic material with time under constant load (traction, compression, twist). 'Creep' can occur during the process of myofascial release or in response to postural or functional patterns of use.

Hysteresis
Process of energy loss due to friction when tissues are loaded and unloaded, which may occur during treatment using stretching or other manual methods.

Load
The degree of force (stress) applied to an area.

Strain
Change in shape as a result of stress.

Stress
Force (load) normalised over the area on which it acts (all tissues exhibit stress–strain responses).

Thixotropy
A quality of colloids in which the more rapidly force is applied (load), the more rigid the tissue response, highlighting the need for sustained and slowly applied force when attempting to modify fascial status.

Viscoelastic
The potential to deform elastically when load is applied, and to return to the original non-deformed state when load is removed.

Viscoplastic
A permanent deformation resulting from the elastic potential having been exceeded, or pressure forces sustained.

---

scene and any muscle left would be a jelly-like structure without form or functional ability.

See Box 1.6 for definitions relating to the characteristic features of connective tissue/fascia.

Functional fascial continuities

Myers (2001) has created a model in which myofascial linkages are described in terms of railway junctions and tracks, which he has termed 'myofascial meridians'. While the interconnectedness of fascia throughout the body has long been understood, Myers' descriptions highlight specific linkages. The myofascial chains, which he describes as 'long functional continuities', are of important clinical value when attempting to identify functional connections between anatomically distant structures, for example the plantar fascia and fascia of the scalp, attaching to the brow ridge, as described in his *superficial back line* (Fig. 1.3), or the anterior compartment of the periosteum of the tibia and the sternocleidomastoid attachment to the temporal bone, as described in his *superficial front line* (Fig. 1.4). These fascial bridges are also of potential clinical importance in application of the progressive inhibition of neuromuscular structures (PINS) method, described by Dennis Dowling in Chapter 11 of this book.

Soft tissue changes – energy and fascial considerations

Taylor (1958) has postulated that tissue changes, apparent to the trained palpating hand, often result from changes in thermodynamic equilibrium. He states that the body is a thermodynamic system and, as such, alterations in the extracellular fluids, viscosity, pH, electrophoretic changes, colloidal osmotic pressure, etc., are subject to thermodynamic laws. One of these laws states that the total energy of such a system and its surroundings must remain constant, although the energy may be changed from one form to another as a result of alterations of the stresses imposed.

For example, through postural stress and gravitational effects, particular changes in the fascia involved would result in energy loss and therefore stasis and stagnation. One of the characteristics of thermodynamics is that of thixotropy, in which gels become more solid with energy loss and more fluid with energy input. Such changes are certainly palpable in soft tissues before and after neuromuscular and other forms of manual treatment. Taylor (1958) has stated that manipulative pressure and stretching are the most effective ways of modifying energy potentials of abnormal soft tissues.

Little (1969) believes that an additional beneficial effect results from the interaction of the bioenergy mechanism of the practitioner with the bioenergy field of the patient.

Eeman (1947) has shown that, after each simple movement that we perform, we retain a

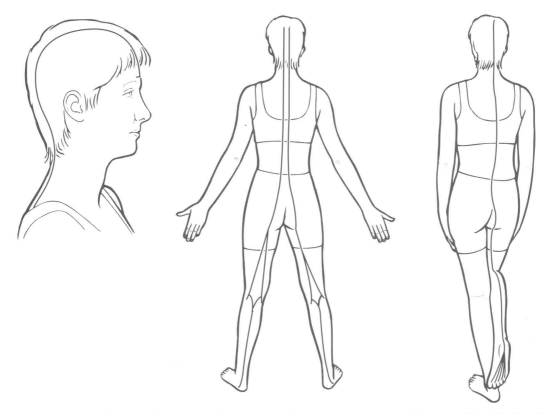

Figure 1.3   Myers' superficial back line. Redrawn from *Journal of Bodywork and Movement Therapies* 1997; 1(2):95, with permission.

degree of unconscious contractile muscular activity. This unconscious continuation of objective contraction is not only wasteful of energy but productive of long-term changes within the tissues involved. He has also shown that unless, and until, neuromuscular relaxation is achieved there cannot be a total resting state of the mind.

Over and above the important factors of posture, functional ability and pain, the musculoskeletal component of the body plays a vital role in the conservation – wastage – of energy and in the attainment, or otherwise, of a truly relaxed mind. Whilst the origins of musculoskeletal dysfunction can be either psychic or physical, the constant interaction of the soma with the mind ensures a degree of psychic stress occurring as a feedback from physically caused chronic muscular tensions.

Rolf (1962) suggests that the human organism, as an energy mass, is subject to gravitational law.

As a plastic medium, capable of change, Rolfing attempts to reorganise and balance the body in relation to gravitational forces. This is done by using pressure and stretch techniques on the fascial tissues in a precise sequence of body areas. The beneficial effects are claimed to be physical, emotional, postural and behavioural.

Rolf (1962) states:

Our ignorance of the role and significance of fascia is profound. Therefore even in theory it is easy to overlook the possibility that far-reaching changes may be made not only in structural contour, but also in functional manifestation, through better organisation of the layer of superficial fascia which enwraps the body. Experiments demonstrate that drastic (beneficial) changes may be made in the body, solely by stretching, separating and relaxing superficial fascia in an appropriate manner.

Osteopaths have observed and recorded the extent to which all degenerative change in the

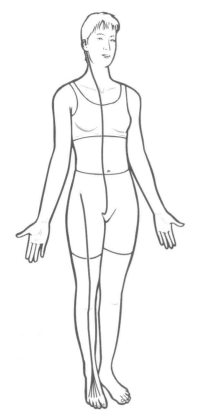

Figure 1.4 Myers' superficial front line. Redrawn from *Journal of Bodywork and Movement Therapies* 1997; 1(2):97, with permission.

body – whether muscular, nervous, circulatory or organic – reflects in the superficial fascia. Any degree of degeneration, however minor, changes the bulk of the fascia, modifies its thickness and draws it into ridges in areas overlying deeper tensions and rigidities. Conversely, as this elastic envelope is stretched, manipulative mechanical energy is added to it, and the fascial colloid becomes more 'sol' and less 'gel' (Greenman 1989). The biophysics of this process have been discussed in a classical paper by R.B. Taylor (1958):

As a result of the added energy, as well as of a directional contribution in applying it, the underlying structures, including the muscles which determine the placement of the body parts in space, and also their relations to each other, have come a little closer to the normal ('normal' as used here must be

differentiated from 'average') – the patient feels 'so much better'.

Without minimising the clinical importance of the structural and biomechanical aspects of the connective tissues, Oschman (2000) has examined and evaluated research, which suggests that far more may be taking place during manual treatment than current understanding can fully explain. See Box 1.7 for a brief summary of aspects of these concepts.

Fascial stress responses and therapeutic opportunities

Changes in the fascia can result from passive congestion, which results in fibrous infiltration and a more 'sol'-like consistency than is the norm. Under healthy conditions a 'gel'-like ground substance follows the laws of fluid mechanics. Clearly, the more resistive drag there is in a colloidal substance, the greater will be the difficulty in normalising this.

Scariati (1991) points out that colloids are not rigid: they conform to the shape of their container, and respond to pressure even though they are not compressible. The amount of resistance they offer increases proportionally to the velocity of motion applied to them, which makes a gentle touch a fundamental requirement if viscous drag and resistance are to be avoided when attempting to produce a release.

When stressful forces (undesirable or therapeutic) are applied to fascia, there is a first reaction in which a degree of slack is allowed to be taken up, followed by what is colloquially referred to as 'creep' – a variable degree of resistance (depending on the state of the tissues). Creep is an honest term which accurately describes the slow, delayed yet continuous, stretch that occurs in response to a continuously applied load, as long as this is gentle enough to not provoke the resistance of colloidal 'drag'.

As the fascia comprises a single structure, the implications for body-wide repercussions of distortions in that structure are clear (Fig. 1.6). An example of one possible negative influence of this sort is to be found in the fascial divisions

---

Box 1.7 Oschman's energy concepts: connective tissue, crystallinity and continuity

---

Peters (2001) discusses Oschman's research into energy phenomena as this relates to health enhancement. He reports that Oschman (2000) makes the point that the intricate traffic of biochemical, structural and electrical information is modulated not only through an electromagnetic flux, and 'clouds' of neuroreceptor traffic, but also as mechanical and rhythmic impulses of sound, heat, gravity, elasticity and pressure.

Oschman (2000) describes the processes:

What we refer to as health is when all the systems, both known and unknown, are functioning collectively, co-operatively . . . The solid state, electronic, photonic and vibratory properties, of this living matrix continuum, play key roles in the integration of function, including injury repair and defence against disease. A debate about whether there is such a thing as 'healing energy' or 'life energy' has been replaced with study of the interaction between biological energy fields, structures and functions . . . There are now instruments sensitive enough to detect the bio-magnetic fields produced by the different organs . . . photometers and thermographs of parallel sensitivity allow us to detect almost infinitesimal variations in light and heat emanating from the body. Previous images of the organism – as being built up of parts – have concealed the most significant attribute of living matter – its continuity.

Oschman (2000) goes on:

The major structural and functional domains of the body are the connective tissues, the cells within them, and the cytoskeletons, nuclei and genetic material within the cells . . . [this] assembly is best described by a single word, continuum . . . Structural and functional continuity has now been confirmed and appreciated by science.

Continuity in living systems is simultaneously mechanical, structural, regulatory, and energetic. A second key to the emerging concepts has come about from recognition of the crystalline properties of living

tissues . . . Crystals have important vibratory characteristics that arise as collective properties of the whole system. When a crystal is broken into its constituents, these unique vibratory phenomena disappear. This is why collective properties such as functional organization and consciousness have been elusive for those who study the system's components piece-by-piece. Molecular arrays or crystals are the dominant structural feature of living matter. Crystallographic techniques such as X-ray diffraction have been essential for determining the structure of nerves, muscles, cell membranes, and connective tissues. From the biophysical perspective, molecular arrays or crystals cannot be described in terms of their constituents alone. (See Fig. 1.5.)

British biophysicist Mae-Wan Ho has developed an elegant quantum theory which describes the organism as a vibrant sentient whole (Ho 1993). Key to Ho's theory (Ho 1997) is the role of the connective tissue as a liquid crystalline material constituting a noiseless excitable vibratory continuum for rapid intercommunication and energy flow, permeating the entire organism and enabling it to function and perceive as a coherent whole.

Oschman (2000) attempts to describe a unitary concept:

The quantum coherence phenomenon, described by biophysicists, may be the origin of Sheldrake's morphogenetic field (Sheldrake 1995). Quantum coherence is a source of measurable light emissions from living systems (Popp et al 1992). Quantum coherence in the living matrix provides a basis for a unitary theory. Water and vibrations of the crystalline molecular lattices play key roles in energy and information storage, transfer, and release.

The conclusion reached by Oschman (2000) is that, almost irrespective of the mode of treatment, a primary interaction occurs between the therapist and the patient, which may involve communication between their energy

---

within the cranium, the tentorium cerebelli and falx cerebri, which are commonly warped during birthing difficulties (too long or too short a time in the birth canal, forceps delivery, etc.) and which are noted in craniosacral therapy as affecting total body mechanics via their influence on fascia (and therefore the musculature) throughout the body (Brookes 1984).

Cantu & Grodin (1992) describe what they see as the 'unique' feature of connective tissue as its 'deformation characteristics'. This refers to a combined viscous (permanent) deformation characteristic as well as an elastic (temporary)

deformation characteristic. This leads to the clinically important manner in which connective tissue responds to applied mechanical force by first changing in length, followed by some of this change being lost while some remains. The implications of this phenomenon can be seen in the application of stretching techniques to such tissues, as well as in the way they respond to postural and other repetitive insults.

Such changes are not, however, permanent, because collagen (the raw material of fascia/connective tissue) has a limited (300–500 days) half-life and, just as bone adapts to stresses

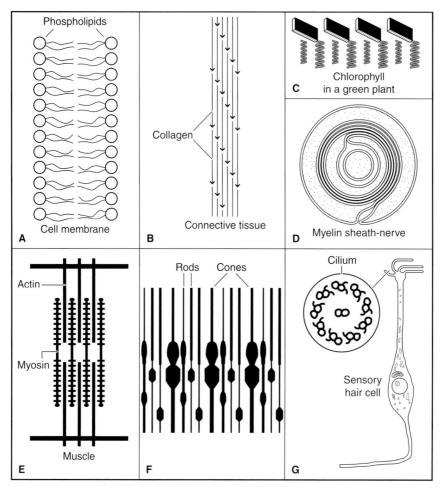

Figure 1.5 Crystalline arrays in living systems. Crystalline arrangements are the rule and not the exception in living systems. (A) Arrays of phospholipid molecules from cell membranes. (B) Collagen arrays form connective tissue. (C) Arrays of chlorophyll molecules in the leaf. (D) The myelin sheath of nerves. (E) The contractile array in muscle is composed of actin and myosin molecules organised around one another. (F) The array of sensory endings in the retina. (G) Arrays of microtubules, microfilaments and other fibrous components of the cytoskeleton occur in nerves and other kinds of cells. The example shown here is the cilia of sensory organs such as those responsible for detecting odours and sound. Reproduced from Oschman (2000) (illustration (D) is reproduced with permission of Arnold).

imposed upon it, so does fascia. Therefore, if negative stresses (posture, use, etc.) are modified for the better and/or positive 'stresses' are imposed (e.g. manipulation and/or exercise), dysfunctional connective tissue can usually be improved over time (Neuberger et al 1953).

Cantu & Grodin (1992), in their evaluation of the myofascial complex, concluded that therapeutic approaches that sequence their treatment protocols to involve the superficial tissues (involving autonomic responses) as well as deeper tissues (influencing the mechanical components of the musculoskeletal system), and which also address the factor of mobility (movement), are in tune with the requirements of the body when dysfunctional. NMT, as it will be presented here, does take this comprehensive approach, and much that it offers seems to be similar to the myofascial release methods currently receiving so much attention in the USA.

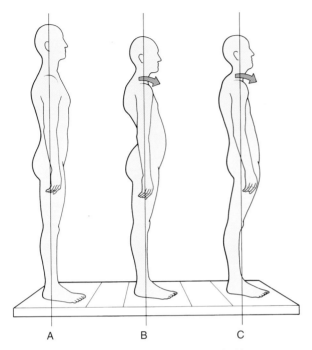

Figure 1.6 Balanced posture (A) compared with two patterns of musculoskeletal imbalance that involve fascial, and general, tissue and joint adaptations.

Cathie (1974) maintains that the contractile phase of fascial activity supersedes all its other qualities. The attachments of fascia, he states, have a tendency to shorten after periods of marked activity that are followed by periods of inactivity, and the ligaments become tighter and thicker with advancing age. The properties of fascia (connective tissue) that he regards as being important to therapeutic consideration are:

1. It is richly endowed with nerve endings.
2. It has the ability to contract and to stretch elastically.
3. It gives extensive muscular attachment.
4. It supports and stabilises, thus enhancing the postural balance of the body.
5. It is vitally involved in all aspects of motion.
6. It aids in circulatory economy, especially of venous and lymphatic fluids.
7. Fascial change will precede many chronic degenerative diseases.
8. Fascial changes predispose towards chronic tissue congestion.
9. Such chronic passive congestion precedes the formation of fibrous tissue, which then proceeds to an increase in hydrogen ion concentration of articular and periarticular structures.
10. Fascial specialisations produce definite stress bands.
11. Sudden stress (trauma) on fascial tissue will often result in a burning type of pain.
12. Fascia is a major arena of inflammatory processes.
13. Fluids and infectious processes often travel along fascial planes.
14. The CNS is surrounded by fascial tissue (dura mater) which, in the skull, attaches to bone, so that dysfunction in these tissues can have profound and widespread effects.

Greenman (1989) describes how fascia responds to loads and stress in both a plastic and an elastic manner, its response depending upon the type, duration and amount of the load. The responses to either acute injury or repetitive microtrauma (e.g. short leg imbalance) are, according to Greenman, likely to follow a sequence of inflammation which subsequently leads to absorption of inflammatory fluids into the superficial fascia, as well as into tight compartmentalised areas in the deep fascia – with this latter event being both palpable and detrimental.

Another variable (apart from the nature of the stress load) that influences the way in which fascia responds to stress, and what the individual feels of the process, relates to the number of collagen and elastic fibres contained in any given region. Neural receptors within the fascia report to the CNS as part of any adaptation process, with the Pacinian corpuscles being particularly important in terms of their involvement in reflex responses.

Other neural input into the pool of activity, and responses to biomechanical stress, involve specialised fascial structures such as tendons and ligaments which contain highly specialised and sensitive mechanoreceptors and proprioceptive reporting stations.

Changes that occur in connective tissue, and which result in such alterations as thickening, shortening, calcification and erosion, may be a painful result of sudden or sustained tension or traction. Cathie (1974) points out that many trigger points (he calls them trigger 'spots') correspond to points where nerves pierce fascial investments. The causes of derangement may, therefore, be seen to result from faulty muscular activity, alteration in bony relationships, visceral positional change (e.g. visceroptosis) and the adoption of unnatural positions. All of these can be sustained repetitive causes or single, violently induced, changes. Chemical (nutritional) factors influencing fascial behaviour should also be considered for, as Pauling (1976) points out, 'Many of the results of deprivation of ascorbic acid involve a deficiency in connective tissue which is largely responsible for the strength of bones, teeth, skin, of the body and which consists of the fibrous protein collagen.'

Pauling goes on to point out that, in deficiency of vitamin C, this binding material becomes less efficient and more fluid. He concludes that the effectiveness of vitamin C in helping the body contain viral particles may to some extent be a result of its strengthening action on connective tissue, which would impede the motion of viral particles through tissue. This illustrates, again, the ubiquitous nature of the musculoskeletal tissues in general and of fascia in particular, and the profound effect on the body's economy of dysfunction in any of its myriad components.

Modern techniques of electron and phase microscopy have been used to study myofascial biochemistry activity, showing that much of the fascia and connective tissue is comprised of tubular structures. Erlinghauser (1959) has shown that lymph and cerebrospinal fluid spread throughout the body via these channels. The implications of this knowledge have not yet been fully realised or investigated by physiologists, but play a large part in the theories (and practice) of cranial and craniosacral therapists (Upledger 1988).

Having briefly scanned the influences of stress, both short and long term, on the musculoskeletal system, and of the varying ways in which the soft tissues respond – acutely, chronically and with variations based on their structure – and before looking more closely at reflex phenomena, notably myofascial trigger points that result from such stress, a brief introduction to neuromuscular technique (see Ch. 2) will provide an indication of its potential for dealing with such soft tissue distress.

REFERENCES

Alexander FM 1957 The use of the self. Educational Publications, London

Baldry P 1993 Acupuncture, trigger points and musculoskeletal pain. Churchill Livingstone, Edinburgh

Barlow W 1959 Anxiety and muscle tension pain. British Journal of Clinical Practice 3(5):339–350

Basmajian J 1974 Muscles alive. Williams & Wilkins, Baltimore

Boadella D 1978 The language of the body in bioenergetic therapy. Journal of the Research Society for Natural Therapeutics

Brookes D 1984 Cranial osteopathy. Thorsons, London

Butler D 1991 Mobilisation of the nervous system. Churchill Livingstone, Edinburgh

Butler D, Gifford L 1989 Adverse mechanical tensions in the nervous system. Physiotherapy 75:622–629

Buzzell K 1970 The physiological basis of osteopathic medicine. Postgraduate Institute of Osteopathic Medicine and Surgery, New York

Cantu R, Grodin A 1992 Myofascial manipulation. Aspen Publications, Gaithersburg, Maryland

Cathie A 1974 Selected writings. Academy of Applied Osteopathy Yearbook 1974. Academy of Applied Osteopathy, Colorado Springs

Chaitow L 1989 Soft tissue manipulation. Thorsons, London

Chaitow L, DeLany J 2000 Clinical applications of neuromuscular technique. Churchill Livingstone, Edinburgh

Chaitow L, Bradley D, Gilbert C 2002 Interdisciplinary approaches to breathing pattern disorders. Churchill Livingstone, Edinburgh

Cyriax J 1962 Textbook of orthopaedic medicine. Cassell, London

Dicke E 1978 A manual of reflexive therapy. Sydney Simons, Scarsdale, New York

DiGiovanna E 1991 An osteopathic approach to diagnosis and treatment. Lippincott, London

Dommerholt J 2000 Posture. In: Tubiana R, Camadio P (eds) Medical problems of the instrumentalist musician. Martin Dunitz, London

Dvorak J, Dvorak V 1984 Manual medicine – diagnostics. Georg Thiem, Stuttgart

Edwards R 1988 Hypotheses of peripheral and central mechanisms underlying occupational muscle pain and injury. European Journal of Applied Physiology 57:275–281

Eeman L 1947 Cooperative healing. Frederick Muller, London

Engel A et al 1986 Skeletal muscle types in myology. McGraw-Hill, New York

Erlinghauser RF 1959 Circulation of CSF through connective tissues. Academy of Applied Osteopathy Yearbook, Carmel, California

Feldenkrais M 1977 Awareness through movement. Harper & Row, New York

Frankel V 1980 Basic biomechanics of the skeletal system. Lea & Febiger, Philadelphia

Gagey 1986 Postural disorders among workers in building sites In: Bles W, Brandt T, eds. Disorders of posture and gait. Elsevier, New York

Gray H 1977 Gray's anatomy. 35th edn. Churchill Livingstone, Edinburgh

Greenman P 1989 Principles of manual medicine. Williams & Wilkins, Baltimore

Grieve G 1985 Mobilisation of the spine. Churchill Livingstone, Edinburgh

Hallgren R, Greenman P, Rechtien J 1993 MRI of normal and atrophic muscles of the upper cervical spine. Journal of Clinical Engineering 18(5):433–439

Henneman E 1957 Relation between size of neurons and their susceptibility to discharge. Science 126:1345–1347

Ho M-W 1993 The rainbow and the worm. The physics of organisms. World Scientific, Singapore

Ho M-W 1997 Quantum coherence and conscious experience. Kybernetes 26:265–276

Horwitz A 1997 Integrins and health. Scientific American 276:68–75

Hynes R 1992 Integrins: versatility, modulation and signalling. Cell 69:11–26

Janda V 1982 Introduction to functional pathology of the motor system. Proceedings of the VIIth Commonwealth and International Conference on Sport. Physiotherapy in Sport 3:39

Janda V 1983 Muscle function testing. Butterworths, London

Janda V 1988 In: Grant R, ed. Physical therapy of the cervical and thoracic spine. Churchill Livingstone, Edinburgh

Janda V 1996 Evaluation of muscle imbalances. In: Liebenson C, ed. Rehabilitation of the spine. Williams & Wilkins, Baltimore

Jokl P 1984 Muscle and low back pain. Journal of the American Osteopathic Association 84(1):64–65

Jones L 1980 Strain and counterstrain. Academy of Applied Osteopathy, Colorado Springs

Kappler R 1997 Thrust techniques. In: Ward R, ed. Foundations for Osteopathic Medicine. Williams & Wilkins, Baltimore

Kolar P 1999 Sensomotor nature of postural functions. Journal of Orthopaedic Medicine 212:40–45

Korr I 1970 The physiological basis of osteopathic medicine. Postgraduate Institute of Osteopathic Medicine, New York

Korr I 1976 Spinal cord as organiser of disease process. Academy of Applied Osteopathy Yearbook, Colorado Springs

Korr I 1978 Neurologic mechanisms in manipulative therapy. Plenum Press, New York

Korr I 1981 Axonal transport and neurotrophic functions in spinal cord as organiser of disease processes (part 4). Academy of Applied Osteopathy March: 451–458

Larsson S-E, Bodegard L, Henriksson KG, Oberg PA 1990 Chronic trapezius myalgia. Morphology and blood flow studied in 17 patients. Acta Orthopaedica Scandinavica 61:394–398

Latey P 1983 Muscular manifesto. P Latey, London

Lederman E 1997 Fundamentals of manual therapy. Churchill Livingstone, Edinburgh

Lewis Sir T 1942 Pain. New York

Lewit K 1985 Manipulation in rehabilitation of the locomotor system. Butterworths, London

Lewit K 1992 Manipulation in rehabilitation of the locomotor system. 2nd edn. Butterworths, London

Lewit K 1999 Manipulation in rehabilitation of the locomotor system. 3rd edn. Butterworths, London

Liebenson C, ed. 1996 Rehabilitation of the spine. Williams & Wilkins, Baltimore

Liebenson C 1999 Muscular imbalance – an update. Dynamic Chiropractic Online. Available: http://www.chiroweb.com/dynamic

Lin J-P, Brown JK, Walsh EG 1994 Physiological maturation of muscles in childhood. Lancet 343:1386–1389

Little KE 1969 Toward more effective manipulative management of chronic myofascial strain and stress syndromes. Journal of the American Osteopathic Association 68:675–685

McConnell C 1962 Osteopathic Institute of Applied Technique Yearbook 1962, London

McPartland J, Brodeur R 1999 Rectus capitis posterior minor. Journal of Bodywork and Movement Therapies 3(1):30–35

Maitland G 1986 Vertebral manipulation. Butterworths, London

Maitland G, Hengeveld E, Banks K, English K 2001 Maitland's vertebral manipulation. 6th edn. Butterworth Heinemann, London

Martin S 2001 Interview with Jeff Bland: lessons from the genome. CAM Magazine November 2001

Mense S, Simons D 2001 Muscle pain. Williams & Wilkins, Philadelphia

Myers T 2001 Anatomy trains. Churchill Livingstone, Edinburgh

Neuberger A et al 1953 Metabolism of collagen. Biochemical Journal 53:47–52

Norris CM 1995a Spinal stabilisation. 1. Active lumbar stabilisation – concepts. Physiotherapy 81(2):61–64

Norris CM 1995b Spinal stabilisation. 2. Limiting factors to end-range motion in the lumbar spine. Physiotherapy 81(2):64–72

Norris CM 1995c Spinal stabilisation. 3. Stabilisation mechanisms of the lumbar spine. Physiotherapy 81(2):72–79

Norris CM 1995d Spinal stabilisation. 4. Muscle imbalance and the low back. Physiotherapy 81(3):127–138

Norris CM 1995e Spinal stabilisation. 5. An exercise program to enhance lumbar stabilisation. Physiotherapy 81(3):138–146

Norris CM 1998 Sports injuries, diagnosis and management. 2nd edn. Butterworths, London

Oschman J 2000 Energy medicine. Churchill Livingstone, Edinburgh

Patterson M, Wurster R 1997 Neurophysiologic system: integration and disintegration. In: Ward R, ed. Foundations for osteopathic medicine. Williams & Wilkins, Baltimore

Pauling L 1976 The common cold and 'flu. WH Freeman

Peck D, Buxton D, Nitz A 1984 A comparison of spindle concentrations in large and small muscles acting in parallel combinations. Journal of Morphology 180:243–252

Peters D 2001 Vitalism revisited. Journal of Bodywork and Movement Therapies 5(3):198–204

Popp FA, Li KH, Gu Q 1992 Recent advances in biophoton research. World Scientific, Singapore

Reich W 1949 Character analysis. Vision Press

Reinert A, Mense S 1993 Inflammatory influence on the density of CGRP- and SP-immunoreactive nerve endings in rat skeletal muscle. Neuropeptides 24:204–205

Richardson C 2000 The muscle designation debate. Journal of Bodywork and Movement Therapies 4(4):235–236

Richardson C, Jull G, Hodges P, Hides J 1999 Therapeutic exercise for spinal segment stabilisation in low back pain. Churchill Livingstone, Edinburgh

Rolf I 1962 Structural dynamics. British Academy of Applied Osteopathy Yearbook 1962. BAAO, New York

Rosenthal E 1987 The Alexander technique and how it works. Medical Problems in the Performing Arts 2:53–57

Rowlerson A 1981 A novel myosin. Journal of Muscle Research and Cell Motility 2:415–438

Scariati P 1991 In: DiGiovanna E, ed. An osteopathic approach to diagnosis and treatment. Lippincott, London

Selye H 1976 The stress of life. McGraw Hill, Philadelphia

Sheldrake R 1995 A new science of life. The hypothesis of morphic resonance. Park Street Press, Rochester, Vermont

Simons D 1987 Myofascial pain due to trigger points. International Rehabilitation Medicine Association Monograph (Series 1), Rademaker, Ohio

Simons D, Travell J, Simons L 1999 Myofascial pain and dysfunction: the trigger point manual. vol. 1: Upper half of body. 2nd edn. Williams & Wilkins, Baltimore

Stiles E 1984 Patient Care 15 May:16–97 & 15 August:117–164

Stoddard A 1969 Manual of osteopathic practice. Hutchinson, London

Taylor RB 1958 Bioenergetics of man. Academy of Applied Osteopathic Yearbook 1958, Carmel, California

Timmons B 1994 Behavioral and psychological approaches to breathing disorders. Plenum Press, New York

Travell J, Simons D 1983 Myofascial pain and dysfunction: the trigger point manual. vol. 1. Williams & Wilkins, Philadelphia

Travell J, Simons D 1992 Myofascial pain and dysfunction: the trigger point manual. vol. 2. Williams & Wilkins, Philadelphia

Upledger J 1988 Craniosacral therapy. Eastland Press, Seattle

Waersted M, Eken T, Westgaard R 1993 Psychogenic motor unit activity – a possible muscle injury mechanism studied in a healthy subject. Journal of Musculoskeletal Pain 1(3/4):185–190

Wall P, Melzack R 1991 Textbook of pain. Churchill Livingstone, Edinburgh

Wang N, Butler JP, Ingbes DE et al 1993 Mechanotransduction across the cell surface and through the cytoskeleton. Science 260:1124–1127

Warwick R, Williams P 1973 Gray's anatomy. 3rd edn. WB Saunders, London

Wolfe F, Simons D 1992 Fibromyalgia and myofascial pain syndromes. Journal of Rheumatology 19(6):944–995

Woo SL-Y et al 1987 Injury and repair of musculoskeletal soft tissues. American Academy of Orthopedic Surgeons Symposium, Savannah, Georgia

2

Introduction to NMT

NMT: A BRIEF HISTORICAL OVERVIEW

Imagine a palpation technique that becomes a means of therapeutic intervention by virtue of the addition of increased pressure.

Imagine also a palpation technique that, in a non-invasive manner, meets and matches the tone of the tissues it is addressing and sequentially seeks out changes from the norm in almost all accessible (to finger or thumb) areas of the soft tissues.

Imagine this approach as systematically providing information regarding tissue tone, induration, fibrosity, oedema, discrete localised soft tissue changes, areas of altered structure, adhesions or pain – and being able to switch from a painless and pleasant assessment mode to a treatment focus that starts the process of normalising the changes it uncovers.

This is neuromuscular technique (NMT).

The developer of European NMT was Stanley Lief, who was born in Lutzen in the Baltic state of Latvia in the early 1890s. He was one of the five children of Isaac and Riva Lief (Riva was the author's grandfather's eldest sister, i.e. her maiden surname was Chaitow). The family emigrated to South Africa in the 1890s where Stanley was given a basic primary school education before starting work in his father's trading store in Roodeport, Transvaal.

Lief's poor health led to an interest in physical culture, one source of which was found in popular health magazines published in the USA. Eventually Lief worked his passage to the USA in order to train under the legendary 'physical culturist' Bernard Macfadden. He qualified in chiropractic and naturopathy before World War I, and was in Britain at its outbreak. After serving in the army he returned to England and worked in institutional 'Nature Cure' (naturopathic) resorts until 1925, when he established his own clinic, Champneys, at Tring in Hertfordshire.

At this world-famous healing resort he established his reputation as a daring and pioneering healer. By using the dietetic, fasting, hydrotherapeutic and physical education and manual methods by which naturopathy aims to restore normality to the sick body, he developed a huge following. It was during his most successful years, before World War II, that he evolved the technique that this book attempts to describe.

Stanley Lief, together with his cousin Boris Chaitow, who worked as his assistant at Champneys before and during World War II, developed and refined the uses of NMT. Boris Chaitow was also born in Latvia and grew up in South Africa in the small mining town of Pilgrim's Rest, now a 'museum town', where the Chaitow trading store-cum-home still stands. He later qualified as an attorney, and was in practice with my father when he became inspired by Stanley Lief's example and, with Lief's help, trained as a chiropractor at National College, Chicago, before joining the staff at Champneys in 1937.

In this book, Lief's basic NMT applications, together with a variety of specialised associated soft tissue manipulation techniques, will be presented. There will also be discussion of various reflex systems that fall within the scope of soft tissue treatment in general, and NMT in particular. For example, detailed reference to, and illustrations of, the neurolymphatic reflexes of Chapman, together with illustrations of other reflex patterns such as myofascial trigger points, have been included. Another of Lief's assistants at Champneys, Tom Moule, continued the development of NMT in health care, and his son, Terry Moule, has contributed his thoughts in Chapter 9, in which his particular focus, the use of NMT in treatment of sports injuries, is briefly outlined. Another evolution of an NMT-like approach, known as Progressive Inhibition of Neuromuscular Structures (PINS), is described by its developer, Denis Dowling, in Chapter 11.

As a modality, NMT complements and may be incorporated into any system of physical medicine. It may – and indeed often should – be used as a means of treatment on its own, or it may accompany (preceding for preference) manipulative and other physical modalities. Its main use up to the present has been in the hands (literally) of the osteopathic profession; however, many physiotherapists, chiropractors, massage therapists and doctors of physical medicine who have studied and used NMT have found it complementary to their own methods of practice.

As it offers a simultaneous diagnostic and therapeutic capability, NMT is time-saving, energy-saving and, above all, efficient.

Other soft tissue manipulative methods such as muscle energy technique (MET) and functional positional release approaches (strain/counterstrain, for example) are commonly used as part of NMT treatment. The key to the successful use of NMT is an ability to sense accurately what it is that the hands are feeling while at the same time having a clear picture of what the particular movement or technique being employed is aimed at achieving. If the practitioner can learn to 'see', with the hands, and by using them let the patient's body 'tell its own tale', then the intelligent application of the methods described has much to offer towards the recovery of normal function.

Holistic methods of healing demand that, in order to create the situation for the maintenance or the restoration of health, the individual must be seen as a totality.

It is necessary, therefore, to attempt to recognise the various factors affecting both the internal and external environment of the individual, because these are part of the complex interacting totality that can influence the individual for good or ill. In the end, the body is self-healing, self-repairing and self-maintaining, if the prerequisites for health are present. Emotional stability, nutritional balance and hygienic considerations all play their part, as do structural and mechanical integrity.

A brief history

In Europe neuromuscular technique has evolved over the past 60 years from the original work of Stanley Lief. In the mid-1930s he was seeking improved means for preparing soft tissue structures for subsequent manipulation. The development of NMT (neuromuscular therapy) in the USA is described at the end of this chapter.

Lief had studied the work of Rabagliatti, whose book *Initis* influenced his interest in connective tissue problems. He also became aware of (and studied) the work of a Dr Dewanchand Varma, a practitioner of Ayurvedic manipulation (Varma called his method 'pranotherapy') who was practising in Paris. In Varma's book *The Human Machine and Its Forces* (Varma 1935), he states:

We have discovered that the circulation of the nervous currents, slows down occasionally because of the obstruction caused by adhesions; the muscular fibres harden and the nervous currents can no longer pass through them. We have demonstrated effective and positive methods designed to restore nervous equilibrium which promotes the healthy circulation of blood, so that new tissues begin to be built up again. Our method of treatment, by the removal of all obstacles to the flow of nervous current, allows energy to proceed unimpeded.

Lief found various of Varma's techniques clinically useful, and from these ideas and methods developed his own soft tissue approach – NMT. Lief's cousin, Boris Chaitow, describes this early development of NMT as follows (B. Chaitow, personal communication, 1983):

In the middle of the 1930s Stanley Lief realised that the integrity of a joint was to a great extent related to the character of the tissues surrounding the joint, related to muscle, tendons, ligaments, blood and nerve supply etc. He felt that in order the better to achieve effective mobility and integrity of function of joints – particularly in the spine but also in all bony articular relationships – it was advisable to normalise, as best one could, the adjacent soft tissues by removing any function-interfering factors, such as tensions, contractions, adhesions, spasms, fibrositic contractures etc., with appropriate application of fingers and hands to those tissues. To this end the neuromuscular technique was evolved to cover every possible type of lesion in whatever part of the body (articular, soft tissue, abdominal, glandular, nervous, vascular etc).

It so happened that at that particular time Stanley Lief had heard of a well-known Indian practitioner named Varma operating in Paris, who was applying an unusual but very effective soft-tissue technique on patients with remarkable benefits. Lief decided to arrange to have a series of treatments on himself from Varma, and finally persuaded the latter to teach him this specialised technique. Much as he appreciated the method used by Varma, he felt it could be improved, and began to develop and subsequently practised the method for which he devised the name of 'Neuromuscular Technique'. This name was an accurate definition of the purpose of the method he evolved from the cruder technique used by Varma. NMT involved an application of hands and fingers to the appropriate areas of soft tissue related to the affected bony articulations, as well as all other areas of soft tissue which his sensitive fingers found to be abnormal in texture. This enables adverse factors in such tissue to be corrected to allow the full function of muscles and nerves to be re-established. In doing so the double benefits are achieved in improving nerve and blood circulation, improving texture of muscle tissue and in being better able to get effective results in manipulating the bony articulations involved, and assuring lasting integrity of their normal function.

Stanley Lief also maintained that joint lesions were not the only factors in the interference in nerve force integrity, but that tensions, contractions, adhesions, muscle spasms and fibrositic contractures in soft tissues could in themselves constitute primary factors in disease (symptom) causation by reducing effective nerve and blood circulation. To this end he developed his diagnostic sensitivity with his fingers so that in a few seconds of palpation over any area of the body, he was able to assess abnormalities present in relation to tensions, adhesions and spasms.

The body's integrity, and its functional efficiency, depends not only on its chemistry influenced by the nature of the food and drink we consume, but also on the effective nerve and blood circulation free of mechanical and functional obstructions. To this second vital purpose there is no formula devised by the osteopathic or chiropractic professions that will more effectively achieve the optimum result than the philosophy and technique devised by Stanley Lief. There is no single part of the body that he was not able to apply his method to to achieve remarkable physiological responses.

Stanley Lief's son, Peter (also a naturopath, chiropractor and osteopath), has described (Lief 1963) the 'neuromuscular' lesion as being associated with:

1. Congestion of the local connective tissues
2. Disturbance of the acid–base balance of the connective tissues

3. Fibrous infiltration (adhesions)
4. Chronic muscular contractions, or hypertrophic or hypotrophic (tone) changes.

The aetiology of the neuromuscular lesion, according to Stanley and Peter Lief, includes a number of causative factors, giving rise to neuromuscular lesions, which may include:

● fatigue, exhaustion, bad posture
● local trauma
● systemic toxaemia
● lack of exercise and oxygen (ischaemia)
● dietetic deficiencies
● psychosomatic causes bringing about muscular tensions.

The presence of a 'lesion' (current terminology would define this as an area of somatic dysfunction) is always revealed by an area of hypersensitivity to pressure. It is remarkable to note just how close Lief came to defining the causes and characteristics of myofascial trigger points, although working many years before the trigger point research of Travell and Simons (Simons et al 1999, Travell & Simons 1992) (see Ch. 3).

TISSUES INVOLVED IN NMT

Boris Chaitow and Peter Lief have both taken part in the development and evolution of the theory and application of NMT as first described by Stanley Lief. Another distinguished British naturopath/osteopath who worked with them, Brian Youngs, has given the following descriptive overview of the tissues involved in NMT (Youngs 1962):

Site of application
As the technique (NMT) operates primarily on connective tissue it will usually be concentrated at those areas where such tissue is most dense, e.g. muscular origins and insertions, especially the broad aponeurotic insertions. The most frequent sites are the superior curved line of the occiput, the numerous insertions and origins of the large, medium and small muscles which attach to the vertebral column; the iliac-crest insertions; the intercostal insertions and abdominal-muscle insertions. Nevertheless, the technique can of course be applied to any area which

requires it – head, face, wrists, etc. Connective tissue is, after all, ubiquitous.

To understand the therapeutic effect of the technique one must have some knowledge of the pathophysiology of the tissue upon which it operates. Connective tissue consists of a matrix containing cells and fibres. It was largely ignored until recently, but has now been made the subject of close study – and even international conferences – in regard to its structure and functions. Dr Rabagliatti, 45 years ago [*Note*: Young was writing in the mid-1960s] was so interested and far-seeing that his book, *Initis*, contained concepts the general truth of which is being proved today. He was, however, a lone voice and because he held unorthodox ideas he was, typically, ignored.

The ubiquity of connective tissue caused Dr Rabagliatti to analogise it to the ether – as the medium for, as he termed it, 'the zoodynamic life force'. [See Box 1.7 for current thinking along these lines.]

Through the connective tissues' planes run the trunks and plexuses of veins, arteries, nerves, and lymphatics. Connective tissue is the support for the structural and, therefore, functional relationships of these systems.

Chemical structure
Briefly, the matrix consists of a jelly-like ground substance in which the fibres, cells, vessels, etc., lie. This ground substance is the 'physical expression of the *milieu interieure*' intervening everywhere between the blood and lymph vessels and the metabolising cells; it plays a major role in the transport, storage and exchange of water and electrolytes. The chemical structure is essentially polysaccharide, hyaluronic acid, chondroitin sulphuric acid, chondroitin sulphate and chondroitin itself, together with proteins which contain a considerable amount of the amino acid tyrosine, which forms the majority of the thyroxine molecule.

The fibres are white fibrous (collagen), yellow (elastin), and reticulin. The collagen fibres are also protein and polysaccharide in composition and are stabilised chemically by the presence of the ground substance constituents. The presence of chondroitin sulphate, for example, renders the enzymatic breakdown of collagen much more difficult. The importance of this point will become more clear later. The formation of fibres appears to be due to a precipitation of fibre constituents by serum glycoproteins under the influence of adrenocorticotrophic hormone.

Reticulin contains more polysaccharide than collagen, and some lipid also. Elastin is also protein and polysaccharide in composition. Sulphur is a constituent of all three. Cells include fibroblasts, mast cells, macrophages and others.

A function of circulation

The nature and composition of connective tissue is a function of circulation. Circulatory efficiency in any area will determine (1) the influx of materials to the area, and (2) the drainage of the area.

Incoming blood leads to the production of lymph and this fluid permeates the ground substance, bringing all the constituents of the blood except the proteins to the connective tissue. Some of these constituents are hormones. Thyroxine, adrenoglucocorticoids and adrenomineralocorticoids are only three of these. Oestrogen and androgens are two more. All these have known effects upon the structure of connective tissue. Thus, a diminution of thyroxine leads to an increase of water retention in most cells and an increase in the quantity of ground substance. The sex hormones also do this, but of most interest to us here are the opposing groups of the adrenocortical hormones. Selye divides these into anti- and pro-inflammatory hormones (A-Cs and P-Cs). These are produced in response to stress situations and they exert both a general and a local effect. By regulating the balance between these two the body can control the ability of the tissues to produce an inflammatory response. But when the A-Cs and the P-Cs are both present in the blood the A-Cs always win the contest, i.e., there is an anti-inflammatory response.

Stressor stimulus

The A-Cs are produced in response to a stimulus – the stressor. The stressor in neuromuscular technique is pain. Effective technique appears to be accompanied by pain in all (I generalise here deliberately) such conditions (and also in the condition without treatment). Pain is probably due to two factors. A much reduced threshold in the area due to circulatory inhibition enabling a build up to just below the threshold level of Lewis pain substance or, alternatively, a disturbance of electrolyte level (e.g., increase of hydrogen ions or disturbance in the calcium/sodium/potassium balance due to the same circumstances). Consequently pain will be produced by even slight stimulus, let alone the heavier movements of neuromuscular technique. Also, pressure and tension proprioceptors may be overstimulated and pain can result from an over application of any ordinary stimulus.

The A-Cs liberated will produce both general effects (general adaptation syndrome) and local effects (local adaptation syndrome) and their effect is anti-inflammatory, both generally and locally, at the area of application of the stressor, i.e., at the areas of technique application. Consequently, there is a breakdown of collagen fibres and a general decrease in water retention in the ground substance; the congested area is decongested.

What Youngs has described tallies closely with what is now known about the biochemical status of tissues under stress, and particularly of the trigger point entity, which will be evaluated in following chapters.

Stanley Lief, albeit inadvertently, provided for the generation of practitioners who were to follow him a tool with which to deal with this pain-producing adaptive end-result of the multiple stresses faced by the modern musculoskeletal system.

In the latter part of the lives of Stanley Lief (d. 1963) and Boris Chaitow (d. 1996), awareness grew as to other applications of use for NMT, most notably its potential to identify and commence elimination of myofascial trigger points.

The principal author has over the past 40 years, since working as assistant to Boris Chaitow in the early 1960s, helped to promote knowledge of NMT – particularly in its diagnostic mode – so that it stands today as a major therapeutic instrument for use by manipulative and massage therapists worldwide. The use of NMT as a broadly applicable sequential assessment and treatment tool was enhanced by exposure to the work of Raymond Nimmo in the late 1960s. Nimmo and his 'receptor-tonus' work seems to be a common link between 'European' NMT and American NMT – as described by Judith Delany in this and other segments of the text devoted to the transatlantic perspective of NMT. Detailed descriptions of Nimmo's findings, with additional insights from Boris Chaitow of the means of application of NMT, in both its assessment and treatment modes, will be found in subsequent chapters.

JUDITH DELANY'S OVERVIEW OF NMT IN THE USA

What has today become neuromuscular therapy in the USA was spawned in the late 1970s from receptor-tonus method (the work of the late Dr Raymond Nimmo). Nimmo, a 1926 graduate of Palmer College of Chiropractic, states in his writings that he questioned many of the philosophical and theoretical teachings of his profession (Nimmo 1959). He studied many aspects of classical chiropractic even though he was convinced that adjustment of the spine was not enough to ensure the health of the individual. He also sought out information as to the role that soft tissues play in pain and dysfunction in an attempt to explain the syndromes he was confronted with in his work.

As Nimmo developed his palpation of the muscles, he noted particular points within the muscles which, when pressed, referred pain to various areas. He called these 'noxious generative points' (NGPs). In 1952 Nimmo purchased *Connective Tissue: Transactions of the Second Conference* (Travell 1952), in which Janet Travell discussed her theories of trigger points. Nimmo found illustrations of referred pain patterns in Travell's work that coincided precisely with his own discoveries. He began working obsessively to develop a sensible treatment plan and states that, as time went by, he learned from others, but probably 80–90% of the techniques he taught were his own work.

Nimmo's constant striving to prove the physiological basis of his work, complete with integration of neurological laws that gave validity and substance to his principles of practice, derived not only from being in the forefront of a newly emerging profession, but also from the fact that his interest in the soft tissue component of the body placed him at the fringes of the teachings of that profession.

He faced peers at a time when they were attempting to validate the principles of chiropractic and asked them to question the very basis of their beliefs. His work endured and many healthcare practitioners who studied with him carried the work forward, under a variety of names (see Box 2.1).

In 1979, Paul St John, who had studied receptor-tonus methodology with Nimmo, published

---

Box 2.1 Chiropractic perspective contribution of Raymond Nimmo

Cohen & Gibbons (1998) have detailed the chiropractic perspective on the work of Nimmo. They point out that, in a survey carried out in 1993 of procedures currently employed by chiropractors in the USA, fully 40% were using Nimmo's receptor tonus methodology, which closely approximates NMT (National Board of Chiropractic Examiners 1993).

Gatterman & Lee (1995) summarise Nimmo's approach:

Nimmo found noxious generative points [trigger points] in muscles that referred pain in characteristic patterns. Viewing these hypersensitive areas, the trigger points of Travell, as abnormal reflex arcs he developed a manual technique designed to reduce the irritable loci. He referred to the inter-relationship of muscle tonus and the central nervous system as 'reverberating circuits', whereby stimulus was self-perpetuating until the cycle was broken . . . This procedure referred to by Travell as ischemic compression offers a noninvasive chiropractic technique instead of the common medical practice of injection of the painful trigger points.

To reach a point where his belief in soft tissue origin of much musculoskeletal pain was widely accepted by his own profession, Nimmo had to contend with, and overcome, the prevailing chiropractic model of 'bone on nerve' concepts. He was certainly an original thinker and his trigger point research was contemporary with, and in some ways ahead of, those of Janet Travell, the major medical researcher into this field. At the very least, Cohen & Gibbons (1998) suggest: 'The similarities are striking and suggest one concept developed concurrently by two outstanding independent researchers.'

There were, nevertheless, distinct differences between the early treatment approaches advocated by Travell, compared with those suggested by Nimmo, in the developmental years of their research into the pain generated by trigger points.

Cohen & Gibbons (1998) explain:

Travell advocated injections to the trigger points and later spray and stretch and 'ischemic compression' to relax the involved muscle. On the other hand Nimmo stated, 'I have found that a proper degree of pressure, sequentially applied, causes the nervous system to release a hypertonic muscle'. Nimmo did not see the trigger points as an object to be injected, stretched, massaged or dissolved by ultrasound.

We should recall that Nimmo's concepts were evolving in the 1950s and that, at that stage of her work, Travell was advocating injection as the primary tool for trigger point deactivation. Over the years, direct compression ('ischemic') – now called 'trigger point release' – has become the preferred method of trigger point treatment, along with stretching (restoring the muscle housing the trigger point to its normal resting length; see Ch. 3).

Nimmo's insistence that trigger points had a neurological origin has not been validated, however, as evaluation of the latest findings of Simons et al (1999) will show (see Ch. 3). This in no way detracts from the enormous contribution made by Nimmo to this area of study.

course manuals relating to similar techniques, which he called neuromuscular therapy (NMT). His concepts were influenced by not only Nimmo (Vannerson & Nimmo 1971), but also Travell & Simons (1983), Mariano Racabado, Leon Chaitow, Rene Cailliet (1977), Aaron Mattes, John Barnes, John Upledger and others, through their writings and seminars. Judith (Walker) Delany's professional association with St John in 1984–1989 led to revisions of previous concepts, with significant changes in treatment techniques and teaching materials, which came to include the influence of posture and craniosacral methods. During this phase, the work of Janet Travell and David Simons had enormous influence. Their book *Myofascial Pain and Dysfunction: The Trigger Point Manual, Volume 1: The Upper Body* (Travell & Simons 1983), and numerous articles by them, began to explain in

greater detail the background to what Nimmo had taught. In 1989, St John and Delany separated their work and both continue to teach neuromuscular therapy. The approaches they have taken, although still containing elements of Nimmo's original work, have now diverged, with the St John Method™ focusing on structural homeostasis of the body and cranium by applying the law of cause and effect, and Delany's NMT American version™ incorporating a systematic approach towards pain relief which addresses six physiological factors: ischaemia, trigger points, nerve compression/ entrapment, postural distortion (biomechanics), nutritional components and emotional wellbeing (stress reduction). Judith Delany provides a detailed overview of NMT American version™ in its current stage of evolution in Chapter 10.

REFERENCES

Cailliet R 1977 Soft tissue pain and disability. FA Davis, Philadelphia

Cohen J, Gibbons R 1998 Raymond L Nimmo and the evolution of trigger point therapy 1929–1986. Journal of Manipulative and Physiological Therapeutics 21(3):167–172

Gatterman M, Lee H 1995 Chiropractic adjusting techniques. In: Peterson D, Weise G, eds. Chiropractic: an illustrated history, pp. 240–261. Mosby, Chicago

Lief P 1963 British Naturopathic Journal 5(10):304–324

National Board of Chiropractic Examiners 1993 Job analysis of chiropractic. Greely, Colorado

Nimmo R 1959 Factor X. The Receptor (1) 4. Reprinted in: Schneider M, Cohen J, Laws S 2001 The collected writings of Nimmo and Vannerson, pioneers of chiropractic trigger point therapy. Self-published, Pittsburgh

Simons D, Travell J, Simons L 1999 Myofascial pain and dysfunction: the trigger point manual, vol. 1: Upper half of body, 2nd edn. Williams & Wilkins, Baltimore

Travell J 1952 Connective tissue: transactions of the second conference. The Josiah Macy Jr Foundation, New York

Travell J, Simons D 1983 Myofascial pain and dysfunction: the trigger point manual. vol. 1: The upper body. Williams & Wilkins, Baltimore

Travell J, Simons D 1992 Myofascial pain and dysfunction: the trigger point manual. vol. 2: The lower body. Williams & Wilkins, Baltimore

Vannerson J, Nimmo R 1971 Specificity and the law of facilitation in the nervous system. The Receptor 2(1). Reprinted in: Schneider M, Cohen J, Laws S 2001 The collected writings of Nimmo and Vannerson, pioneers of chiropractic trigger point therapy. Self-published, Pittsburgh

Varma D 1935 The human machine and its forces. Health for All, London

Youngs B 1962 Physiological background of neuro-muscular technique. British Naturopathic Journal 5(6):176–190

3

Myofascial trigger points and other reflex phenomena

PAIN PATTERNS

The radiating and/or referred symptoms deriving from myofascial trigger points are a major cause of sustained pain and dysfunction, according to Wall & Melzack (1989), the leading researchers into pain. Trigger points are indeed stated by them to be a part of all chronic pain conditions, often the major part. To be sure there are many other descriptions and classifications of reflex pain patterns – many of which are outlined in the following chapters – and these demand a brief review of the possible mechanisms involved.

A priority involves the need to differentiate between pain and referred symptoms that are of a spinal, nerve root, origin and those that have different aetiologies.

Difference between referred phenomena and radicular pain

Pain and other root syndrome effects deriving from damaged or dysfunctional vertebral or intervertebral structures need to be differentiated from the non-radicular pain and symptoms that derive from reflexogenic activity, such as myofascial trigger points.

The key characteristics of radicular dysfunction from, for example, a herniated disc, will include (Dubs 1950, Dvorak & Dvorak 1984):

- pain located in the regions supplied by the nerve roots from the segment (s) involved

- a loss of sensitivity in the appropriate dermatomes related to the segment(s) involved
- a loss of motor power – possibly to the point of paralysis – of the muscle innervated by the nerve roots involved, and possible atrophy
- disturbances of the deep tendon reflexes in the related areas. Diagnosis of the presence of such dysfunction requires expert neurological assessment; however, practitioners and therapists should be aware of these key signs, which alert them to the possibility that nerve root syndromes may be a feature of the patient's problem.

Non-radicular patterns of referred pain

Dvorak & Dvorak (1984) have described five variations on the theme of referred symptomatology, different ways of seeing the same phenomena, aside from nerve root syndromes. These are:

1. Referred pain – which includes the findings described by researchers such as Lewis (1938), Kellgren (1938), Hockaday & Whitty (1967), who demonstrated that mechanical and chemical stimulation to various spinal structures produces referred pain. This is discussed further in this chapter.
2. Myofascial trigger points, which are discussed extensively in this chapter, and which form the major focus of neuromuscular technique application in North America.
3. Pseudoradicular syndromes, which Brugger (1962) describes as being quite distinct from root syndromes and which derive from a 'nociceptive somatomotoric blocking effect' occurring in tissues such as joint capsules, tendon origins and other local (to joint) tissues. These painful reflex effects are noted in muscles and their tendinous junctions as well as the skin – which Brugger calls 'tendomyosis' – defined as, 'the reflexogenic functional change in the muscle in the presence of concurrent functionally dependent muscle pain'. Dvorak & Dvorak (1984) include in this category of referred pain

and symptoms the phenomena of viscerosomatic and somatovisceral influences, in which, for example, organ dysfunction is said to produce tendomyotic changes (Korr 1975). Some aspects of these phenomena form part of the discussion of facilitation in this chapter.

4. Tender points, as described by Jones (1981), which Dvorak & Dvorak equate with the tender points described by Kellgren (1938) (see Ch. 4 for more on Jones' work), are seen to be spontaneously arising areas of tenderness related to acute or chronic strains, usually located in those soft tissues shortened at the time of the strain. These seem to equate with so-called 'Ah shi' points in traditional Chinese acupuncture methodology (i.e. points not necessarily present on acupuncture meridian maps, but occurring spontaneously in association with strain in the region).

5. Spondylogenic reflexes, knowledge of which Dvorak & Dvorak describe as being based on empirical clinical observation that demonstrates relationships between the axial skeleton and the peripheral soft tissues which 'are not easily explained on the basis of radicular, vascular or humoral reasoning'. The effects of these reflexes include 'demonstrable zones of irritation . . . which are painful swellings, tender upon pressure, located in the musculofascial tissue in topographically well-defined sites' (Sutter 1975).

Dvorak & Dvorak (1984) suggest that these different classifications and descriptions are focusing on the same phenomena, with terminology and interpretations being the variables, rather than there being a host of different physiological patterns of response to stress and trauma.

In this context, earlier research into referred pain is worth re-evaluating, because it highlights basic facts – of which many have lost sight.

Speransky

Speransky, in his classic book *A Basis for the Theory of Medicine* (Speransky 1943), demonstrated clearly that 'From any nerve point it is easy to bring into action nerve mechanisms, the functioning of which terminates at the periphery, in changes of a bio-physico-chemical character.' And further: 'Justification exists for the thesis that any nerve point, not excluding peripheral nerve structures, can become the originator of neurodystrophic processes, serving as the temporary nerve centre of these processes.'

Speransky continued: 'It is obvious from this [evidence] that the irritation of any point of the complex network of the nervous system, can evoke changes, not only in the adjacent parts, but also in remote regions of the organism.'

 Kellgren

Following on from the pioneering work of Sir Thomas Lewis, the researcher J. H. Kellgren performed a series of studies in the late 1930s which deserve our attention (Kellgren 1938, 1939, Lewis 1938).

Kellgren (1938) effectively showed (using himself and volunteers) that by irritating fascia and muscle he could produce referred sensations in other structures. For example, among his early findings was evidence that a saline injection into the occipital muscles would produce a headache, while similar irritation to the masseter muscle produced a toothache.

Kellgren (1939) concluded that such distribution of pain usually followed segmental pathways, although he modified this position when he applied his studies to clinical work, at which time he not only identified localised, exquisitely painful spots that referred painful symptoms to distant areas, but also noted that the distribution of pain from such spots did not in fact always follow peripheral neural pathways. He also showed that a local anaesthetic injection into such spots could obliterate the referred pain sensations.

Kellgren (1939) stated:

Superficial fascia (of the back) and supraspinous ligaments induce local pain when stimulated, while stimulation of the superficial portions of the interspinous ligaments and superficial muscles results in diffuse pain. Deep muscles, ligaments and periostium of the apophyseal joints as well as the joints themselves can cause referred pain according to segmental innervation when stimulated [saline solution or mechanical stimulus].

Additional research at that time (1940s) indicated that there was not always a predictable pattern of pain distribution from such experiments (Feinstein et al 1954) (Fig. 3.1).

Research by many others in the 1940s, continuing up to the present, has further investigated referred patterns of pain that do not seem to follow neurological pathways, or even known patterns of viscerally caused pain – or, for that matter, the common acupuncture pathways as described in traditional Chinese medicine – myofascial trigger points.

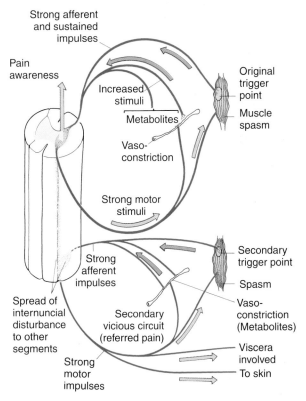

Figure 3.1 Schematic representation of the secondary spread of neurologically induced influences deriving from acute or chronic soft tissue dysfunction and involving trigger point activity and/or spasm.

Evans

Evans, in discussing reflex pain, describes the mechanism as follows:

A prolonged bombardment of pain impulses sets up a vicious circle of reflexes spreading through a pool of many neuron connections upward, downward and even across the spinal cord and perhaps reaching as high as the thalamus itself. Depending upon the extent of the pool (internuncial pool), we detect the phenomena of pain and sympathetic disturbances a long distance from the injured (trigger) area of the body and occasionally even spread to the contralateral side.

Dittrich

Dittrich (1954) has shown a constant pattern of fibrosis of subfascial tissue, with adhesions between this and the overlying muscle fascia, in a number of distinctive and common pain patterns. For example, in what he calls the 'mid-sacral syndrome' which develops from sacral lesions, referred pain is almost always present in the buttock and sometimes in the thigh, leg or foot. Referred tenderness is elicited in the lower part of the buttock. The fibrous adhesions (trigger area) are found at the level of the 3rd sacral vertebra, near the spine.

In the 'mid-lumbar syndrome', Dittrich showed that there is referred pain and tenderness in the lower lumbar, upper sacral and sacroiliac regions. The trigger point is found over the lateral third of the sacrospinalis muscle at the level of the upper margin of the iliac crest.

The 'latissimus dorsi syndrome' could result from irritation of the aponeurosis of this muscle at either of the sites of injury, sacral or lumbar, mentioned above. Referred pain would develop in the sclerotonic distributions of the 6th, 7th and 8th cervical nerves.

Dittrich pointed out that pathological changes at the two sites had been discovered by operative findings. His technique was to remove these triggers surgically or to obliterate the triggers by injection of local anaesthetic. (No concern is expressed as to the mechanical, postural or other reasons that may have produced them, nor any mention made of more conservative manipulative methods of normalisation.)

The presence of 'fibrosed subfascial tissue' supports the theories of Stanley Lief and Boris Chaitow, and their use of NMT in treating such problems (see Ch. 2). The locale of these, close to bony insertions, further supports the rationale behind neuromuscular technique application.

It seems that soft tissue lesions, characterised by fibrosis of subfascial tissue (fat, etc.) with fibrous connections between the structure and the overlying fascia, can initiate sensory irritation that produces referred pain and tenderness. In addition, autonomic nervous involvement may be activated to produce vasomotor, trophic, visceral or metabolic changes. Symptoms will disappear when the offending lesion is normalised, by whatever method. However, a system that both corrects the offending trigger and attempts to prevent its recurrence would seem to offer greater clinical benefits. Before surveying some of the other reflex patterns that are pertinent to this text, a brief summary of current thinking on the aetiology of muscle pain, as described by Mense & Simons (2001) is provided in Box 3.1.

Other reflexogenic models

Gutstein

Gutstein (1956) showed that conditions such as ametropia may result from changes in the neuromuscular component of the craniocervical area, as well as from more distant conditions involving the pelvis or shoulder girdle. He states:

Myopia is the long-term effect of pressure of extra-ocular muscles in the convergence effort of accommodation involving spasm of the ciliary muscles, with resultant elongation of the eyeball. A sequential relationship has been shown between such a condition and muscular spasm of the neck.

Normalisation of these muscles by manipulation relieves eye symptoms as well as fascial, dorsolumbar and abdominal tenderness. Gutstein terms these reflexes 'myodysneuria' and suggests that the reference phenomena of such spots or triggers would include pain, modi-

---

Box 3.1 Mense & Simons perspective on muscle pain

In Chapter 1 a brief overview (see 'Modern pain concepts') was provided of how muscle pain evolves, as described by Mense & Simons (2001). In this section some of the major causes of muscle pain are outlined, based on the same researchers' descriptions and discussions.

Local muscular pain
Local muscular pain is defined as deriving from local pain receptors, in the muscle, rather than via neural or central neurons. These free nerve endings (nociceptors) may be sensitized by mechanical (blows, repetitive or single strain injuries, rupture of fibres, etc.) and chemical (e.g. bradykinin) influences that either irritate or increase nociceptor sensitivity, leading to tenderness and soreness (such as occurs following unaccustomed exercise). Non-steroidal anti-inflammatory drugs decrease the degree of such sensitisation. The types of situation that bring about such sensitisation include trauma, inflammation and ischaemic circulatory deficit (such as that resulting from intermittent claudication or prolonged voluntary contraction, especially if this involves an already ischaemic muscle).

Local muscle pain involving inflammation may additionally lead to feelings of weakness and dysaesthesia. Local muscle pain may also be caused by the influence of a trigger point within the painful muscle, or referring to it from a distant muscle.

Metabolic causes of local muscle pain include enzyme deficiencies and hypothyroid status that 'compromise oxidative metabolism in the muscle mitochondria' (Mense & Simons 2001). Inflammatory process may result from injury or infection (e.g. *Staphylococcus aureus*) or infestation (e.g. trichinosis caused by *Trichinella spiralis* deriving from undercooked meat such as pork).

Local muscle pain resulting from compartment syndrome may result from development of a haematoma, oedema or infection in a muscle surrounded by a fascial envelope (such as flexor digitorum longus muscle in the deep posterior compartment). Surgical intervention may be called for to relieve the pressure before irreparable tissue damage occurs. A similar scenario may result from a plaster cast applied too tightly. Rarely toxicity-induced myalgic pain may derive from contaminated tryptophan, a sleep-inducing and pain-relieving amino acid, useful in the treatment of fibromyalgia. As pure tryptophan is no longer available because of contamination in the manufacturing process following a Japanese attempt to modify genetically the bacteria used in its production, tryptophan is now available in a plant-derived form, free of contaminants, as 5-hydroxytryptophan (Chaitow 2000).

Nerve lesion or dysfunction
Neuropathic muscle pain derived from a nerve lesion or dysfunction in the cranial (spinal) or dorsal root nerves. Causes may be mechanical (trauma) or entrapment (see notes on Maitland, Butler and Gifford in Ch. 1), or as a result of the development of a neuroma, which can lead to phantom pain. Pain from a herniated disc is an example of radicular pain. Peripheral neuropathies may occur in conditions such as diabetes. The causes of widespread pain conditions, which also involve autonomic symptoms, such as complex regional pain syndrome (previously called reflex sympathetic dystrophy), are thought to involve the sympathetic nervous system in an as yet unknown way.

Referred pain
Pain that is referred to and from muscles can be confusing. Mense & Simons (2001) use the term 'mislocalization of pain', in which 'the muscle in which the pain is felt serves only as a starting point for finding the source of pain, which is really what requires treatment'. The mechanisms are not clear, although the phenomenon is at the very heart of the pain often found to derive from distant trigger point activity. Mense & Simons indicate that there are confusing influences from trigger points when they reflexly influence other structures: 'Why trigger points cause reflex spasm in one situation and reflex inhibition in another is not at all clear. One possibility is that the distinction between muscles prone to tightness [postural – see Ch. 1] and muscles prone to weakness [phasic – see Ch. 1] may be of fundamental physiologic significance.' What is known is that specific dermatome and myotome distribution of sensations is not constant in relation to the symptoms produced by an active trigger point. Discussion in this chapter on the phenomena of local and segmental facilitation, and also of viscerosomatic reflex activity, covers aspects of this form of reflexogenic and referred pain.

Muscular tension
Pain deriving from muscular tension may involve biomechanical rather than neural influences. Factors such as the viscoelastic tone and the colloidal nature of soft tissues involving thixotropic qualities, as well as non-neurologically mediated contractures, may be present (see notes on fascia in Ch. 1, and also Fig. 3.2).

This topic is complex and the reader is referred to Mense & Simons (2001, Ch. 5) for greater detail.

Aspects of the influence on muscular pain deriving from organ dysfunction, postural imbalances, the presence of active trigger points, and conditions such as fibromyalgia are all discussed in this and later chapters.

---

fications of pain, itching, hypersensitivity to physiological stimuli, spasm, twitching, weakness and trembling of striated muscles; hypertonus or hypotonus of smooth muscle of blood vessels, and of internal organs; hypersecretion or hyposecretion of visceral, sebaceous and sudatory glands. Somatic manifestations may also occur in response to visceral stimuli

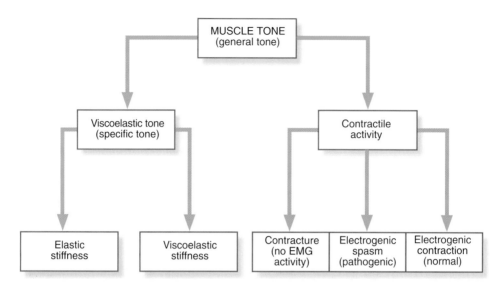

Figure 3.2 Diagram showing terminology used in describing tightness of muscles. Redrawn from Mense S & Simons D, Muscle pain, Williams & Wilkins, 2001, with permission.

of corresponding spinal levels (Gutstein 1944).

Many such trigger areas are dormant and asymptomatic. Gutstein's method of treatment was the injection of an anaesthetic solution into the trigger area. He indicated, however, that, where accessible (e.g. muscular insertions in the cervical area), the chilling of these areas combined with pressure yielded good results. This is in line with Mennell's work (1975), and fits into the field of NMT.

Amongst the patterns of vasomotor sebaceous, sudatory and gastrointestinal dysfunction mentioned by Gutstein (1944a) are the following, all of which relate to reflex trigger points or 'myodysneuria' (fibrositis/fibromyalgia):

1. Various patterns of vasomotor abnormality such as coldness, pallor, redness, cyanosis, etc. These variations in response to stimulation relate to the fact that most organs respond to weak stimuli by an increase in activity and to very strong stimuli by inhibiting activity. Menopausal hot flushes are one example, and these seem often to be linked to musculoskeletal pain. Gutstein found that obliteration of overt and silent triggers in the occipital, cervical, interscapular, sternal and epigastric regions was accompanied by years of alleviation of premenopausal, menopausal and late menopausal symptoms. Proponents of NMT have long emphasised the importance of normalising these very structures.

2. Gutstein maintains that normalisation of skin secretion, and therefore of hair and skin texture and appearance, may be altered for the better by the removal of active trigger areas in the cervical and interscapular areas.

3. The conditions of hyperhidrosis, hypohidrosis and anhidrosis may accompany vasomotor and sebaceous dysfunction. Gutstein noted that abolition of excessive perspiration as well as anhidrosis followed adequate treatment.

4. Gutstein quoted a number of practitioners who have achieved success in treating gastrointestinal dysfunctions by treating trigger areas. Some of these were treated by procaine injection, others by pressure techniques and massage. The abdominal wall lends itself to the latter procedure, as evidenced by the work of Cornelius (1909), whose treatment was not dissimilar to Lief's NMT.

Among the conditions that have responded to such treatment are pylorospasm, bad breath, heartburn, regurgitation, nausea, abdominal distension, constipation and nervous diarrhoea. Gutstein (1944b) tried to denote localised functional sensory and/or motor abnormalities of musculoskeletal tissue (comprising muscle, fascia, tendon, bone and joint) as myodysneuria (now known as fibromyalgia; formerly known as 'fibrositis' and 'muscular rheumatism'). He viewed the causes of such changes as multiple; among them are:

1. Acute and chronic infections which, it is postulated, stimulate sympathetic nerve activity via their toxins.
2. Excessive heat or cold, changes in atmospheric pressure, and draughts.
3. Mechanical injuries, both major and repeated minor microtraumas. Postural strain, unaccustomed exercises, etc., which may predispose towards future changes by lowering the threshold for future stimuli (facilitation).
4. Allergic and endocrine factors, which can cause imbalance in the autonomic nervous system.
5. Inherited factors that make adjustment to environmental factors difficult.

6. Arthritic changes – because muscles are the active components of the musculoskeletal system it is logical to assume that their circulatory state has influence over bones and joints. Spasm in muscle may contribute towards osteoarthritic changes, and such changes may produce further neuromuscular changes, which themselves produce new symptoms.
7. Visceral diseases may intensify and precipitate somatic symptoms in the distribution of their spinal and adjacent segments.

In these examples of Gutstein's concept, we can see strong echoes of the facilitation hypothesis in osteopathic medicine, and it seems likely that they are describing the same set of circumstances leading to hyperreactive responses – and all that this leads to in terms of pain and dysfunction.

Diagnosis of myodysneuria was made according to some of the following criteria:

● A varying degree of muscular tension and contraction is usually present, although

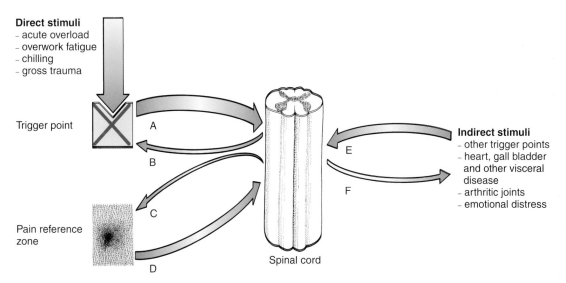

Figure 3.3 Direct stress influence can affect the hyperreactive neural structure of a myofascial trigger point, leading to increased activity (A–B) as well as referring sensations (pain, paraesthesia, increased sympathetic activity) to a target area (C–D) that feed back into the cord to increase the background stress load. Other stimuli reach the cord from distant trigger points and additional dysfunctional areas (E–F).

sometimes adjacent, apparently unaffected, tissue is more painful.

- Sensitivity to pressure or palpation of affected muscles and their adjuncts.

Marked hypertonicity may require the application of deep pressure to demonstrate tenderness.

Travell and Bigelow

Travell & Bigelow (1947) produced evidence to support much of what Gutstein had reported. They indicated that high-intensity stimuli from active trigger areas produced, by reflex, prolonged vasoconstriction with partial ischaemia in localised areas of the brain, spinal cord or peripheral nerve structures (Fig. 3.3). A wide pattern of dysfunction might result, affecting almost any organ of the body. The phenomenon of hysteria, with symptoms as varied as disordered vision, respiration, motor power and cutaneous sensation, was often mediated by afferent neural impulses from trigger areas in skeletal muscle. These triggers, when similarly located, produced the same pattern of clinical effects, whether activated in one patient by psychogenic factors or in another by different factors (e.g. mechanical or traumatic).

It is worth noting that Travell (1981) has shown that the effect of a trigger point on the muscle housing it is to produce weakness of contraction without atrophy, and that this is often accompanied by a decreased range of movement in associated joints.

Dowling

Dowling (2000) has described a variation on the use of inhibitory pressure (see Box 3.5), which allies itself closely with the methods of NMT and other soft tissue approaches utilising the effects of compression in a physiologically useful manner. Using two points of contact, progressive, sequential pressure applications are used to inhibit pain and modify function. Dowling's work fits well with other approaches (acupressure, strain/counterstrain, use of neurolymphatic reflexes, etc.) that depend on the underlying mechanisms that allow manual input to modify neuromuscular function and pain. See Chapter 11 for a full explanation of progressive neuromuscular inhibition technique (PINS).

UNDERSTANDING FACILITATION

If we are to make sense of the phenomenon of myofascial trigger points there is a need to grasp the processes that lead to hyperirritability and hyperreactivity of specific neural structures – facilitation. Trigger points are localised areas of soft tissue dysfunction that negatively influence distant target areas, and that evolve in a manner similar to that observed when spinal segments become facilitated as a result of stress of one sort or another.

To understand trigger points, we need to understand spinal facilitation first. Facilitation occurs in both spinal and paraspinal tissues (segmental facilitation) as well as in discrete local areas of muscles, mainly near their origins and insertions but also close to their bellies and in areas where fascial stress occurs due to external influences and forces (myofascial trigger points). Understanding facilitation helps us to see how the different classification systems, all describing variations on the same phenomenon of referred pain – listed by Dvorak & Dvorak (1984) and described earlier in this chapter – are held together aetiologically.

Patterson (1976) explains segmental (spinal) facilitation as follows:

The concept of the facilitated segment states that because of abnormal afferent or sensory inputs to a particular area of the spinal cord, that area is kept in a state of constant increased excitation. This facilitation allows normally ineffectual or subliminal stimuli to become effective in producing efferent output from the facilitated segment, causing both skeletal and visceral organs innervated by the affected segment to be maintained in a state of overactivity. It is probable that the 'osteopathic lesion', or somatic dysfunction with which a facilitated segment is associated, is the direct result of the abnormal segmental activity as well as being partially responsible for the facilitation.

A facilitated segment therefore emerges from a prolonged period during which abnormal or altered inputs from a single source (or more than one source) of irritation, impinging on the spinal cord, keep the interneurons or motor neurons of that spinal segment in a constant state of excitement, thus allowing normally ineffectual inputs to produce outputs to all organs receiving innervation from the excited area. This concept implies that the spinal cord is a relatively passive mediator of the influences imposed on it and that the neural paths act as communicators of that activity (Denslow et al 1949).

Research on spinal functions seems to indicate, however, that the spinal cord, besides being the determiner of where abnormal activity is sent, by virtue of predetermined pathways, may participate actively in either controlling abnormal or unusually intense inputs, or amplifying and retaining such inputs in certain circumstances (Korr 1986).

Initially, only intensities of afferent input above a certain level would result in increased sensitivity of the spinal pathway. Inputs of lower intensity would either produce no alterations, or would cause an actual decrease in sensitivity as a protective mechanism against undue changes in homeostatic processes. It is apparent that the potential for sensitisation by different types of afferent inputs may differ widely. Thus, inputs from pain receptors may sensitise the pathway at low levels because of the properties of the initial synapses between pain afferent fibres and interneurons. In this event an initially protective increase in response might occur, followed eventually by detrimental facilitation of a segment. On the other hand, inputs from joint receptors seem to have a less dramatic effect at similar input levels (Dowling 1991).

It is now known that emotional arousal would also affect the susceptibility of the pathways to sensitisation (Baldry 1993). The increase in descending influences from the emotionally aroused subject would result in an increase in toxic excitement in the pathways and allow all additional inputs to produce sensitisation at low intensities. Thus, highly emotional people, or those in a highly emotional situation, would be expected to show a higher incidence of facilitation of spinal pathways.

As the higher brain centres influence the tonic levels of the spinal paths, it might also be expected that physical training and mental attitudes would tend to alter the tonic excitability, reducing the person's susceptibility to sensitisation from everyday stress. Thus the athlete would be expected to withstand a comparatively high level of afferent input before experiencing the self-perpetuating results of sensitisation.

A further corollary of the hypothesis is that slowly developing conditions, or slowly increasing inputs, would result in less sensitisation at high levels than sudden inputs. The slow development of a chronic source of increased sensory input initially would cause habituation, resulting in resistance to sensitisation until the input level was abnormally high. On the other hand, sudden increases in input, such as a sudden mechanical stress, would be expected to produce sensitisation of the neural pathways most rapidly.

Korr

The premier researcher into facilitation over the past half-century has been Irwin Korr (Korr 1970, 1976). In early studies he demonstrated, for example, that if readings were taken of resistance to electricity in the paraspinal skin of an individual there were often marked differences, with one side showing normal resistance and the other showing reduced resistance (facilitated area).

When 'stress' was applied elsewhere in the body and the two areas of the spine were monitored, it was the area of facilitation, where electrical resistance was reduced, that showed a dramatic rise in electrical (i.e. neurological) activity. In one experiment, volunteers had pins inserted into one calf muscle in order to gauge the effect in the paraspinal areas under investigation – with the spinal areas being monitored for electrical activity. Almost no increase occurred in the normal region, but the facilitated area showed enormously enhanced neurological activity after 60 seconds (Korr 1977) (Fig. 3.4).

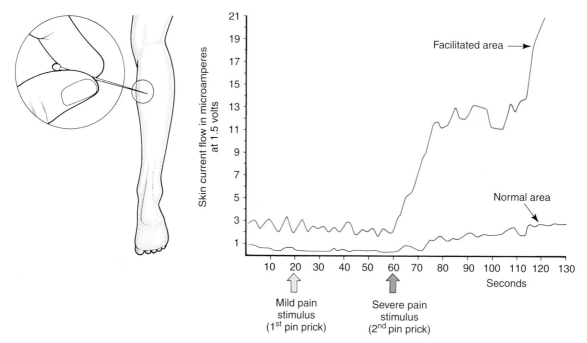

Figure 3.4 Pain stimuli produce a marked reaction in the facilitated area (red line) and little reaction in the normal area (black line).

The implications of this and hundreds of similar studies are that any form of stress impacting the individual, be it climatic, chemical, emotional, physical or anything else, would produce just such a rise in neurological output from facilitated areas.

In many instances involving spinal segmental facilitation there is a chronic degree of neurological bombardment resulting from internal organ dysfunction. For example, it is almost always possible to predict that cardiovascular disease is present (or will soon be present) when two or more segments of the spine in the region of T2, T3 and T4 display tense, rigid, 'board-like' characteristics on palpation, especially if these tissues do not respond to normal efforts to reduce their hypertonicity (Beal 1983).

Tension headaches and facilitation

Danish research (Bendtsen 2000) suggests that there exists:

. . . a pathophysiological model for tension-type headache [resulting from] central sensitization [facilitation] at the level of the spinal dorsal horn/trigeminal nucleus due to prolonged nociceptive inputs from pericranial myofascial tissues. The increased nociceptive input to supraspinal structures may in turn result in supraspinal sensitization. The central neuroplastic changes may affect the regulation of peripheral mechanisms and thereby lead to, for example, increased pericranial muscle activity, or senstization may be maintained even after the initial eliciting factors have been normalized, resulting in conversion of episodic into chronic tension-type headache.

This research demonstrates the need to understand how, over time, a reversible problem may become entrenched and chronic. It is knowledge of facilitation and sensitization that also explains how multiple stress elements affecting the person as a whole (climatic, emotional, postural, nutritional, etc.) might feed into the sensitized structures, exacerbating symptoms, despite apparently not directly impacting the involved structures.

Viscerosomatic reflexes

Many of the various systems involving reflexively active points described in this and the next chapter, such as connective tissue zones, Chapman's reflexes and Bennett's reflexes, as well as trigger points, may involve viscerosomatic reflex activity.

Beal

Myron Beal (1985) has described this phenomenon as resulting from afferent stimuli, arising from dysfunction of a visceral nature. The reflex is initiated by afferent impulses arising from visceral receptors, which are transmitted to the dorsal horn of the spinal cord, where they synapse with interconnecting neurons. The stimuli are then conveyed to sympathetic and motor efferents, resulting in changes in the somatic tissues, such as skeletal muscle, skin and blood vessels.

Abnormal stimulation of the visceral efferent neurons may result in hyperaesthesia of the skin, and associated vasomotor, pilomotor and sudomotor changes. Similar stimuli of the ventral horn cells may result in reflex rigidity of the somatic musculature. Pain may result from such changes.

The degree of stimulus required, in any given case, to produce such changes will differ, because factors such as prior facilitation of the particular segment, as well as the response of higher centres, will differ from person to person.

In many cases it is suggested, by Korr and others, that viscerosomatic reflex activity may be noted before any symptoms of visceral change are evident, and that this phenomenon is therefore of potential diagnostic and prognostic value.

The first signs of viscerosomatic reflexive influences are vasomotor reactions (increased skin temperature), sudomotor (increased moisture of the skin), skin textural changes (e.g. thickening), increased subcutaneous fluid and increased contraction of muscle. The value of light skin palpation in identifying areas of facilitation cannot be too strongly emphasised (Lewit 1992).

These signs disappear if the visceral cause improves. When such changes become chronic, however, trophic alterations are noted, with increased thickening of the skin and subcutaneous tissue, and localised muscular contraction. Deep musculature may become hard, tense and hypersensitive. This may result in deep splinting contractions, involving two or more segments of the spine, with associated restriction of spinal motion. The costotransverse articulations may be significantly involved in such changes.

Patterns of somatic response will be found to differ from person to person, and to be unique, in terms of location, the number of segments involved, and whether or not the pattern is unilateral or bilateral. The degree of intensity will also differ, and is related to the degree of acuteness of the visceral condition (Hix 1976). Research involving animals, as well as observations in humans, using regional nerve blocks, has helped to define site locations of response, in various forms of visceral dysfunction. Beal (1985) notes that, when the voluminous research into segmental associations with organ dysfunction is compounded, three distinct groups of visceral involvement are found in respect of particular sites:

1. T1–T5: heart and lungs
2. T5–T10: oesophagus, stomach, small intestine, liver, gall bladder, spleen, pancreas and adrenal cortex
3. T10–L2: large bowel, appendix, kidney, ureter, adrenal medulla, testes, ovaries, urinary bladder, prostate gland, uterus.

There appears to be a consensus as to sidedness being apparent, in reflexes of unpaired organs. Thus, left-sidedness is noted in conditions involving the small intestine and heart, and right-sidedness for gall bladder disease and appendix. The stomach may produce reflex activity on either, or both, sides. Many studies have been concerned with the identification of viscerosomatic reflexes. One 5-year study involved more than 5000 hospitalised patients (Beal 1985), and concluded that most visceral disease appeared to influence more than one spinal region, and that the number of spinal segments involved seemed to be related to the duration of the disease. Kelso noted in this study that there was an increase in the number of palpatory findings in the cervical region, related to patients with sinusitis, tonsillitis, diseases of the oesophagus and liver complaints. Soft tissue changes were noted in patients with gastritis, duodenal ulceration, pyelonephritis, chronic appendicitis and cholecystitis, in the region of T5–T12.

Palpating facilitated spinal tissues

Somatic dysfunction is usually assessed by means of palpatory investigation, and Beal (1983) insists that investigation should pay attention to the various soft tissue layers:

The skin for changes in texture, temperature and moisture; the subcutaneous tissue for changes in consistency and fluid; the superficial and deep musculature for tone, irritability, consistency, viscoelastic properties, and fluid content; and the deep fascial layers for textural changes.

He advises that 'Special attention [should] be given to the examination of the costotransverse area, where it is felt that autonomic nerve effects are predominant', and notes that tests for the quality and range of joints have not been found to differentiate between visceral reflexes and somatic changes, which confirms the importance of the soft tissue assessment in order to elicit such information.

Beal (1983) notes that the supine position is ideal for assessment of paraspinal tissues – the hand being gently inserted under the region, and pressure, or springing techniques applied (Fig. 3.5). He has not investigated the use of patient examination in the prone position, as he suggests that this position is precluded in acutely ill patients. Nevertheless, since Beal notes the difficulty of applying diagnostic measures with the patient supine when the mid to lower thoracic area is under review, a prone position is suggested, unless the patient cannot manage this. The availability of a couch with a split head-piece would make this more comfortable. As we will see, the methods employed by those using connective tissue massage involve the

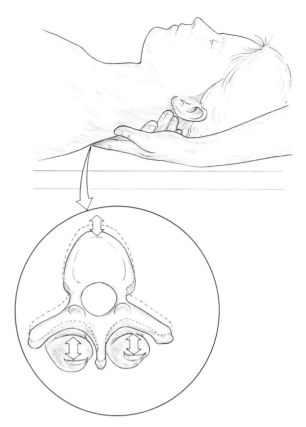

Figure 3.5 Beal's 'springing' assessment for paraspinal facilitation rigidity associated with segmental facilitation.

patient being seated. This helps in assessing skin and superficial tissue status, but is not really suitable for deeper penetration.

Beal suggests that the diagnosis of a paraspinal viscerosomatic reflex be based on two or more adjacent spinal segments showing evidence of somatic dysfunction, and being located within the specific autonomic reflex area. There should be deep confluent spinal muscle splinting, and resistance to segmental joint motion. Skin and subcutaneous tissue changes that are consistent with the acuteness or chronicity of the reflex should be noted.

Specific identification of the origin of the reflex is, he suggests, difficult.

The usefulness of understanding the nature of such reflexes often involves clinical frustration when, for instance, localised soft tissue dysfunction fails to respond to treatment. Suspicion may then be alerted to possible visceral activity maintaining the muscular or joint dysfunction.

According to Beal, treatment of the acute stage should be aimed primarily at breaking into the reflex arc. In cases of serious illness the treatment may consist of gentle digital pressure, of short duration, to effect a local change in superficial tissues. When relaxation has been accomplished in the subcutaneous and superficial paraspinal musculature, the deep muscle contraction can be addressed. The duration of treatment is dependent upon the patient's condition and perceived energy level. Beal suggests that acute conditions that are not life threatening may be addressed in a more aggressive manner (asthma is given as an example).

It is suggested that NMT is also an ideal method of addressing soft tissue manifestations of such reflex activity, because it offers a diagnostic as well as a therapeutic opportunity to address both superficial and deep tissues. Viscerosomatic reflex changes are just one of the many reasons for altered tissue findings, which may be noted in the general NMT assessment. Awareness of the possibility that what is being noted is of reflex origin adds to the potential for accurate diagnosis. In Chapter 4 a variety of other reflex systems are evaluated.

Causes of local facilitation

Melzack & Wall (1989), in their exhaustive investigation of pain, are clear in their statement that all chronic pain has myofascial trigger point activity as at least a part of its aetiology, and that in many instances trigger points are the major contributors to the pain.

A trigger point is a localised, palpable area of soft tissue that is painful on pressure and that refers symptoms, usually including pain, to a predictable target area some distance from itself. It is an area of local facilitation that has developed following a very similar aetiological pathway to that occurring in segmental (spinal) facilitated areas.

Facilitation paraspinally and in general muscle tissue can be the result of repetitive minor or single major traumatic influences or stress factors (as described in Ch. 1). The form of facilitation that is our main focus in this chapter is a localised area of hyperirritability – the trigger point.

Travell and Simons

Much research and clinical work has been done in recent years in this field by Janet Travell (Travell 1957, Travell & Simons 1983, 1992), who is on record as stating that if a pain is severe enough to cause a patient to seek professional advice (in the absence of organic disease) referred pain is likely to be a factor, and therefore a trigger area is probably involved. She maintains that patterns of referred pain are constant in distribution in all people; only the intensity of referred symptoms or referred pain will vary.

Among the effects of an active trigger point, apart from pain, there may be numbness, tingling, weakness, lack of normal range of movement. The aetiological myofascial trigger point for a particular pain pattern is always located in a particular part of a particular muscle (Webber 1973). While eradication of the trigger, by whatever appropriate means, can remove all symptoms, treatment of the target or reference area is useless.

 TRIGGER POINTS (Fig. 3.6)

Trigger points are localised areas of deep tenderness and increased resistance, and digital pressure on such a trigger will often produce twitching and fasciculation (see Fig. 3.6). Pressure maintained on such a point will produce referred pain in a predictable area. If there are a number of active trigger points, the reference areas may overlap.

What is distinctive about active trigger points (myofascial trigger points) is that, when active, they also refer sensations or symptoms to a distinct target area, and this target area is more or less reproducible in other individuals, when trigger points are located in similar positions. No other soft tissue dysfunction has this particular attribute.

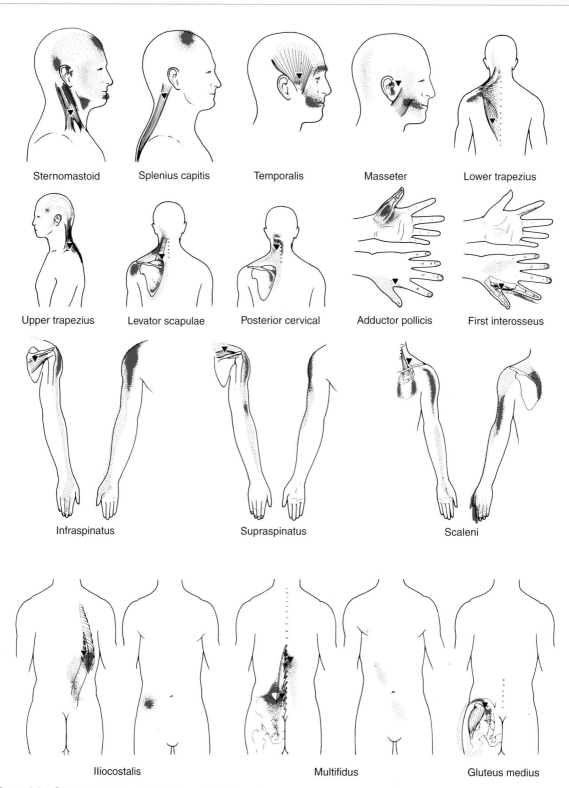

Figure 3.6 Some common trigger points and their target areas.

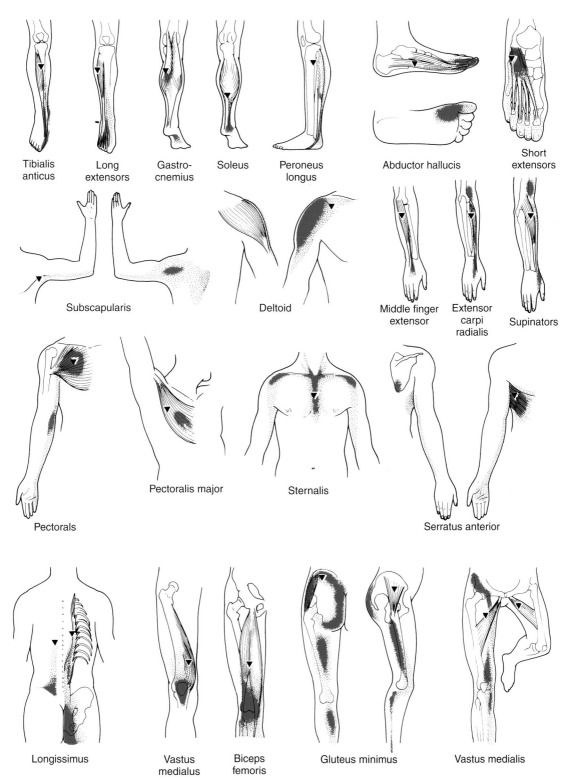

Tibialis anticus

Long extensors

Gastro-cnemius

Soleus

Peroneus longus

Abductor hallucis

Short extensors

Subscapularis

Deltoid

Middle finger extensor

Extensor carpi radialis

Supinators

Pectorals

Pectoralis major

Sternalis

Serratus anterior

Longissimus

Vastus medialus

Biceps femoris

Gluteus minimus

Vastus medialis

Figure 3.6 *continued*

Before an active trigger point exists there needs to be a period of evolution towards that unhappy state. This involves the development of soft tissue changes that are palpable and probably sensitive, or painful, but that, until sufficient localised stress has been involved, will not refer symptoms onwards. In other words, many localised muscular areas of sensitivity or pain, which do not refer pain or other symptoms, may be considered to be embryonic or evolutionary trigger points. A single trigger may refer pain to several reference sites and can give rise to embryonic, or satellite, triggers in those target areas. Travell (1981) describes, for example, how a trigger in the distal areas of the sternomastoid muscle can give rise to new triggers in the sternalis muscle, the pectoral muscle and/or serratus anterior.

Travell's description of a trigger point is:

It lies in skeletal muscle, and is identified by localised deep tenderness, in a palpable firm band of muscle (muscle hardening); and at the point of maximum deep hyperalgesia, by a positive 'jump sign', a visible shortening of the part of the muscle which contains the band. To elicit the jump sign most effectively, one must place the relaxed muscle under moderate passive tension, and snap the band briskly with the palpating finger.

The trigger point must also refer symptoms or sensations, which are familiar to the patient, to a target area. Otherwise, rather than being active, it may be a latent trigger point, which could be activated by stress or strain on the tissues in which it lies (Box 3.2). The difference between most other areas of discrete palpable soft tissue dysfunction and an active trigger is this quality of referring symptoms. All other points may be prospective triggers, but are not active (Fig. 3.7).

STAR OR TART (see also p. 234)

In osteopathic medicine an acronym 'STAR' is used as a reminder of the characteristics of somatic dysfunction, which would include those relating to myofascial trigger points:

- Sensitivity (or 'Tenderness')
- Tissue texture change
- Asymmetry
- Range of motion reduced.

> **Box 3.2** Active and latent trigger points defined (see Fig. 3.6)
>
> An active trigger point, when mechanically stimulated by compression, needling, stretch or other means, will refer to, or intensify, a target zone (referral pattern, usually of pain) which the person recognises as being part of their current symptom picture.
>
> When a latent trigger point is stimulated, it refers a pattern that may be unfamiliar to the person, or that is an old pattern which they used to have but have not had for a while (previously active, reverted to latent).
>
> All the same characteristics that denote an active trigger point may be present in the latent trigger point, with the exception of the person's recognition of their active pain pattern. The same signs as described for segmental facilitation, such as increased hydrosis, a sense of 'drag' on the skin, loss of elasticity, etc., can be observed and palpated in these localised areas as well.
>
> Travell & Simons (1983, 1992) use the term 'essential pain zone' to describe a referral pattern that is present in almost every person when a particular trigger point is active. Some trigger points may also produce a 'spill-over pain zone', beyond the essential zone or in place of it, where the referral pattern is usually less intense. These target zones should be examined, and ideally palpated, for changes in tissue 'density', temperature, hydrosis and other characteristics associated with satellite trigger point formation. Any appropriate manual treatment, movement or exercise programme that encourages normal circulatory function is likely to modulate these negative effects and reduce trigger point activity.

The acronym is modified in some texts to 'TART' (Tenderness – Asymmetry – Range of movement modified – Tissue texture change).

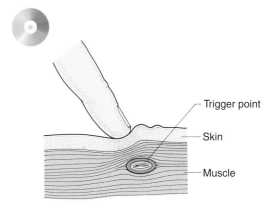

Figure 3.7 Trigger points are areas of local facilitation that can be housed in any soft tissue structure, most usually muscle and/or fascia. Palpation from the skin or at depth may be required to localise them.

Box 3.3   Understanding and treating central and attachment trigger points (Chaitow & DeLany 2000, Simons et al 1999)

Simons, Travell and Simons' (1999) model of central trigger points

- Central trigger points form almost directly in the centre of the muscle's fibres, close to the motor endplate (neuromuscular junction).
- This formation is probably due to dysfunctional endplate activity.
- A metabolic crisis occurs and acetylcholine (ACh) is excessively released at the synapse, usually associated with overuse or strain, leading to release of calcium.
- The resulting ischaemia in the area creates an oxygen/nutrient deficit and a local energy crisis.
- Without available adenosine triphosphate (ATP), the calcium ions, which are keeping the gates open for ACh to keep flowing, cannot be removed.
- A chemically sustained contracture occurs. This is involuntary without motor potentials, and should be distinguished from a contraction, which is voluntary and involves motor potentials, and spasm, which is involuntary with motor potentials.
- As the endplate keeps producing this ACh flow, the actin/myosin filaments shorten and bunch in the immediate area of the motor endplate (centre of fibre).
- A contracture 'knot' forms the characteristic trigger point nodule.
- The remainder of the sarcomeres of that fibre are stretched, creating the equally characteristic taut band, which is usually palpable.
- When massage, stretch applications, injection or other modalities are applied, which disturbs the sarcomeres, alters the chemistry or possibly damages the endplate, the cycle is disrupted and the tissue relaxes, often in seconds – often permanently.

Simons, Travell and Simons' model of attachment trigger points

- Attachment trigger points form at junctures of myofascial and tendinous or periosteal tissues.
- Tension from taut bands on periosteal or connective tissues can lead to enthesopathy or enthesitis, as recurring concentrations of muscular stress may provoke inflammation, with a strong tendency towards subsequent fibrosis and calcific deposition.

Processes

- Central and attachment trigger points can both lead to referred and/or radiating pain; however, the local processes seem to be different and the two types of trigger point seem to respond to different therapeutic approaches.
- Until they have been examined thoroughly and tissue reactions noted, attachment trigger points should be addressed, with their tendency towards inflammation in mind.

- Central trigger points should be addressed with their contracted central sarcomeres and local ischaemia in mind.
- As the end of that taut band is likely to create enthesopathy, stretching the muscle before releasing its central trigger point might further inflame the attachments.
- Techniques should first be applied to relax the taut fibres before manual stretching (such as gliding strokes or myofascial release) is attempted.
- Stretches, particularly those involving active range of motion, should be applied gently until reaction is noted, to avoid further tissue insult.
- When passive stretching is applied, care should be taken to assess for tendinous or periosteal inflammation, in order to avoid placing more tension on already distressed connective tissue attachments.

Treatment choices for central trigger points

- Elongation of the tissue to its full length is, according to Simons et al (1999), critical to abolish the mechanism sustaining a trigger point.
- This may be achieved manually by application of gliding strokes from the centre of the fibres out to the attachment sites, stretching the tissue passively through its range of motion, or by having the person perform active range of motion, both during the treatment session and at home.
- Proprioceptive neuromuscular facilitation (PNF) techniques can be used to override the mechanisms causing the condition.
- Reciprocal inhibition (RI) and post-isometric relaxation (PIR) can accompany or precede range of motion movements and stretches to augment the benefits (see MET notes in Ch. 8).
- Central trigger points seem to respond well to heat.
- When compression techniques are used, local chemistry can change as a result of induced ischaemia, followed by flushing of the tissues when the compression is released (see Box 3.5).
- The effects of thermal or other applications (skin irritants such as capsaicin, moxibustion, dry or wet needling, etc.) may induce the contracture to release.
- Contrast hydrotherapy, employing alternating ice and heat, can be effective via its circulatory and/or neurological (reflex) influences.

Treatment choices for attachment trigger points

- Attachment trigger points seem to respond to ice applications rather than heat.
- Gliding techniques should be applied from the centre of the fibres out towards the attachments, unless contraindicated (as in some extremity tissues).
- By elongating the tissue toward the attachments, sarcomeres that are shortened at the centre of the fibre will be lengthened, and those that are overstretched near the attachment sites will have their tension released.

While the 'tenderness' and range of motion characteristics, as listed in the STAR acronym, hold true for trigger points, the following refinements have been detailed by Simons et al (1999):

- The soft tissues housing the trigger point will demonstrate a painful limit to stretch range of motion.
- A palpable taut band with exquisitely tender nodule should be located.
- Pressure on the tender spot elicits pain familiar to the patient and often a pain response ('jump sign').

Baldry (1993) noted that the commonest sites for trigger points are close to:

- muscular origins and insertions
- free borders of muscle
- muscle belly
- motor end-point
- body tissues other than muscle, including skin, fascia, ligament, joint capsule and periosteum, and also in scar tissue.

Simons et al (1999), in their latest research, place great emphasis on the distinct differences in treatment protocols for so-called 'attachment' and 'central' trigger points (see Box 3.3).

Trigger points: symptoms other than pain

While pain is the commonest symptom arising from the activity of trigger points, other symptoms may be noted, including lymphatic stasis and reduced mobility of joints.

Lymphatic stasis

Travell & Simons (1983, 1992) have identified triggers that impede lymphatic function.

The scalenes (in particular anticus) can entrap structures passing through the thoracic inlet. This is aggravated by the 1st rib (and clavicular) restriction, which can be caused by triggers in anterior and middle scalenes. Scalene trigger points have been shown reflexly to suppress lymphatic duct peristaltic contractions in the affected extremity, whereas triggers in the posterior axillary folds (subscapularis, teres major, latissimus dorsi) influence lymphatic drainage affecting the upper extremities and breasts. Similarly, triggers in the anterior axillary fold (pectoralis minor) can be implicated in lymphatic dysfunction affecting the breasts (Kuchera 1997).

Autonomic effects
(Travell & Simons 1983, 1992)

- Vasoconstriction (blanching)
- Coldness
- Sweating
- Pilomotor response
- Ptosis
- Hypersecretion.

Clinical symptoms other than pain
(Kuchera & McPartland 1997)

- Diarrhoea, dysmenorrhoea
- Diminished gastric motility
- Vasoconstriction and headache
- Dermatographia
- Proprioceptive disturbance, dizziness
- Excessive maxillary sinus secretion
- Localized sweating
- Cardiac arrhythmias (especially pectoralis major triggers)
- Goose flesh
- Ptosis, excessive lacrimation
- Conjunctival reddening.

Linking symptoms to specific trigger points
(Simons 2002)

- Tension-type headache may derive from active triggers located in sternocleidomastoid, upper trapezius, posterior cervical musculature or temporalis.
- Frozen shoulder symptoms may be associated with trigger points in subscapularis, supraspinatus, pectoralis major and minor, and in the deltoid muscles.

- Epicondylitis may derive from trigger points present in the extensors of the fingers and hand, supinator and triceps brachii.
- Carpal tunnel syndrome may be associated with triggers in the scaleni and finger extensors.
- Atypical angina pectoris pain may be associated with active trigger points in left side pectoralis major or in the intercostals.
- Low back pain may involve trigger points in quadratus lumborum, iliopsoas, thoracolumbar paraspinals, rectus abdominis, piriformis, gluteus maximus and/or medius.

Reduced mobility

Joint restrictions have been noted as deriving from trigger point activity; for example, Kuchera (1997) has listed trigger points associated with shoulder restriction as shown in Table 3.1.

Production of trigger points

The causes of trigger point presence can relate to any combination of physical or psychic stress factors that result in alterations in normal tone in muscles, fascia and other soft tissues which, in turn, can effect changes in joint play, breathing, posture, etc. (Fig. 3.8). The progression from hypertonicity to retained metabolic wastes and relative ischaemia, in muscles affected by, for example, poor posture, has been discussed previously (see Ch. 1). The feature of ischaemia and prolonged stress seems to be a major pre-

Table 3.1 Trigger points associated with shoulder restriction (Kuchera 1997)

Restricted motion	Muscle housing trigger point
Flexion	Triceps
Abduction	Subscapularis Infraspinatus Supraspinatus Teres major Levator scapulae
Internal rotation	Teres major Infraspinatus
External rotation	Subscapularis Pectoralis minor

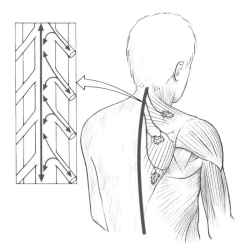

Figure 3.8 Trigger points evolve in specific areas of stressed myofascial tissue. As these tissues compensate progressively towards an ever more dysfunctional fibrotic state, so the activity of associated trigger points increases.

disposing condition in the production of trigger points and their referred pain and dysfunction. Travell's research has shown that a series of embryonic trigger points develops in target/referred areas so that, in time, a chain reaction of triggers may be present.

Identifying trigger points

Kuchera & McPartland (1997) have described the major clinical characteristics of trigger points, based largely on the work of Travell and Simons. They report that, due to an apparent metabolic crisis involving impaired circulation and neural hyperreactivity (facilitation), a number of palpable signs are usually apparent:

- Altered cutaneous temperature (increased or decreased) (see Box 3.4)
- Altered cutaneous humidity (usually increased)
- Small nodular or spindle-shaped thickening representing trigger point locality
- A 'jump' sign (or exclamation !) may accompany palpation because of extreme sensitivity
- A local twitch response may be elicited by stroking across the long axis of taut band housing trigger

---

Box 3.4 Thermography and trigger points (Baldry 1993)

Various forms of thermography have been used to identify trigger point activity, including infrared electrical or liquid crystal.

Swerdlow & Dieter (1992) found, after examining 365 patients with clinically demonstrable trigger points in the upper back, that 'although thermographic "hot-spots" are present in the majority, the sites are not necessarily where the trigger points are located.'

Is it possible that 'old' triggers lie in ischaemic tissue leading to 'cold spots' being noted?

Thermal examination of reference zones (target areas) usually shows that skin temperature is raised – but not always. Simons (1987) attributes this anomaly to different effects of triggers on the autonomic nervous system.

Barrall (1996) has shown that manual–thermal diagnosis is accurate with respect to 'heat' only 70% of the time. Apparently, when heat is noted during off-the-body scanning as when the hand moves over a truly warm area and then over a cooler area, the difference between the two areas' provokes a sensation of 'heat', even though the area being scanned when this is noted may be appreciably cooler than surrounding tissues. This remains a valuable tool, however, as 'different' – whether hot or cold – suggests direct palpation of the area to be a useful next step.

● Local trophic changes or 'goose-flesh' may be evident overlying the trigger site.

Palpation might therefore involve (see Ch. 5 for a fuller presentation of assessment methods when using skin characteristics as a feature):

1. Off-body scan (manual thermal diagnosis), which may offer evidence of variations in local circulation; trigger point activity is more likely in areas of greatest 'difference' (see Box 3.4).
2. Movement of skin on fascia – resistance indicates the general locality of reflexogenic activity – a 'hyperalgesic skin zone' such as a trigger point (Lewit 1992).
3. Local loss of skin elasticity – refines definition of the location (Lewit 1992).
4. Light stroke, seeking 'drag' sensation (increased hydrosis), offers pinpoint accuracy of location (Lewit 1992).

5. Digital pressure (angled rather than perpendicular) into tissues seeks confirmation of active trigger (recognisable referred symptoms) or inactive, latent, trigger (local pain or unfamiliar referral pattern).
6. Use of NMT in its assessment mode (see Chs 5, 6, 11).

Obstacles to direct palpation of myofascial trigger points

Using skin characteristics (see Ch. 5) and thermal assessments (see Box 3.4) it is usually possible to identify the location of soft tissue somatic dysfunction. To establish whether the form that dysfunction takes involves a myofascial trigger point, palpatory pressure into the tissues is required (as in assessment mode NMT; see Chs 5 and 6 in particular). Apart from undeveloped, or unrefined, palpation skills, Simons (2002) suggests various reasons for failing to achieve direct palpation of myofascial trigger points, including:

● supervening layer(s) of fat
● intervening muscle(s), which may be hypertonic, indurated, fibrotic or simply too thick to allow palpation pressure to achieve contact with the trigger point
● intervening aponeurosis
● tense, thick, subcutaneous tissue
● spasm.

 Trigger point features

The pathways that allow particular triggers to produce symptoms in target areas do not follow known neurological patterns, nor do they precisely mimic the pathways of traditional Chinese medicine meridians – although there is some overlap. Wall & Melzack (1989) have shown that approximately 80% of major trigger point sites are on established acupuncture points.

Travell & Simons (1983) have described the trigger point as follows:

In the core of the trigger lies a muscle spindle that is in trouble for some reason. Visualise a spindle like a strand of yarn in a knitted sweater . . . a metabolic crisis takes place which increases the temperature locally in the trigger point, shortens a minute part of the muscle (sarcomere) – like a snag in a sweater, and reduces the supply of oxygen and nutrients into the trigger point. During this disturbed episode an influx of calcium occurs and the muscle spindle does not have enough energy to pump the calcium outside the cell where it belongs. Thus a vicious cycle is maintained and the muscle spindle can't seem to loosen up and the affected muscle can't relax.

Simons (1994) has reviewed the work of others who have tested this concept and found that at the centre of the trigger points there is indeed a lack of oxygen compared with that in the muscles surrounding it (Simons 1994).

Travell & Simons (1983, 1992) have confirmed that the following factors can all help to maintain and enhance trigger point activity:

- nutritional deficiency, especially vitamins C, B complex and iron
- hormonal imbalances (low thyroid hormone production, menopausal or premenstrual situations)

Box 3.5 Compression: method and effects (see Fig 3.9)

Method 1

1. Apply firm digital compression to the trigger point sufficient to produce localised discomfort or pain, as well as symptoms in the target area.
2. Maintain this compression for 5 seconds.
3. Release for 2–3 seconds.
4. Reapply pressure (same level) and keep repeating '5 seconds on, 2–3 seconds off' until the patient reports a reduction in local or referred pain *or* an increase in pain (which is rare) *or* until 2 minutes have passed with no change in the pain level.
5. If using the INIT sequence (see Ch. 9), the next phase involves the positional release component.

Method 2

1. Apply firm digital pressure to the trigger point, sufficient to produce localised discomfort or pain, as well as symptoms in the target area.
2. Maintain the pressure for approximately 10 seconds.
3. Increase the degree of pressure slightly and maintain for a further 10 seconds.
4. Increase the degree of pressure once more and maintain for approximately 10 more seconds.
5. Slowly release pressure and, if utilising the INIT sequence, the positional release component follows (see Ch. 9).

Manual contacts with trigger points
Tendons should be ignored when locating central trigger points. Only the actual length of the fibre is considered; for instance, the long tendon of either biceps brachii head is not included when assessing for central trigger points in this muscle; only the length of its belly is taken into account.

Central trigger points are usually palpable, with either flat palpation (against underlying structures), flat compression (between thumb and fingers like a clothes-peg) or pincer compression (between thumb and fingers like a C-clamp) (see upper trapezius treatment in Ch. 11).

A general thickening in the central portion of a muscle's belly will usually soften when a broad general pressure is applied by using a flat compression. Compressions may be applied wherever the tissue may be lifted without compressing neurovascular bundles.

A precise compression of individual fibres is possible by using the more specific pincer palpation or flat palpation, both of which capture specific bands of tissue.

Underlying structures, including neurovascular courses which might be impinged or compressed, and sharp surfaces such as foraminal gutters, determine whether pincer or flat palpation is more appropriate.

Compression techniques, between fingers and thumb, have the advantage of offering information from two or more of the examiner's digits simultaneously, whereas flat palpation against underlying tissues offers a more solid and stable background against which to assess the tissue.

Effects
The following effects are probable or possible during the application of sustained or intermittent digital compression of tissues:

- Ischaemia, which is reversed when pressure is released (Simons et al 1999).
- 'Neurological inhibition' results from sustained efferent barrage (Ward 1997). See Chapter 12 for details of the use of inhibitory pressure in a sequential manner when treating localised pain.
- A degree of mechanical stretching occurs as 'creep' of connective tissue commences (Cantu & Grodin 1992).
- Piezoelectric effects modify the 'gel' state of tissues to a more solute ('sol') state (Barnes 1997).
- Rapid mechanoreceptor impulses interfere with slower pain messages ('gate theory') (Wall & Melzack 1989).
- Pain-relieving endorphin and enkephalin release occurs (Baldry 2001).
- Taut bands associated with trigger points release spontaneously (Simons et al 1999).
- Traditional Chinese medicine suggests modification of energy flow through tissues following pressure application (Zhao-pu 1991).

- infections (bacteria, viruses or yeast)
- allergies (wheat and dairy in particular)
- low oxygenation of tissues (aggravated by tension, stress, inactivity, poor respiration).

Box 3.6 Algometrics: using appropriate pressure

When applying digital pressure to a tender point in order to ascertain its status ('Does it hurt?', 'Does it refer?', etc.), or when treating a trigger point, it is important to have some way of knowing that the pressure being applied is uniform.

It has been shown that, using a simple technology (bathroom scales), physical therapy students can be taught accurately to produce specific degrees of pressure on request. The students were tested applying posteroanterior pressure force to lumbar tissues. After training, using bathroom scales to evaluate pressure levels, the students showed significantly reduced error, both immediately after training and 1 month later (Keating et al 1993).

The term 'pressure threshold' is used to describe the least amount of pressure required to produce a report of pain and/or referred symptoms (Hong et al 1996). It is obviously useful to know how much pressure is required to produce pain and/or referred symptoms, and whether this degree of pressure is different before and after treatment, or at a subsequent clinical encounter. Without a measuring device such as an algometer there would be no means of standardised pressure application.

Use of an algometer is not really practical in everyday clinical work, but it becomes an important tool in research, as an objective measurement of a change in the degree of pressure required to produce symptoms. An algometer is also a useful tool for a practitioner to use in training themselves to apply a standardised degree of pressure when treating, and to 'know' how hard they are pressing.

An algometer is a hand-held, spring-loaded, rubber-tipped, pressure-measuring device, which offers a means of achieving standardised pressure application. Using an algometer, sufficient pressure to produce pain is applied to points, at a precise 90° angle to the skin. The measurement is taken when pain is reported.

Baldry (referring to research by Fischer) discusses algometer use (he calls it a 'pressure threshold meter') and suggests it should be employed to measure the degree of pressure required to produce symptoms 'before and after deactivation of a trigger point, for when this is successful, the pressure threshold over the trigger point increases by about 4 kg' (Baldry 1993, Fischer 1988).

Digital pressure at 45° angle introduces ischaemic, inhibitory pressure.

Various models exist:

- [✓] Temporarily cuts off circulation, 'flushing' tissues when released
- [✓] Inhibition of neural activity
- [✓] Local mechanoreceptors stimulated, producing gating of pain messages
- [✓] Release of local endorphins and brain enkephalins
- [✓] Mechanical stretching of tissues
- [✓] Alters gel-like tissues to softer 'sol' state
- [✓] Taut bands associated with trigger points release
- [✓] Enhanced energy flow according to TCM (Traditional Chinese Medicine)

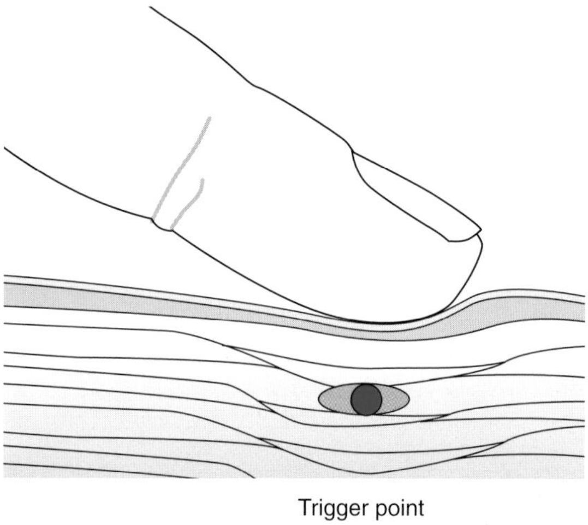

Trigger point

Figure 3.9 Schematic representation of myofascial trigger point.

Trigger point deactivation

A number of methods exist for the deactivation of such trigger points, ranging from use of pharmacological agents such as novocaine or xylocaine, to coolant sprays and acupuncture techniques. It is noteworthy that direct digital pressure techniques can also effectively deactivate trigger points – if only temporarily in many instances. Clinical experience has shown that an absolute requirement for trigger point deactivation (apart from removal of the causes) involves the need to restore the muscle in which the trigger point lies to its normal resting length.

Trigger point deactivation may be achieved by (Chaitow & DeLany 2000, Kuchera 1997, Travell & Simons 1992):

- inhibitory compression as used in osteopathic soft tissue manipulation, neuromuscular therapy and massage (see Boxes 3.5 and 3.6)
- chilling techniques (spray, ice, possibly combined with stretching – 'spray & stretch')
- acupuncture, injection, etc. (Baldry 1993)
- positional release methods such as strain/counterstrain (Chaitow & Delany 2000, Jones 1981)
- muscle energy (stretch) techniques (Simons et al 1999)
- myofascial release methods (Barnes 1997)
- combination sequences such as integrated neuromuscular inhibition technique (INIT) (Chaitow 1994)
- correction of associated somatic dysfunction possibly involving high-velocity thrust (HVT) adjustments and/or osteopathic or chiropractic mobilisation method (Liebenson 1996)
- education and correction of contributory and perpetuating factors (posture, diet, stress, breathing habits, etc.) (Bradley 1999)
- self-help strategies (stretching, etc.) (Simons et al 1999)
- microcurrent applications (McMakin 1998)
- ultrasound (Lowe & Honeyman-Lowe 1999).

Clinical experience suggests that failure to restore the muscle containing the trigger point to its normal resting length means that treatment is likely to provide only short-term relief. It is vital to remember that a trigger point is self-perpetuating, unless it is treated correctly and sufficiently. This means that, once symptoms have been relieved, the muscle containing the trigger should be stretched gently to its longest resting length. Failing this, symptoms will return, irrespective of the technique used (chilling, pressure, injection, acupuncture, etc.).

Such stretching should be gradual and gentle, and the recommendation of Lewit (1992) and Travell & Simons (1992) is that muscle energy

technique (MET), in which gentle isometric contractions followed by stretch are employed (see Ch. 8), is the method of choice to achieve that stretching. Lewit (1992) suggests that, in many instances, stretching is adequate in itself for deactivating trigger point activity.

Other views on trigger points

In order to gain further understanding of the significance of these widespread noxious entities, it is essential to be aware of the process of facilitation, as well as Selye's general and local adaptation syndromes (see Chs 1 and 9 on clinical applications of NMT). We need, also, to be aware of views of others who have tried to make sense of the myriad systems that have identified patterns of reflex activity in surface tissues (as discussed in Ch. 4).

Mennell

Mennell (1975) agrees that a muscle that can attain and maintain its normal resting length is a pain-free muscle. One that cannot (a muscle in spasm) is usually a source of pain, regardless of whether the source of the spasm is in that muscle or not. Whatever the means used to 'block' the trigger activity, and whatever the neuropathological routes involved, the critical factor in the restoration of pain-free normality is that, during any relief from the state of spasm or contraction, the affected muscle should have its normal resting length restored by stretching. Mennell defines trigger points as localised palpable spots of deep hypersensitivity from which noxious impulses bombard the central nervous system to give rise to referred pain. Mennell favours chilling the trigger area by vapocoolant or ice-massage – an approach supported by Travell and Simons, who now both advocate MET as well. Details of their recommended methods are given in Chapter 8.

Chaitow

Chaitow (1994) has proposed that a sequence of treatment to achieve trigger point deactivation – commencing with palpation/identification utilising NMT, followed by ischaemic compression (also NMT), followed by adoption of a positional release posture (such as is used in osteopathic functional technique or strain/counterstrain; see Ch. 8) – should be followed by a stretching of the tissues housing the trigger point. The stretching in this sequence can follow a focused (to activate the fibres involved) isometric contraction, or be applied at the same time as the contraction – introducing an isolytic muscle energy approach into the methodology (see Ch. 8).

This sequence has been dubbed 'integrated neuromuscular inhibitor technique' (INIT) and is considered further in the chapters that deal with treatment.

Chaitow and Delany

Chaitow & Delany (2001) have hypothesised that there are times when the activity of a trigger point might be regarded as serving a useful physiological role, and that in such circumstances deactivation would be counterproductive. Treatment of trigger points may then best be left until after correction of the adaptational mechanisms that have

caused their formation. An example involves the stabilisation of the sacroiliac joint during the gait cycle. As the right leg swings forward, the right ilium rotates backwards in relation to the sacrum (Greenman 1996). Simultaneously, sacrotuberous and interosseous ligamentous tension increases to brace the sacroiliac joint in preparation for heel strike. Just before heel strike, the ipsilateral hamstrings are activated, thereby tightening the sacrotuberous ligament (into which they merge) to further stabilise the sacroiliac joint. In the case of an unstable or dysfunctional sacroiliac joint, a persistent bracing mechanism, involving a hypertonic biceps femoris, possibly including trigger point activity, might represent a potentially useful attempt to maintain stability in the joint. Deactivation of the trigger point, and/or release of the tight hamstring, could in such circumstances reduce stability, with undesirable results (van Wingerden et al 1997).

Bradley

New Zealand physiotherapist Dinah Bradley epitomises those practitioners who use trigger

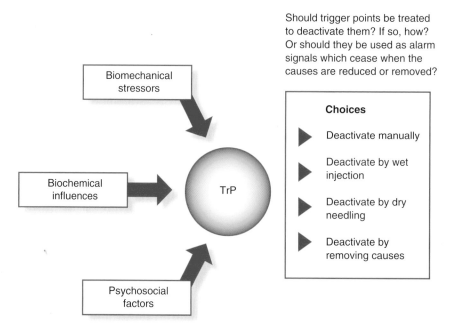

Figure 3.10 Schematic representation of trigger point deactivation choices.

points as monitors, rather than treating them. Bradley, an expert in breathing rehabilitation, palpates and identifies key trigger points in the intercostals and upper trapezius as a rule, at the outset of the patient's course of breathing rehabilitation. She asks them to ascribe a value out of 10 to the trigger point, while it is under digital pressure, before they commence their exercise and treatment programme (no direct treatment is given to the trigger points themselves), and periodically during the rehabilitation course, as well as at the time of discharge.

Bradley (1999) states:

I use trigger point testing as an objective measurement. Part of [the patient's] recovery is a reduction in musculoskeletal pain in these overused muscles. I use a numeric scale to quantify this. Patients themselves feel the reduction in tension and pain [over time], a useful subjective marker for them, and an excellent motivator.

This use of trigger points, in which they are not directly deactivated but are used as monitors of improved breathing function, highlights several key points. [Fig. 3.10]

It is possible to draw various conclusions from this approach:

● As function and oxygenation improves, trigger points become less reactive and painful.
● Enhanced breathing function represents a reduction in overall stress, reinforcing the concepts associated with facilitation: as stress (of whatever kind) reduces, trigger points react less actively.
● Direct deactivation tactics are not the only way to reduce trigger point activity.
● Trigger points can be seen to be acting as 'alarm' signals, virtually quantifying the current levels of adaptive demand being imposed on the individual, or on the specific tissues.

The stress burden and trigger points

One of Selye's most important findings is commonly overlooked when the concurrent impact of multiple stressors on the system is being considered (Selye 1974). Shealy (1984) summarises as follows:

Selye has emphasized the fact that any systemic stress elicits an essentially generalized reaction, with release of adrenaline and glucocorticoids, in addition to any specific damage such stressor may cause. During the stage of resistance (adaptation), a given stressor may trigger less of an alarm; however, Selye insists that adaptation to one agent is acquired at the expense of resistance to other agents. That is, as one accommodates to a given stressor, other stressors may require lower thresholds for eliciting the alarm reaction. Of considerable importance is Selye's observation that concomitant exposure to several stressors elicits an alarm reaction at stress levels which individually are sub-threshold. That is, one-third the dose of histamine, one-third the dose of cold, one-third the dose of formaldehyde, elicit an alarm reaction equal to a full dose of any one agent.

In short, therefore, as adaptation to life's stresses and stressors continues, pain thresholds drop, and a lesser stress load is required to produce responses (pain, etc.) from facilitated structures, whether paraspinal or myofascial.

HYPERVENTILATION: AN EXAMPLE OF COMPOUND STRESS INFLUENCES

There are few more complex functional stress influences than those that arise from altered breathing patterns, such as are manifest when upper chest breathing and/or hyperventilation is habitual. Chaitow et al (2002) have expressed this as follows:

Consider someone who is habitually breathing in an upper chest mode (for postural, habitual, emotional or other reasons), the stress of which will place adaptive demands on the accessory breathing muscles, with consequent hypertonicity, shortness, reciprocal inhibition, malcoordination, stiffness and pain, almost certainly involving trigger point activity, as well as joint dysfunction.

● The biomechanical changes which evolve from this functional chaos will modify the structure of the breathing apparatus to the extent that normal breathing function becomes difficult or impossible.
● In addition the individual will probably display evidence of anxiety as a direct result of respiratory alkalosis, deriving from CO_2 imbalance . . . caused by the breathing pattern. Or the breathing pattern may have been created because of a predisposing anxiety (Timmons 1994).

● This pattern of breathing, and the anxiety it encourages, feeds back into a cycle of aggravated upper chest breathing, reinforcing the pattern.

● What may have started as an emotional state will have evolved into a chronic biochemical imbalance and a state of relative biomechanical rigidity.

It is easy to see how [therapeutic] interventions which focus on the anxiety would be helpful, as would focus on the biomechanical/structural imbalances: Interventions which reduce anxiety will help all associated symptoms. Such interventions might also involve biochemical modification (medication etc.), stress coping approaches or psychotherapy.

Interventions which improve breathing function, probably involving easing of soft tissue distress (including deactivation of trigger points) and/or joint restrictions, should also help to reduce the symptoms by allowing, with retraining, a more normal breathing pattern to be practiced.

The most appropriate approach will be the one which most closely deals with causes rather than effects, and which allows for long term changes which will reduce the likelihood of recurrence. Biochemistry, biomechanics and the mind are seen, in this example, to be inextricably bonded with each other.

The lesson to be learned from this all-too-common example is that treating pain and dysfunction in the neck, shoulders and thorax of such an upper chest breather, with trigger points as major features, might usefully involve manual methods, or relaxation/psychotherapy (if appropriate), or rebeathing retraining, or a combination of methods.

PATHOPHYSIOLOGY OF FIBROMYALGIA/FIBROSITIS/ MYODYSNEURIA

The changes that occur in tissue involved in the onset of myodysneuria/fibromyalgia, according to Gutstein, are thought to be initiated by localised sympathetic predominance, associated with changes in the hydrogen ion concentration and calcium and sodium balance in the tissue fluids (Petersen 1934). This is associated with vasoconstriction and hypoxia/ischaemia. Pain results, it is thought, from these alterations affecting the pain sensors and proprioceptors.

Muscle spasm and hard nodular localised tetanic contractions of muscle bundles (Bayer 1950), together with vasomotor and musculomotor stimulation, intensify each other, creating a vicious cycle of self-perpetuating impulses. There are varied and complex patterns of referred symptoms that may result from such 'trigger' areas, as well as local pain and minor disturbances.

Such sensations as aching, soreness, tenderness, heaviness and tiredness may all be manifest, as may modification of muscular activity due to contraction resulting in tightness, stiffness, swelling, etc.

Recent research has resulted in strict guidelines for a diagnosis of fibromyalgia from the American College of Rheumatology (Wolfe et al 1990):

1. History of widespread pain.

Pain is considered widespread when all of the following are present: pain in the left side of the body, pain in the right side of the body, pain above the waist and pain below the waist. In addition there should be pain in the spine or the neck or front of the chest, or thoracic spine or low back.

2. Pain in 11 of 18 palpated tender point sites.

There should be pain on pressure (around 4 kg of pressure maximum) on not less than 11 of the following sites (Fig. 3.11):

—Either side of the base of the skull where the suboccipital muscles insert

—Either side of the side of the neck between the 5th and 7th cervical vertebrae – technically described as between the 'anterior aspects of inter-transverse spaces'

—Either side of the body on the midpoint of the muscle that runs from the neck to the shoulder (upper trapezius)

—Either side of the body on the origin of the supraspinatus muscle that runs along the upper border of the shoulder blade

—Either side, on the upper surface of the rib, where the 2nd rib meets the breast bone, in the pectoral muscle

—On the outer aspect of either elbow just below the prominence (epicondyle)

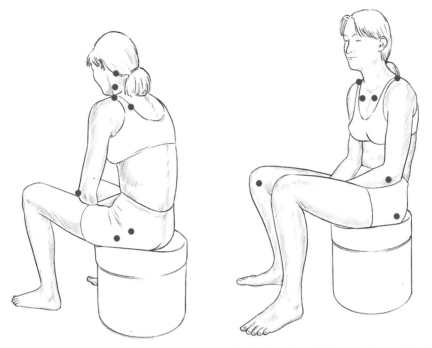

Figure 3.11   Sites of the 18 fibromyalgia tender points as defined by the American College of Rheumatologists.

—In the large buttock muscles, either side, on the upper outer aspect in the fold in front of the muscle (gluteus medius)

—Just behind the large prominence of either hip joint in the muscular insertion of piriformis muscle

—On either knee in the fatty pad just above the inner aspect of the joint.

A puzzle

The question is often asked: Is fibromyalgia the same as myofascial pain syndrome (pain problems in which trigger points are clearly involved)?

Do trigger points actually cause fibromyalgia?

The condition called myofascial pain syndrome (MPS) – a disorder in which pain of a persistent aching type is referred to a number of target areas by triggers lying some distance away – has long been recognised as a cause of severe and chronic pain. Since many experts insist that the 'tender' points that are palpated when diagnosing fibromyalgia need to refer pain elsewhere if they are to be taken seriously in the diagnosis (making them trigger points by definition), the question needs to be asked whether MPS is not the same thing as fibromyalgia syndrome (FMS)? The answer is: not quite.

Scandinavian researchers showed in 1986 that around 65% of people with fibromyalgia had identifiable trigger points, and it is clear, therefore, that there is an overlap between FMS and MPS.

D. P. Baldry, a leading British physician/acupuncturist, has summarised the similarities and differences between these two conditions (Baldry 1993) as follows:

The two conditions are *similar* or identical in that both fibromyalgia and MPS:

- are affected by cold weather
- may involve increased sympathetic nerve activity and may involve conditions such as Raynaud's phenomenon
- have tension headaches and paraesthesia as a major associated symptom

- are unaffected by anti-inflammatory pain-killing medication, whether of the cortisone type or standard formulations.

Fibromyalgia and MPS are *different* in that:

- MPS affects males and females equally; fibromyalgia mainly involves females.
- MPS is usually local to an area such as the neck and shoulders, or low back and legs, although it can affect a number of parts of the body at the same time, whereas fibromyalgia is a generalised problem, often involving all four 'corners' of the body at the same time.
- Muscles containing areas that feel 'like a tight rubber band' are found in around 30% of people with MPS, but in more than 60% of people with FMS.
- People with FMS have poorer muscle endurance than people with MPS.
- MPS can sometimes be bad enough to cause disturbed sleep, whereas in fibromyalgia the sleep disturbance has a more causative role, and is a pronounced feature of the condition.
- MPS produces no morning stiffness whereas fibromyalgia does.
- Fatigue is not usually associated with MPS, while it is common in fibromyalgia.
- MPS can sometimes lead to depression (reactive) and anxiety, whereas, in a small proportion of fibromyalgia cases, depression/anxiety can be the trigger for the start of FMS.
- Conditions such as irritable bowel syndrome, dysmenorrhoea and a feeling of swollen joints are noted in fibromyalgia, but seldom in MPS.
- Low-dosage tricyclic antidepressant drugs are helpful in dealing with the sleep problems, and many of the symptoms of fibromyalgia, but not of MPS.
- Exercise programmes (cardiovascular fitness) can help some patients with fibromyalgia, according to experts, but this is not a useful approach in MPS.
- The outlook for people with MPS is excellent because the trigger points usually respond quickly to massage, manipulative or acupuncture techniques, whereas the outlook for those with fibromyalgia is less positive, with a lengthy treatment and recovery phase being the norm.

Schneider (1995) reports:

It is now clear that there are several important differences between fibromyalgia (FM) and myofascial pain syndrome (MFPS) . . . local treatment applied to tender points [in FM] is ineffective, yet specific treatment of trigger points [in MFPS] is dramatically effective.

Simons (2002) has summarised the main differences between MPS and fibromyalgia (Table 3.2).

CONCLUSION AND HYPOTHESIS

We have seen how hyperreactive local (trigger point) and spinal areas can arise and be main-

Table 3.2 Differences between MPS and fibromyalgia (Simons 2002)

Myofascial trigger points	Fibromyalgia
Muscular origin	Systemic or central nervous system origin
Female : male ratio 1:1	Female : male ratio 4–9 : 1
Local or regional pain	Widespread, general pain
Focal tenderness	Widespread tenderness of most of body
Muscle feels tense (taut bands)	Muscle feels soft and doughy
Restricted stretch range of motion	Commonly hypermobile
Examination for trigger points anywhere	Examination for prescribed tender points
Immediate response to trigger point injection	Delayed response to trigger point injection
May also have fibromyalgia	Nearly all also have myofascial trigger points
All myofascial trigger points are tender	Not all tender points are myofascial trigger points

tained and/or aggravated as a result of repetitive and continuous stress of one sort or another.

What we see in fibromyalgia is that areas of the brain behave in a facilitated manner, and that this hyperreactive brain activity could well be another version of this same phenomenon (facilitation). If so, we can learn much about fibromyalgia from our experience of handling localised facilitation processes such as trigger points.

Korr's studies, discussed previously, show that facilitated areas act as 'neurological lenses', focusing whatever stress impacts on the person as a whole through these sensitised tissues.

If that 'tissue' happens to be (a part of) the brain, we have a situation in which it becomes imperative for stress of all sorts (climatic, emotional, structural/postural, nutritional, toxic, infective, allergenic, etc.) to be minimised, and this includes tailoring therapeutic interventions

to be as non-invasive as possible (deep massage causes increased muscle pain in fibromyalgia, whereas light massage does not).

Constitutional therapeutic approaches such as deep relaxation, non-stressful hydrotherapy, wellness massage and similar methods are more likely to be helpful than anything that makes adaptive demands on an already compromised individual.

Summary. Trigger points are certainly often part – in some cases the major part – of the pain suffered by people with fibromyalgia. When they are present (as they certainly are if pressure on the 'tender point' produces pain somewhere else in the body), we need to know more about them and how they can be treated successfully.

In the next chapter an overview is presented of other reflex systems, awareness of which should add to our comprehensive understanding of myofascial trigger points.

REFERENCES

Baldry P 1993 Acupuncture trigger points and musculoskeletal pain. Churchill Livingstone, Edinburgh

Baldry P 2001 Myofascial pain and fibromyalgia syndromes. Churchill Livingstone, Edinburgh

Barnes M 1997 The basic science of myofascial release. Journal of Bodywork and Movement Therapies 1(4):231–238

Barrall J-P 1996 Manual–thermal diagnosis. Eastland Press, Seattle

Bayer H 1950 Pathophysiology of muscular rheumatism. Zeitschrift für Raeumaforschung 9:210

Beal M 1983 Palpatory testing of somatic dysfunction in patients with cardiovascular disease. Journal of the American Osteopathic Association 82(11):73–82

Beal MC 1985 Viscerosomatic reflexes: a review. Journal of the American Osteopathic Association 85(12):786–801

Benatsen L 2000 Central sensitization in tension-type headache – possible pathophysiological mechanisms. Cephalalgia 20(6):603–610

Bradley D 1999 Breathing retraining advice from three therapists. Journal of Bodywork and Movement Therapies 3(3):159–167

Brugger A 1962 Pseudoradikulare syndrome. Acta Rheumatologica 19:1

Cantu R, Grodin A 1992 Myofascial manipulation. Aspen Publications, Gaithersburg, Maryland

Chaitow L 1994 Integrated neuro-muscular inhibition technique in treatment of pain and trigger points. British Osteopathic Journal XIII:17–21

Chaitow L 2000 Fibromyalgia syndrome – a practitioner's guide to treatment. Churchill Livingstone, Edinburgh

Chaitow L, DeLany J 2000 Clinical applications of neuromuscular technique. vol. 2: Lower body. Churchill Livingstone, Edinburgh

Chaitow L, Bradley D, Gilbert C 2002 Multidisciplinary approaches to breathing pattern disorders. Churchill Livingstone, Edinburgh

Cornelius A 1909 Die neurepunkt lehre. vol. 2. George Thins, Leipzig

Denslow J, Korr I et al 1949 Quantitative studies of chronic facilitation. American Journal of Physiology 150:229–238

Dittrich RJ 1954 Somatic pain and autonomic concomitants. American Journal of Surgery

Dowling D 1991 In: DiGiovanna E, ed. An osteopathic approach to diagnosis and treatment. Lippincott, Philadelphia

Dowling D 2000 Progressive neuromuscular inhibition technique (PINS). Journal of the American Osteopathic Association 100(5):285–298

Dvorak J, Dvorak V 1984 Manual medicine diagnostics. Georg Thieme, Stuttgart

Dubs R 1950 Beitrag zur anatomie der lumbosakralen region. Fortschritte der Neurologie – Psychiatrie 18:69

Feinstein B, Longton J, Jameson R, Schiller F 1954 Experiments on pain referred from deep somatic tissues. Journal of Bone and Joint Surgery 36A:981

Fischer A 1988 Documentation of muscle pain and soft tissue pathology. In: Kraus H, ed. Diagnosis and treatment of muscle pain. Quintessence, Chicago

Greenman PE 1996 Principles of manual medicine. 2nd edn. Williams & Wilkins, Baltimore

Gutstein R 1944a A review of myodysneuria (fibrositis). American Practitioner and Digest of Treatments 6(4):114–124

Gutstein R 1944b The role of abdominal fibrositis in functional indigestion. Mississippi Valley Medical Journal 66:114–124

Gutstein R 1956 The role of craniocervical myodysneuria in functional ocular disorders. American Practitioner's Digest of Treatments November

Hix E 1976 Reflex viscerosomatic reference phenomena. Osteopathic Annals 4(12): 496–503

Hockaday M, Whitty CW 1967 Patterns of referred pain in the normal subject. Brain 90: 481–496

Hong C-Z, Chen Y-N, Twehouse D, Hong D 1996 Pressure threshold for referred pain by compression on trigger point and adjacent area. Journal of Musculoskeletal Pain 4(3):61–79

Jones L 1981 Strain and counterstrain. Academy of Applied Osteopathy, Colorado Springs

Keating J, Matuyas T, Bach T 1993 The effect of training on physical therapists' ability to apply specified forces of palpation. Physical Therapy 73(1):38–46

Kellgren J 1938 Observations on referred pain coming from muscle. Clinical Science 3:175–190

Kellgren J 1939 On the distribution of pain arising from deep somatic structures. Clinical Science 4:35–46

Korr I 1970 Physiological basis of osteopathic medicine. Postgraduate Institute of Osteopathic Medicine and Surgery, New York

Korr I 1975 Proprioceptors and somatic dysfunction. Journal of the American Osteopathic Association 74:638

Korr I 1976 Spinal cord as organiser of disease process. Academy of Applied Osteopathy Yearbook 1976

Korr I, ed. 1977 Neurobiological mechanisms in manipulation. Plenum Press, New York

Korr I 1986 Somatic dysfunction. Journal of the American Osteopathic Association 86(2):109–114

Kuchera M 1997 Travell & Simons myofascial trigger points. In: Ward R, ed. Foundations of Osteopathic Medicine. Williams & Wilkins, Philadelphia

Kuchera M, McPartland J 1997 Myofascial trigger points. In: Ward R, ed. Foundations of Osteopathic Medicine. Williams & Wilkins, Philadelphia

Lewis T 1938 Suggestions relating to the study of somatic pain. British Medical Journal 1:321–325

Lewit K 1992 Manipulative therapy in rehabilitation of the locomotor system. Butterworths, London

Liebenson C 1996 Rehabilitation of the spine. Williams & Wilkins, Baltimore

Lowe J-C, Honeyman-Lowe G 1999 Ultrasound treatment of trigger points. Medecine du Sud-est April–May–June no. 2:12–15

McMakin C 1998 Microcurrent treatment of myofascial pain in head, neck and face. Topics in Clinical Chiropractic 5(1):29–35

Melzack R, Wall P 1989 Textbook of pain. 2nd edn. Churchill Livingstone, London

Mennell J 1975 The therapeutic use of cold. Journal of the American Osteopathic Association 74:1146–1158

Mense S, Simons D 2001 Muscle pain. Williams & Wilkins, Philadelphia

Patterson M 1976 Model mechanism for spinal segmental facilitation. Academy of Applied Osteopathy Yearbook 1976

Petersen W 1934 The patient and the weather: autonomic disintegration. Edward Bros, Ann Arbor

Schneider M 1995 Tender points – fibromyalgia vs. trigger points – myofascial pain syndrome. Journal of Manipulative and Physiological Therapeutics 18(6):398–406

Selye H 1974 Stress without distress. Lippincott, Philadelphia

Shealy CN 1984 Total life stress and symptomatology. Journal of Holistic Medicine 6(2):112–129

Simons D 1987 Myofascial pain due to trigger points. International Rehabilitation Medicine Association, monograph 1

Simons D 1994 Myofascial pain syndromes. Journal of Musculoskeletal Pain 2(2):113–121

Simons D 2002 Understanding effective treatments of myofascial trigger points. Journal of Bodywork and Movement Therapies 6(2) (81–88).

Simons D, Travell J, Simons L 1999 Myofascial pain and dysfunction: the trigger point manual. Vol. 1: Upper half of body. 2nd edn. Williams & Wilkins, Baltimore

Speransky A 1943 A basis for the theory of medicine. International Publishers, New York

Sutter M 1975 Versuch einer Wesensbestimmung pseudoradikularer syndrome. Schweizerische Rundschau für Medizin Praxis 63:42

Swerdlow B, Dieter N 1992 Evaluation of thermography. Pain 48:205–213

Timmons B 1994 Behavioral and psychological approaches to breathing disorders. Plenum Press, New York

Travell J 1957 Symposium on mechanism and management of pain syndromes. Proceedings of the Rudolph Virchow Medical Society

Travell J 1981 Identification of myofascial trigger point syndromes. Archives of Physical Medicine 62:100

Travell J, Bigelow N 1947 Role of somatic trigger areas in the patterns of hysteria. Psychosomatic Medicine 9(6):353–363

Travell J, Simons D 1983 Myofascial pain and dysfunction: the trigger point manual. Vol. 1: Upper half of body. 1st edn. Williams & Wilkins, Baltimore

Travell J, Simons D 1992 Myofascial pain and dysfunction: the trigger point manual. Vol. 2: The lower extremities. Williams & Wilkins, Baltimore

Van Wingerden J-P, Vleeming A, Kleinvensink G, Stoekart R 1997 The role of the hamstrings in pelvic and spinal function. In: Vleeming A, Mooney V, Dorman T, 1997

Wall P, Melzack R 1989 Textbook of pain. Churchill Livingstone, Edinburgh

Ward R 1997 Foundations of osteopathic medicine. Williams & Wilkins, Philadelphia

Webber TD 1973 Diagnosis and modification of headache and shoulder-arm-hand syndrome. Journal of the American Osteopathic Association 72:697–710

Wolfe F, Simons D 1992 Fibromyalgia and myofascial pain syndromes. Journal of Rheumatology 19(6):944–951

Wolfe F, Smythe HA, Yunus MB et al 1990 The American College of Rheumatology 1990 Criteria for the Classification of Fibromyalgia. Arthritis and Rheumatism 33:160–172

Zhao-Pu W 1991 Acupressure therapy. Churchill Livingstone, Edinburgh

4

The variety of reflex points

REFLEX PATTERNS AND AREAS

In this chapter some of the major systems that have identified and classified reflex areas on the body surface will be discussed, because many of the 'points' that these identify are bound to be accessed during the application of NMT in an assessment or a treatment mode.

Osteopathic physician Eileen DiGiovanna (1991) states: 'Today many physicians believe there is a relationship among trigger points, acupuncture points and Chapman's reflexes. Precisely what the relationship may be is unknown.' She quotes from a prestigious osteopathic pioneer, George Northup, who stated as far back as 1941:

One cannot escape the feelings that all of the seemingly diverse observations (regarding reflex patterns) are but views of the same iceberg the tip of which we are beginning to see, without understanding either its magnitude or its depth of importance.

Awareness of the reflex potential of the body surface widens the therapeutic potential of NMT, although deciding which of the many possible applications of reflex activity to utilise in diagnosis or treatment can be a daunting task. The discussion in this text of these reflex systems and classifications should not be taken as indicating recommendation for their use, merely recognition of the fact that they are widely used, and that NMT offers an additional means of access and employment of their potential.

Felix Mann (1983), one of the pioneers of acupuncture in the West, has entered the controversy as to the existence, or otherwise, of acupuncture meridians (and indeed acupuncture points). Mann, in an effort to alter the emphasis that traditional acupuncture places on the specific charted positions of points, stated:

McBurney's point, in appendicitis, has a defined position. In reality it may be 10 cms higher, lower, to the left or right. It may be one centimetre in diameter, or occupy the whole of the abdomen, or not occur at all. Acupuncture points are often the same, and hence it is pointless to speak of acupuncture points in the classical traditional way. Carefully performed electrical resistance measurements do not show alterations in the skin resistance to electricity, corresponding with classical acupuncture points. There are so many acupuncture points mentioned in some modern books, that there is no skin left which is not an acupuncture point. In cardiac disease, pain and tenderness may occur in the arm however this does not occur more frequently along the course of the heart meridian, than anywhere else in the arm.

Hence, Mann concludes, meridians do not exist, or – more confusingly perhaps – the whole body is an acupuncture point!

Leaving aside the validity of Mann's comment, it is true to say that if all the multitude of points described in acupuncture, traditional and modern, together with those points described by Travell and co-workers, Chapman, Jones and Bennett (see later in this chapter), were to be placed together on one map of the body surface, we would soon come to the conclusion that the entire body surface is a 'potential acupuncture point'. This realisation is supported by Speransky's findings from the 1930s, as discussed in Chapter 3.

Are all tender points trigger points?

A number of respected researchers and clinicians are frequently in error when they describe localised soft tissue areas that palpate as sensitive but that do not refer symptoms elsewhere, as do trigger points. Certainly a trigger point will always be palpable, and will always be sensitive to pressure, but then so will most other 'points', whether these be Chapman's reflexes, Gutstein's myodysneuria points, Jones's tender

points or acupuncture alarm points. These, however, will not necessarily refer painful symptoms to distant sites in the obvious manner displayed by trigger points. This is not to say that any 'tender' or sensitive point cannot become a trigger point, since, clearly, before it is active, a trigger point has to evolve and in its earlier stages will be painful, sensitive or tender, but may at the time of palpation not be sufficiently sensitised and hyperreactive to refer pain and other symptoms. If a point 'belonging' to any of the various classifications discussed below does refer symptoms in the manner of trigger points, then it can be so classified and treated.

Distinguishing features of myofascial trigger points
(modified from Simons 2002)

- Active myofascial trigger points produce regional pain complaints and not bodywide pain and tenderness.
- Not all tender points are myofascial trigger points, but all myofascial trigger points are tender.
- Referred tenderness, as well as referred pain, is characteristic of a myofascial trigger point.
- All myofascial trigger points are associated with a taut band.
- Not all taut bands are palpable (requires sufficient palpation skill and accessibility).
- All active myofascial trigger points cause a clinical pain (sensory disturbance) that is familiar to the patient.
- Only an active myofascial trigger point, when compressed, reproduces the clinical sensory symptoms that are familiar to the patient.
- However, a latent myofascial trigger point produces no clinical sensory (pain or numbness) complaint that is familiar to the patient.

Some of the major 'point' classifications involving reflex activity and with a diagnostic potential are considered in this chapter, in alphabetical order (not in order of apparent importance).

ACUPUNCTURE POINTS

Soft tissue changes often produce organised discrete areas that act as generators of secondary problems. It would be advantageous to examine briefly another aspect of 'trigger' points: the existence of a network of points that is supposedly constantly capable of reflex activity. This network is, of course, the pattern of acupuncture points (Fig. 4.1). What is of interest is that the location of these fixed anatomical points is capable of corroboration by electrical detection, each point being evidenced by a small area of lowered electrical resistance.

When 'active', due presumably to reflex stimulation, these points become even more detectable, as the electrical resistance lowers further. The skin overlying them also alters and becomes hyperalgesic and not difficult to palpate as differing from surrounding skin. Active acupuncture points also become sensitive to pressure and this is of value to the therapist because the finding of sensitive areas during palpation or treatment is of diagnostic importance. Sensitive and painful areas that do not have detectable tissue changes as part of their make-up may well be 'active' acupuncture points (or *tsubo*, which means 'points on the human body' in Japanese). Not only are these points detectable and sensitive, but they are also amenable to treatment by direct pressure techniques. They are, therefore, well worth studying.

One of the leading oriental experts on pressure techniques is Katsusuke Serizawe, who discusses a 'nerve reflex' theory for the existence of these points (Serizawe 1976):

The nerve reflex theory holds that, when an abnormal condition occurs in an internal organ, alterations take place in the skin and muscles related to that organ by means of the nervous system. These alterations occur as reflex actions. The nervous system, extending throughout the internal organs, like the skin, the subcutaneous tissues, and the muscles, constantly transmits information about the physical condition to the spinal cord and the brain. These information impulses, which are centripetal in nature, set up a reflex action that causes symptoms of the internal organic disorder to manifest themselves in the surface areas of the body. The reflex symptoms may be classified into the following three major groups: (a) sensation reflexes; (b) interlocking reflexes; (c) autonomic system reflexes.

(a) Sensation reflexes. When an abnormal centripetal impulse travels to the spinal cord, reflex action causes the skin at the spinal column affected by the impulse to become hypersensitive. This sensitivity to pain is especially notable in the skin, subcutaneous tissues, and muscles located close to the surface, since these organs are richly supplied with sensory nerves.

(b) Interlocked reflexes. An abnormality in an internal organ causes a limited contraction, stiffening, or lumping of the muscles in the area near the part of the body that is connected by means of nerves to the affected organ. Stiffness in the shoulders, back, arms, and legs are symptoms of this kind. In effect, the interlocked reflex actions amount to a hardening and stiffening of the muscles to protect the ailing internal organ from excess stimulus. When the abnormality in the organ is grave, however, the stiffening of the muscles is not limited to a small area, but extends over large parts of the body.

(c) Autonomic system reflexes. Abnormalities in the internal organs sometimes set up reflex action in the sweat glands, the sebaceous glands, the pilomotor muscles, and the blood vessels in the skin. The reflex action may cause excess sweat or drying of the skin as the consequence of cessation of sweat secretion. Its effect on the pilomotor muscles may be to cause the

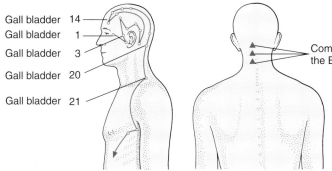

Gall bladder 14
Gall bladder 1
Gall bladder 3
Gall bladder 20
Gall bladder 21

Common trigger point sites on the Bladder meridian

Figure 4.1A, B Location of some important acupuncture points on the head and neck. Research indicates that over 75% of defined acupuncture points are also sites of common trigger points.

condition known as goose flesh. The sebaceous glands may be stimulated to secrete excess sebum, thus causing abnormal oiliness in the skin; or they may stop secreting sebum, thus making the skin abnormally dry. The reflex action may cause chills or flushing because of its effects on the blood vessels in the skin.

I have discussed the ways in which abnormalities in internal organs cause changes in the conditions of the surface organs of the body however the intimate relation between internal organs and external ones has a reverse effect as well; that is, stimulation to the skin and muscles affects the condition of the internal organs and tissues. For instance, stimulation transmitted to the spinal cord from the body surface sets up a reflex action in the internal organ that is controlled by the nerves at the level of the spinal column receiving external stimuli. Stimuli of this kind instigate peristaltic motion or contraction in the organ. The effect of such external stimulation on blood vessels and on the secretion of hormones has been scientifically verified.

The reader will note a conceptual link between the forces underlying *tsubo* usage and our understanding of facilitation as explained in Chapter 3. Quite obviously, there may be more effective ways of dealing with organ dysfunction than by pressure techniques to *tsubo*/acupuncture points. However, because our study is concerned basically with manual treatment, it is worth taking account of the knowledge accumulated by the Chinese and Japanese over many centuries.

Acupuncture points and their morphology

Melzack, and other researchers, maintain that there is little, if any, difference between acupuncture points and most trigger points (Travell & Simons 1992, Wall & Melzack 1989) and, because all sensitive points are capable of becoming trigger points, any research into the structure of acupuncture points should enhance our understanding of trigger point activity.

The morphology of acupuncture points has been studied, notably by Jean Bosey (1984), Professor of Anatomy at Montpellier University, France. Some of his major conclusions, in summary, are as follows:

Points are situated in palpable depressions ('cupules'). The skin (epiderm) over the point is a little thinner at the cupule level, under which lies a fibrous cone in which there is frequently found either a neurovascular formation, or simply a cutaneous neurovascular bundle. Free nerve endings are noted, and the presence, beneath the point, of Golgi endings and Pacini corpuscles is common. Connective tissues lie below at varying depths. Fascia and aponeurosis are noted and, it is stated: 'A passage of vessels and nerves, through the fascia, is very often found under the acupuncture point.'

An anatomical study of 100 acupuncture points showed that they overlay large nerve trunks in 42% of cases, large veins in 40% and cutaneous neurovascular pedicals in 18%. In deeper structures the effect of stimulation (by needling or pressure) of muscle and tendon receptors is noted, but this is thought to be indirect, rather than direct, because of the extremely small size of, for example, muscle spindles and Golgi tendon organs. The practice of manipulating the needle, thus imposing a degree of traction on the underlying (muscular) tissue, is noted, and this would, it is observed, impose stimulation on such receptor organs. Fat is also a common factor in the morphology of points, and this, and the connective tissue, is thought to be a key factor in the achievement of the 'acupuncture sensation' that accompanies successful treatment. The conclusion reached is that a number of tissues are simultaneously affected by any particular acupuncture needle (and, the author stresses, by strong finger pressure).

Some points, when dissected, showed that neurovascular structures lie immediately below the point, which could account for the particular effects noted by such points being treated. This is of interest to those using Bennett's neurovascular points. The implications for those practitioners not employing needles, and who rely on pressure techniques in order to provide stimulus or sedation to such areas, is that, if accurately applied, the effects of pressure should be identical (to needle acupuncture), especially in relation to pain control.

Acupuncture and applied kinesiology

An attempt to correlate the various reflex systems and methods has been made by the American chiropractor George Goodheart. His system of applied kinesiology involves testing muscle groups for weaknesses and then, depending upon the results of such tests, using various massage and pressure techniques applied to specific locations (points) in order to normalise function. These points correspond to Chapman's reflexes, acupuncture points and other less well known reflex systems. Many of Goodheart's techniques, theories and methods support and utilise methods that are in line with NMT.

Acupressure and pain thresholds

It has been shown that pain thresholds can be dramatically raised by pressure techniques applied to specific points. Researchers at the Peking Medical College conducted complex experiments which demonstrated that finger pressure acupuncture produced a rise of 133% in pain threshold of rabbits (using radiant heat as the painful stimulus). When cerebrospinal fluid was perfused from one rabbit to another after such experiments, the recipient rabbit was found to have achieved a rise in pain threshold of up to 80%. This suggested the presence of hormone-like substances produced by the brain in response to the original acupressure stimulus. These substances are now known to be enkephalins and endorphins, and these play a role in NMT pain control. The point used in these tests was equivalent to the acupuncture point known as Bladder 60, posterior to the ankle (externally) and just anterior to the Achilles tendon.

Acupuncture points and trigger points: are they the same phenomenon?

Because they spatially occupy the same positions in at least 75% of cases (Wall & Melzack 1989) there is often a coincidence of treatment in that a trigger point could be 'mistaken' for an active acupuncture point, and vice versa. Wall & Melzack (1989) have concluded that 'trigger points and acupuncture points when used for pain control, though discovered independently and labelled differently, represent the same phenomenon'.

Baldry (1993) does not agree, however, claiming differences in their structural make-up. He states:

It would seem likely that they are of two different types, and their close spatial correlation is because there are A-delta afferent-innervated [fast transmitting receptors with a high threshold and sensitive to sharply pointed stimuli or heat produced stimulation] acupuncture points in the skin and subcutaneous tissues immediately above the intramuscularly placed, predominantly C afferent-innervated [slow transmitting, low threshold, widely distributed and sensitive to chemicals – such as those released by damaged cells – mechanical or thermal stimulus] trigger points.

Clearly, stimulation of an area that has, beneath the contacting instrument or digit, both an acupuncture and a trigger point will influence both types of neural transmission and both 'points'. Which route of reflex stimulation is producing a therapeutic effect, or whether other mechanisms altogether are at work – endorphin release, for example – is therefore open to debate. This debate can be further widened if we include the vast array of other reflex influences identified by other systems and workers, as discussed later in this chapter.

Whereas traditional oriental concepts focus on 'energy' imbalances in reaction to acupuncture points, there exist also a number of Western interpretations.

Melzack et al (1977) have assumed that acupuncture points represent areas of abnormal physiological activity, producing a continuous low-level input into the central nervous system (CNS). They suggested that this might eventually lead to a combining with noxious stimuli deriving from other structures, innervated by the same segments, to produce an increased awareness of pain and distress. They found it reasonable to assume that trigger points and acupuncture points represented the same phenomenon, having found that the location of trigger points on Western maps, and acupuncture points used commonly in painful conditions, showed a remarkable 75% correlation in position.

It is interesting that the link between the source of pain or tender points, and the referred area of pain noted in trigger points, in many instances seems to travel along the routes of traditional acupuncture meridians, but certainly not always. Spontaneous pain in such a point, according to acupuncture tradition, indicates the need for urgent attention. It is not the intention of this book to provide instruction in acupuncture methodology, nor necessarily to endorse the views expressed by traditional acupuncture in relation to meridians and their purported connection with organs and systems. However, it would be short-sighted to ignore the accumulated wisdom that has led many thousands of skilled practitioners to ascribe particular roles to these points, for example Alarm, Associated and Akabane points as described in this chapter. As far as a manual therapy is concerned, there seems to be value in having awareness of the reported roles of particular acupuncture points, and of incorporating this into diagnostic and therapeutic settings.

As we palpate and search through the soft tissues, in basic neuromuscular technique, we are bound to come across areas of sensitivity that relate to these points. They are also often found to overlap with neurolymphatic and neurovascular points, as described elsewhere in this text.

For example, reflex number 19 in Chapman's reflexes, which relates to the urethra, is identical to the neurovascular point of the bladder, and the acupuncture alarm point of the Bladder meridian. Careful comparison will show many such overlaps. General guidance as to how to treat acupuncture points, which are sensitive, must relate to whether a stimulating or sedating effect is desired. The body often seems to utilise therapeutic stimulation to its best advantage. Selye has shown us (see Ch. 1) that homoeostatic mechanisms are at work, so that any stimulus, if appropriate and not excessive, can result in a beneficial response. In accord with the methods used in treating neurolymphatic and neurovascular points (described elsewhere in this chapter) it is suggested that, to some extent, the 'feel' of the tissues be allowed to guide the practitioner. A change (in the sense of a release of tension, or a softening, or a sensing of a gentle pulsation in the tissues) is often an indication of an adequate degree of therapy. In order to sedate what is an overactive point, up to 5 minutes of sustained or intermittent pressure, or rotary contact, may be required.

For stimulation, the timing could involve between 20 seconds and 2 minutes. By this time, some degree of change should be palpable. As must be clear, if pressure is sustained beyond a certain point quite the opposite effect will be achieved. This is a common natural phenomenon which occurs in response to all factors in life that are initially stimulating. If prolonged, they become enervating or exhausting, and in terms of therapy this is undesirable unless anaesthesia is required.

A short cold (water) application, for example, will stimulate, whereas a long one will sedate, and too much can kill. The words of Speransky and Selye should be recalled and the minimum effort used, consistent with achieving a response.

We have noted previously that many of the different reflex systems have points that seem to be interchangeable, and that many of these are traditional acupuncture points. In terms of local pain, the view of Chifuyu Takeshige (Takeshige 1985), Professor of Physiology at Showa University, is that 'The acupuncture point of treatment of muscle pain is the pain-producing muscle itself.'

Respected acupuncture clinicians, such as George Ulett, suggest that 'acupuncture points are nothing more than time honoured muscle motor points'. Professor C. Chan Gunn, however, finds this too simple an explanation, and states: 'Calling acupuncture points "motor points" or "myofascial trigger points" is too simple. They are Golgi tendon organs.' These, and other researchers, are quoted by Stephen Botek, Assistant Professor of Clinical Psychiatry, New York Medical College (Ernst 1983). He believes that 'myofascial needling' is the term of choice to define the type of acupuncture that dispenses with traditional explanations as to the effects of acupuncture. The points utilised in a specific study (Botek 1985) were Large Intestine 4 (Hoku) in the web between thumb and the first finger, and Stomach 36 (Tsu san li) below the knee. The study recorded skin temperature of the face, hands and feet. It was found that, compared with a resting period, both manual and electrical stimulation of both points induced a general warming effect. This was immediate in the face (Lewith & Kenyon 1984) and appeared after 10–15 minutes in hands and feet. The temperature increase was notably more marked after manual acupressure than after electrical stimulation. Manual stimulation of these points was shown to be more effective than other forms of stimulation.

Lewith & Kenyon (1984) point to a variety of suggestions having been made as to the mechanisms via which acupuncture, or acupressure, achieves pain-relieving results. These include neurological explanations such as the 'gate control theory'. This, and variations on this theme, look at the various structures of the CNS and the brain in order to define the precise mechanisms involved in acupuncture's pain-relieving action.

This, in itself, is seen to be an incomplete explanation, and humoral (endorphin release, etc.) and psychological factors are also shown to be involved in modifying the patient's perception of pain.

A combination of reflex and direct neurological elements, as well as the involvement of a variety of secretions, such as enkephalins and endorphins, is thought to be the modus operandi of acupressure, and probably of all of the various systems of reflex activity discussed in this section (neuro-lymphatics, etc.).

Many of the points of referred pain and tenderness used in Western medical diagnosis are also acupuncture points, for example:

- Head's zones could be shown to include most acupuncture points, especially the Alarm and Associated points (given below).

- The points noted as being 'tender' in appendicitis, such as McBurney's, Clado's, Cope's, Kummel's, Lavitas's, are on the Stomach, Spleen and Kidney meridians of traditional acupuncture, and these are used by acupuncturists in treating appendicitis.
- Patients with a gastric ulcer produce tenderness at a site known as Boas' point, and this is sited precisely on Bladder point 21, which is the Associated point of the Stomach meridian.
- Brewer's point, in Western medicine, is noted in kidney infection, and this is Bladder point 20, the Associated point for the Spleen (in traditional acupuncture this has a controlling role over water, the element of the kidneys).

The degree of overlap between these well known points can also be noted when comparing other classification systems of points.

Ah Shi points

Acupuncture methodology also includes the treatment of points that are not listed on the meridian maps, and that are known as Ah Shi points. These include all painful points that arise spontaneously, usually in relation to particular joint problems or disease. For the duration of their sensitivity they are regarded as being suitable for needle or pressure treatment. These points may therefore be thought of as identical to the 'tender' points described by Lawrence Jones in his strain/counterstrain method, discussed later in this chapter.

Alarm points, Associated points, Akabane points

There are, in traditional acupuncture, a number of key points that are most likely to become painful in relation to particular visceral dysfunction. These have been classified as Alarm points. They are presented below, and the following general information may make their employment easier:

- The Alarm points are found only on the ventral surface of the body, each point being associated with one of the 12 meridians and its functions. Six of the points are on the midline, the others are bilateral. Tenderness elicited by palpation of an Alarm point may indicate dysfunction of the organ related to the point. In traditional acupuncture, if sensitivity is noted on light pressure, there is an associated energy deficiency. If heavy pressure is required, the condition relates to an energy excess.

● Associated points lie on the back of the body, and these are all on the Bladder meridian, which runs parallel to the spine, bilaterally. Each Associated point is related to one of the meridians and its function. The same assumed relationship with energy deficit or excess exists, as in Alarm points (sensitivity on light pressure = deficiency, and on heavy pressure = excess). There are also a few extra Associated points, as

illustrated (see Fig. 4.3). Spontaneous pain at any of these listed points indicates a disorder in that meridian, and in its associated organ or function.

Table 4.1 Alarm points

			Acupuncture point
Point 1	Lung		LU1
Point 2	Liver		LV14
Point 3	Gall bladder		GB24
Point 4	Kidney	Bilateral	GB25
Point 5	Spleen		LV13
Point 6	Large intestine		ST25
Point 7	Heart constrictor		VC17
Point 8	Heart		VC14
Point 9	Stomach		VC12
Point 10	Triple heater		VC5
Point 11	Small intestine		VC4
Point 12	Bladder		VC3

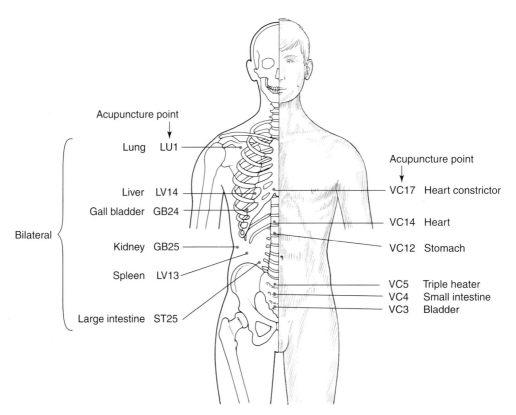

Figure 4.2 Location of Alarm points, which lie on the anterior surface of the body. If spontaneous pain develops in any alarm point, the associated meridian is thought to be involved. If light pressure produces tenderness, an 'energy deficiency' is considered to exist; if heavy pressure produces tenderness, an 'energy excess' is assumed. An understanding of the organs and functions associated with particular meridians is necessary in order to utilise these points therapeutically or diagnostically.

● Akabane points are found on the fingers and toes, being the terminal points of the meridians. Sensitivity of any of these is said to relate to dysfunction and imbalance of energy in that meridian. Electronic measurement of these points (Melzack et al 1977) is performed in a number of modern electroacupuncture systems such as electroacupuncture according to Voll (EAV). Manual testing is common, and was obviously the method used before electrical methods arrived on the scene. These points are all bilateral.

Location of Alarm points

Alarm points (Table 4.1, Fig. 4.2) are on the anterior surface of the body. Spontaneous pain at any point is considered to indicate a disorder of the affiliated meridian. If tenderness is elicited on light pressure, a deficiency of energy in the meridian is assumed, whereas tenderness elicited on heavy pressure indicates an excess of energy in the meridian.

These are reflex points for meridian function, and awareness of the roles apparently played by the various meridians in body energy economics

Table 4.2 Associated points

Meridian		Bladder meridian point
Point 1	Lung	B13
Point 2	Heart constrictor	B14
Point 3	Heart	B15
Point 4	Governor vessel	B16
Point 5	Liver	B18
Point 6	Gall bladder	B19
Point 7	Spleen	B20
Point 8	Stomach	B21
Point 9	Triple heater	B22
Point 10	Kidney	B23
Point 11	'Sea of Energy'	B24 (extra associated point)
Point 12	Large intestine	B25
Point 13	Small intestine	B27
Point 14	Bladder	B28

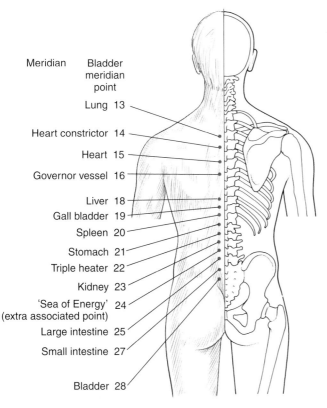

Figure 4.3 Location of Associated points, which lie on the dorsal surface of the body slightly lateral to the median line bilaterally. If spontaneous pain develops in any associated point, the allied meridian is thought to be involved. If light pressure produces tenderness, an 'energy deficiency' is considered to exist; if heavy pressure produces tenderness, an 'energy excess' is assumed. An understanding of the organs and functions associated with particular meridians is necessary in order to utilise these points therapeutically or diagnostically.

is necessary to evaluate the significance of reactions that produce tenderness in Alarm points.

Location of Associated points

Associated points are on the dorsum of the body (Fig. 4.3). Spontaneous pain is thought to indicate a disorder in the meridian associated with it. Tenderness elicited on light pressure indicates a deficiency in energy in that meridian, and tenderness elicited on heavy pressure indicates an excess of energy in the associated meridian. These points are all on the Bladder meridian and their associations are given in Table 4.2. The points are slightly lateral to the median line bilaterally and are also reflex points for the meridians with which they are associated.

Location of Akabane points

Akabane points (Table 4.3, Fig. 4.4) represent the terminal points of the meridians. Sensitivity of these is thought to relate to imbalance in the energy of the meridian. Comparative sensitivity shows relative imbalance in organ (energy) systems. Manual or electronic testing is possible.

BENNETT'S NEUROVASCULAR REFLEX POINTS
(Martin 1977)

A wide degree of clinical experience resulted in an American chiropractor, Terrence Bennett, reaching the conclusion that there was a group of previously unknown reflexes available for diagnostic and therapeutic use, which he termed neurovascular reflexes. He described his work in

Table 4.3 Akabane points

Points on feet	Points on hands
1. Spleen	7. Large intestine
2. Liver	8. Heart constrictor
3. Stomach	9. Triple heater
4. Gall bladder	10. Heart
5. Kidney	11. Small intestine
6. Bladder	12. Lung

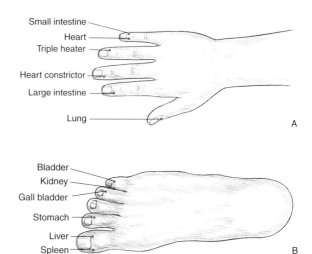

Figure 4.4A, B Location of Akabane points, which represent the terminal points of the 12 meridians. Sensitivity of the points is thought to relate to imbalance in related organs (energy) systems. Both manual and electronic testing of these points is possible.

a series of lecture notes, which were compiled and published by Ralph Martin, after Bennett's death, as *Dynamics of Correction of Abnormal Function* (Martin 1977). The major points are listed in Chapter 5, which deals with diagnostic procedures.

Bennett describes the tissues that are palpated as altered in texture, being contracted or indurated, in much the same way as Chapman's reflexes (described below). His method of treatment calls for a slight degree of pressure, which he describes as 'only minimal, enough to render the tissues semi-anaemic, which is adequate stimulus'.

Experience indicates that the light pressure should be accompanied by slight stretching of the skin. In accordance with the views of Karel Lewit (1992), gentle stretching of the skin induces reflex activity when hyperalgesic (sensitised) skin zones are used therapeutically (see Ch. 5). When hyperalgesia occurs, skin becomes less elastic, with greater adherence to the underlying fascia and with lowered resistance to electricity. In Bennett's system the skin is stretched with the minimum of force, so as to take up the slack, by the fingertips being drawn lightly apart. In most cases, if the area involves any degree of soft tissue dysfunction, a lack of anticipated elasticity will be noted in the skin as this distraction takes place. By maintaining the slight stretch on the tissues (in effect a 'mini' myofascial release), a yielding occurs, and it is after this that a pulsation sensation should normally be felt. John Thie (1973) describes this pulsation sensation thus:

A few seconds after contact is made, a slight pulse can be felt, at a steady rate of 70 to 74 beats per minute. This pulse is not related to the heartbeat, but is believed to be the primitive pulsation of the microscopic capillary bed, in the skin.

Bennett insisted that the contact be maintained until a response was noted in the form of the tissue altering, relaxing and, most importantly, until the operator became aware of the presence of pulsation. This could arrive within a few seconds or take some minutes to emerge, depending on the patient and his or her condition. Bennett termed the pulsation felt as the 'arteriole pulse' because, he stated: 'It is the beginning of the system, at the junction of the artery and the arteriole, that controls the metabolism. The sensation of pulsation is essential . . . It has to be there, or else we are not accomplishing anything.' Together with this, the change in tissue feel is important: 'The tissues under your fingers begin to relax as you work for a few moments; you sense the degree of tension releasing. When it releases that is all you can do.'

Some points are purely diagnostic, others are used for treatment, and some are both. For example, the coronary reflex in the 2nd thoracic interspace on the left, which is a palpable area of tissue change and which is sensitive to the patient, is only diagnostic (not illustrated). Awareness of Bennett's reflex areas may be found to be a useful addition to the range of available therapeutic and diagnostic knowledge. In using NMT in its diagnostic mode, the tissues being evaluated will yield a multitude of sensitive points. Some of these may correlate with Bennett's findings, and they may then be used as part of an overall assessment of the nature of the dysfunction affecting the patient. They may, of course, also be used, as Bennett intended, as a system in their own right, for assessing and

treating visceral and functional physiological changes and pathology. A number of Bennett's points have been incorporated into the methods of applied kinesiology, notably the points on the cranium, which are used for treating emotional disturbances.

Among the cautions issued by Bennett are:

- Do not overtreat the points on the cranium (2–3 minutes is a maximum).
- In hyperthyroid patients, do not treat the thyroid and pituitary reflexes at the same visit (one should be treated, and alternated with the other at a subsequent visit).
- If the heart is enlarged then the 3rd rib, at the mid-clavicular line, should not be treated.
- Aortic sinus reflex should be treated before any of the brain reflexes are contacted.
- If the ovary is being treated, the thyroid should receive prior attention.

A list of Bennett's reflex points can be found in Chapter 5, which considers diagnostic applications of NMT.

CHAPMAN'S REFLEXES
(Kuchera 1997, Mannino 1979, Owens 1980, Patriquin 1997, Walther 1988)

In the 1930s, Chapman and Owens described a 'neurolymphatic' reflex pattern, now widely used in osteopathic and chiropractic methodology. Chaitow (1965) discussed these reflexes as follows:

The reflexes of Chapman that I intend to discuss are not the whole picture – being only a part of the visible portion of the iceberg – but of immense value nonetheless. Drs Chapman and Owens first reported on Chapman's original findings in the late 1930s. A revised edition of their work has been published by the Academy of Applied Osteopathy.

The surface changes of a Chapman's reflex are palpable. They may best be described as contractions located in specific anatomical areas and always associated with the same viscera. In describing each organ reflex Chapman normally indicated tissue reflex areas, occurring anteriorly and posteriorly. These reflexes found in the deep fascia are described as 'gangliform' contractions. These contractions vary in size from a pellet to a large bean and are located anteriorly in the intercostal spaces near the sternum.

Similar tissue changes are found in those reflexes occurring on the pelvis. The tissue changes found in reflexes located on the lower extremities are described as 'stringy masses' or 'amorphous shotty plaques'. Those reflexes occurring posteriorly along the spine, midway between the spinal processes and the tips of the transverse processes are of a more oedematous nature.

Characteristics

Patriquin (1997) describes the characteristics of Chapman's reflexes as:

- small
- smooth
- firm
- discretely palpable
- approximately 2–3 mm in diameter

Sometimes described as feeling like small pearls of tapioca, lying, partially fixed, on the deep aponeurosis or fascia.

Clinical value of the reflexes

Because the location of these palpable tissue changes is relatively constant in relation to specific viscera, it is possible to establish the location of pathology without knowing its nature. The value of these reflexes is threefold:

1. As diagnostic aids – Patriquin (1997) points out that some of the reflexes, such as that for appendix (tip of 12th rib on the right; see point 38 on Fig. 5.8B) are invaluable in helping with differential diagnosis when faced with right lower abdominal pain: 'Today, Chapman's reflexes are more likely to be used as an integral part of osteopathic physical examination than as a specific therapeutic intervention.'
2. They can be utilised to influence the motion of fluids, mostly lymph.
3. Visceral function can be influenced through the nervous system. '[The] reflexes can be clinically manipulated to specifically reduce adverse sympathetic influence on a particular organ or visceral system . . . patients with frequent bowel movements from the effects of IBS report they have normal or near normal function for days to months after soft tissue treatment over the iliotibial bands and/or the lumbosacral para-

spinal tissues and associated Chapman's reflexes' (Patriquin 1997). (See point 24, anterior and posterior, in Figs 5.8A and 5.8C.)

Mechanism of the reflexes

Regarding the mechanism whereby these reflexes act, it would appear that, in so far as the intercostal reflexes are concerned, stimulation of the receptor organs that lie between the anterior and posterior layers of anterior intercostal fascia acts through the intercostal nerve, which enervates the external and internal intercostal muscles and thus, through the sympathetic fibres, affects the intercostal arteries, veins, lymph nodes, etc. Stimulation thus causes afferent and efferent vessels draining these tissues to increase or decrease, permitting lymph flow to be increased or decreased, thus affecting the drainage of the entire lymph system in the area. Through the sympathetic fibres associated with these tissues, the lymph nodes of the vital organs are also affected.

Explaining results of neuromuscular technique

These reflexes seem to offer explanations for the sometimes startling results obtained through neuromuscular technique. Stanley Lief placed great emphasis on normalising the tissues of the intercostal spaces and the paravertebral areas – sites of many major neurolymphatic reflexes. He also stressed the importance of not overtreating, a consideration that cannot be repeated too often.

Research evidence supports Chapman's reflex usefulness

In a trial conducted to assess the effects of forms of manipulation on blood pressure, one of the methods used was stimulation of a Chapman's reflex (Mannino 1979). A specific effect attributable to this treatment was noted. The point chosen for treatment was the one related to adrenal function. The trial involved treatment of this point, or a sham point, in which pressure was applied to either the real or a false point, for a total of 2 minutes, in a make-or-break circular motion. The point is located in the intertransverse space, on both sides of the 11th and 12th thoracic vertebrae, midway between the spinous processes and the tips of the transverse processes (see point 37 on Fig. 5.8F). The sham treatment involved the area between the 8th and 9th thoracic vertebrae, which relates to small intestine problems, and would have no effect on the sort of condition being assessed in these trials.

The results showed no immediate effect on blood pressure, but did indicate fascinating alteration in aldosterone levels and subsequent blood pressure drop. Abnormalities in aldosterone levels have been shown in populations with essential hypertension. Following treatment of the reflexes there was a demonstrable and consistent fall in aldosterone levels within 36 hours of stimulation of the Chapman reflex for the adrenals, but no change at all in the levels when the sham points were stimulated. A drop of 15 mmHg systolic and 8 mmHg diastolic was noted some 36 hours after treatment of the adrenal points. The delay in response suggested that the treatment had a tendency to interrupt, or damp down, a feedback to the adrenal medulla by the sympathetic nervous system (Patriquin 1997).

Nimmo's dismissal of the Chapman reflexes

An element of disinformation has emerged regarding Chapman's neurolymphatic reflexes.

Vannerson & Nimmo (1971) writing in *The Receptor* – the journal of the organisation that used (in the 1960s) to teach Nimmo's receptor-tonus technique (see Ch. 2) – stated:

Research has not borne out the presumption [by Chapman] of a neurolymphatic reflex. Muscle fibres, which alone have the specific function of constricting vessels, do not exist in the walls of lymph vessels, except for a few fibres in the thoracic duct, and a few large trunks. These are sparsely located, and have little effect in lymph fluid propulsion.

These two authors then deride Chapman's assertion that the reflexes could exist at specific sites, an idea that they call 'fantastic'.

Nimmo & Vannerson's first point is in contradiction to *Gray's Anatomy* (Gray 1973), which tells us that lymph moves in a number of ways. Filtration occurs, generated by filtration of fluid from the capillaries. There is also a degree of movement engendered by contraction of surrounding muscles, which compress lymph vessels, the movement of which is determined by the presence of valves. This muscular contraction is dependent upon normal activity, and muscular contraction–relaxation sequences. Lymph is further capable of being moved, in such regions, according to Gray, by massage movements. Pulsating arterial vessels, in close proximity, also assist lymph movement, as does respiratory movement. Also in contradiction of Nimmo & Vannerson, Gray states: 'The smooth muscle in the walls of the lymphatic trunks is most marked just proximal to the valves; stimulation of sympathetic nerves accompanying the trunks, results in contraction of the vessels; the intrinsic muscle of the vessels thus probably aids the flow of the lymph.'

In 1979, rhythmic pulse waves were recorded from the lymphatic vessels of five healthy, upright, motionless males at a rate of 8–10 per minute, asynchronous with respiration or leg movement (Oszeweski & Engeset 1979). Degenhardt & Kuchera (1996) describe the process as follows: 'The regulation of the intrinsic contractility of the lymphatic system is based on transmural distension of the vessel walls and neural and humoral mediators.' They comment:

The physiology of the lymphatic system is quite complex. Research has only begun to demonstrate the many factors that influence lymphatic flow. The extrinsic compression of the myofascia on the lymphatics has been the focus of many manipulative techniques . . . Studies now consistently demonstrate contractility in the lymphatic vessels. This intrinsic pumping has been shown to be under autonomic control, modulated locally by soft tissue chemicals and systemically produced hormones. Currently it appears that intrinsic contractions have more influence on lymph flow that extrinsic forces.

This evidence, therefore, suggests that the term 'neurolymphatic reflex', as described by Chapman, may indeed be an accurate description of the phenomenon. Nimmo & Vannerson's second observation (relating to the specificity of the reflex sites) may be more valid, especially if anatomical individuality is taken into account. Points of the body surface are never likely to be precisely identifiable by description of anatomical position. However, a general identification as to site is possible. McBurney's point, for example, if present in appendicitis, is usually located within a few degrees of its commonly described location. There are exceptions, of course, and in the inscrutable manner of the Orient, the Chinese have taken this well into account, in describing the locations of acupuncture points. The invention of the 'human inch', which takes account of the individual anatomical proportions of each person, allows for such individualisation. In terms of the charts and maps to be found in this text, the same factor should be borne in mind. The positions are approximate, because variations exist from person to person.

Dysfunction in soft tissues is, however, palpable, and not dependent upon maps. Thus, the general guidelines provided by charts are useful, but cannot take the place of palpatory skills.

A complete illustrated list of Chapman's reflexes is found in Chapter 5, which deals with diagnosis and treatment using NMT.

Palpating for, and treating, the neurolymphatic points

Kuchera (1997) suggests: 'If Chapman's [neurolymphatic] myofascial tender points are to be tested, palpate them early in the examination because motion of the myofascial tissues in their area decreases their sensitivity. In this case their diagnostic clue, tenderness with palpation, may not be evident.'

If, during NMT assessment mode application to the anterior thorax and abdominal region (see Ch. 7) unusual tenderness is noted in the region of the umbilicus, this may relate to bladder, kidney or adrenal dysfunction (see points 15, 16 and 37 on Figs 5.8A & 5.8B); similarly, tenderness in the area if an anterior point is noted in the left fifth or sixth intercostal interspace (see points 13 and 14 on Fig. 5.8A), the patient may

usefully be asked about, for example, stomach or digestive symptoms. Treatment of the lymphatic aspects of these dysfunctional organs or functions (should their existence be corroborated by other clinical evidence) might usefully include gentle applications of rotary pressure to the posterior points, in the sequence described in Chapter 5.

Arbuckle (1977) writes of Chapman's reflexes:

The diagnostic value of these reflexes is amazing. For instance, a female having severe pain in the right lower quadrant of the abdomen, presents several possibilities, but the offending organ may well be located by means of the reflexes, the positive one showing whether the disturbance is due to appendix, cecum, tube or ovary. With a degree of understanding of the interrelation of the endocrine glands, and of the importance of the lymphatics and the autonomic distribution, the therapeutic value of these considerations can be shown clinically. There is a definite sequence, which must be followed, in the management of these reflexes, to produce desired results, and, if not so applied, just as surely as the misapplication of any other therapy, further confusion of the body mechanism will result.

CONNECTIVE TISSUE MASSAGE

Another system that uses reflex effects diagnostically as well as therapeutically is connective tissue massage (CTM). CTM involves 'rolling' the tissues in order to achieve reflex and local effects. According to Ebner (1962), the palpable reflex tissue changes utilised in diagnosis and treatment in CTM methodology can take any of the following forms:

- drawn-in bands of tissue
- flattened areas of tissue
- elevated areas, giving the impression of localised swelling
- muscle atrophy or hypertrophy
- osseous deformity of the spinal column.

The strokes pull and stretch the tissues, and it is suggested that the method's effectiveness is based on a viscerocutaneous reflex. Bischof & Elmiger (1960) explain:

The specific mechanical stimulation of the pull on connective tissue seems to be the adequate stimulus to elicit the nervous reflex. Connective tissue massage acts first on the sympathetic terminal reticulum in the skin. The smallest branches of the autonomic nervous system contact the impulses activated by the pulling strokes to the sympathetic trunk and the spinal cord. The impulses travel from the skin either through a somatosensory spinal nerve via a posterior root ganglion to the grey matter or over the vascular plexus to the same segmental sympathetic ganglion or to the ganglion of the neighbouring segment, through the ramus communicans albus to the posterior root and grey matter of the spinal cord. They terminate either directly or by means of the internuncial neurons at the efferent autonomic root cells.

In the efferent pathway the impulses travel from the autonomic lateral horn, or the intermediolateral column, over the anterior root, ramus communicans albus, to the segmental sympathetic ganglion or to the ganglion of the neighbouring segment and finally to the diseased organ. The origin of the connective tissue reflex zones and the influence of the CTM depend on the relationship between the function of the internal organs, vessels, and nerves as well as the tissues of the locomotor apparatus, which descend from the same metamere.

Clara reminds us that the human embryo is composed of many homogeneous primitive segments (metameres) that are arranged serially. This arrangement is concerned with the mesoderm and the tissue regions derived from it: sclerotomes, myotomes, dermatomes, (ectoderm), angiotomes and nephrotomes. Second, the ectoderm participates in the segmentation (metamerism), as in each of the primitive segments or metameres one corresponding spinal nerve enters. The skin over the segment is also innervated, and in this way the segmentation is projected to the skin. This embryonal connection between the primitive segment and the spinal nerve (dermatome) develops early and remains unchanged postembryonically. Head was the first to point out that the internal organs that develop from the entoderm correspond to certain spinal cord segments, although the entoderm does not participate in the segmentation. The relationship between tissues and their spinal root innervation is the scientific foundation for CTM and other forms of segmental therapy.

Most investigators differ little in their reports concerning the segmental connections of the internal organs. Different schemes have been proposed by Hansen, Keegan, Dejerine and others to relate skin topography with the internal organs, and reference to the cited texts on the subject (Bischof & Elmiger 1960, Ebner 1962) is suggested for further information.

During and after CTM there are a number of reflex reactions including vasodilatation and diffuse or localised sweating. Some of these reflexes do not seem to be segmental in nature. For example, dilatation of the upper extremity blood vessels occurs when the pelvis is treated by CTM. The maximal skin temperature increase occurs about half an hour after massage is discontinued and persists for an hour or so. It is of interest that the vasodilatory effect of CTM is as pronounced, or even more pronounced, following lumbar sympathectomy.

Some of the reactions to CTM are normal autonomic responses such as pleasant fatigue, bowel movements and diuresis. Oedema is markedly reduced and hormonal distribution is seen to achieve a degree of balance. Aspects of CTM are similar to those of NMT, and the 'skin rolling' methods used in some body areas are virtually identical in application. The effects are therefore interesting from a comparative point of view.

Research evidence into clinical effectiveness of CTM in cases of anxiety

A Scottish hospital undertook a trial in which a small group of patients attending a general psychiatric outpatient clinic were treated with CTM (JPR 1983). The research was carried out at Bangour Village Hospital, near Broxburn in West Lothian.

The group selected presented with symptoms of impaired peripheral circulation, muscular tension and pain. A frequent complaint was of sleep impairment, which was not associated with any particular pathology, and which was resistant to even large doses of hypnotic drugs. Those selected for the trial responded poorly to drugs, and were unable to learn standard relaxation techniques.

CTM was applied. An initial diagnostic assessment was made, using a specific massage stroke, applied systematically to the back. This was a form of subdermal traction, or deep stroking, which stimulates the autonomic branch of the nervous system. Patients reported a slight sensation of scratching or cutting. Where tissues were particularly tense when treated in this way, the sensation was stronger, being described as deep dull pressure or a sharp cutting sensation, both unrelated to the actual pressure being applied. A flare reaction of the tissues followed, and in some cases a weal developed, which sometimes persisted for some hours. The treatment proper consisted of a series of strokes that moved systematically through the back, each treatment lasting some 30–45 minutes, followed by a period of rest. Patients reported a feeling of warmth and of being 'peaceful', and frequently fell asleep immediately. The night's sleep following treatment was reported generally to be deep and refreshing. The usual length of a course was 10 treatments, and these ceased either when patients reported the disappearance of symptoms or when no further improvement was seen to be forthcoming. A positive response often involved profuse sweating during treatment, and this was sometimes unilateral.

A number of measurements and tests were conducted during the rest phase, after treatment. Arousal was tested by the playing, over a period, of 20 loud noises. The physiological responses of the patients were recorded. Among the findings were that four out of five patients had a reduction in response to stress (randomly occurring loud noises) after CTM. This was of significant proportions. EMG activity, recorded on the frontalis muscle, showed that there was a significant decrease in response in three cases. Skin resistance was measured every minute during the rest period, and during the periods of stimulation with noise. EMG measurements were also recorded on the forearm extensor muscles. The findings were that in two subjects there was a significant increase in skin resistance, indicating lowered arousal, and two other subjects showed reduction in forearm extensor EMG activity. The other patient showed inconclusive effects. All subjects showed a significant response in one or more of the psychophysiolog-

ical parameters. After cessation of treatment, three out of five patients ceased use of drugs completely, and the other two required diazepam in only small doses. All reported diminution of symptoms. The researchers report that the differences noted in response, between EMG findings in the frontalis muscle and forearm extensor, is of interest because the former is more reactive in depressive illness and the latter is more so in cases of agitation.

It is significant that patients responded in their own way. There were no consistent findings, apart from overall reduction in evidence of symptoms and better sleep patterns. This supports the hypothesis that each individual has a unique pattern of response to stress, and that this pattern is consistent, regardless of the type of stress endured. The response to nonspecific therapy, such as CTM, allows the response of the individual to continue to be individual. They therefore utilise the beneficial aspects of the therapy in their own way, to meet the needs of their unique physiology.

The evidence resulting from this trial is that CTM is a useful tool in dealing with the consequences of psychiatric disturbances, anxiety and agitation. Clinical experiences indicates that similar results may be derived from treatment utilising NMT. This is particularly relevant to problems involving sleep disturbance, such as is common in chronic fatigue syndrome and fibromyalgia – especially where anxiety forms one of the causal features (or results) of these widespread problems.

Jones' tender points (Fig. 4.5)
(Jones 1980)

In his evolution of the 'strain and counterstrain' (SCS) functional manipulative approach to the normalisation of hypertonicity, Lawrence Jones described a series of 'points' that he had identified. These sensitive areas were, Jones discovered, related to specific strains and stresses in the musculoskeletal system, and were used by the therapist as monitors while the areas was being guided into a position of ease, during which process there was both a reduction in sen-

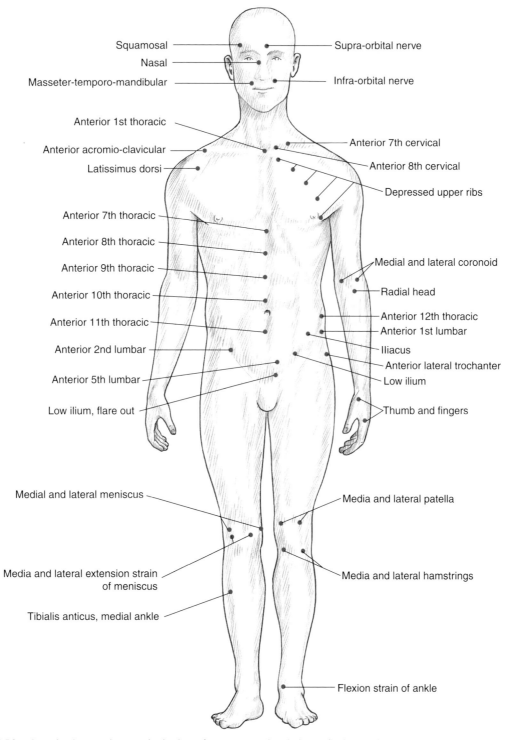

Figure 4.5A   Jones' points on the anterior body surface, commonly relating to flexion strains.

Figure 4.5   Location of Jones' tender points, which are bilateral in response to specific strain (acute or chronic) but are shown on only one side of the body in these illustrations. The point locations are approximate and will vary within the indicated area, depending upon the specific mechanics and tissues associated with the particular trauma or strain.

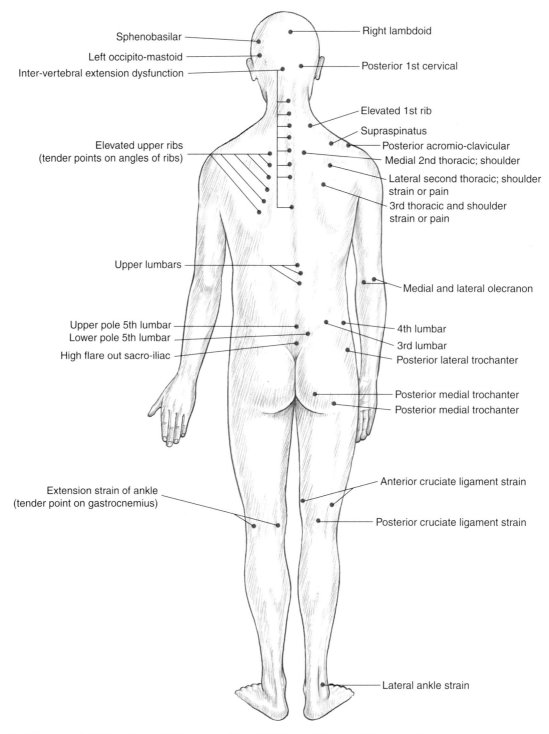

Figure 4.5B Jones' points on the posterior body surface, commonly relating to extension strains.

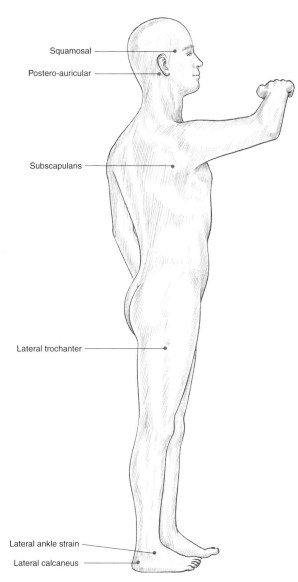

Squamosal

Postero-auricular

Subscapularis

Lateral trochanter

Lateral ankle strain

Lateral calcaneus

Figure 4.5C   Jones' points on the lateral body surface, commonly relating to strains involving side-bending or rotation.

rated into the integrated (INIT) sequence for trigger point deactivation, as described in Chapter 9.

In many ways these 'tender' points, while sensitive to palpation, are not usually areas in which the patient was previously aware of pain. They are therefore similar to Ah Shi – spontaneously tender – points in traditional Chinese medicine (Chaitow 1991).

Significantly perhaps, as the area being treated is positioned in 'ease' so that tenderness vanishes from the tender point, a degree of ischaemic compression/inhibitory pressure/ acupressure would be taking place. It is worth considering that the benefits noted, in terms of pain relief and reduction in contraction or spasm, could relate in some part to the resulting inhibitory/endorphin release action as well as to the subsequent improvement in circulation and possible neural influences, through the tissues and neurological modulation produced by the placing of the tissues into a situation of 'ease'.

Periosteal pain points
(Adapted from Lewit 1992)

These painful areas (Table 4.4) usually relate to acute or chronic contraction of associated muscles and tendons.

Felix Mann, pioneer acupuncture researcher and author, describes periosteal acupuncture as being more effective than ordinary acupuncture in a number of conditions (Mann 1963). He lists the sites given in Table 4.5 amongst the common sites usefully employed in this approach. Clinical experience indicates that NMT ischaemic compression techniques and muscle energy methods are as likely as traditional needling to produce benefit when treating these points.

CONFUSION?

The soft tissues are of major importance to the body's economy, structural integrity and wellbeing. They are also a major source of pain and dysfunction and, as must now be obvious, of reflex disturbances.

sitivity in the palpated tender point as well as a relaxation (increased ease) of the stressed tissues associated with it. The tender points as described by Jones and the methods of treating them fall within the umbrella term 'positional release techniques' (Chaitow 2001, D'Ambrogio & Roth 1997, Deig 2001). The methodology of SCS is summarised in Chapter 8, and is incorpo-

Table 4.4 Periosteal pain points (adapted from Lewit 1992)

Site	Muscular/joint implication
Pain on head of metatarsals	Dropped arch, flat foot
Spur on calcaneum (pain on pressure)	Tight plantar aponeurosis
Pain on tubercle of tibia	Tight long adductor/possible hip dysfunction
Pain on head of fibula	Biceps femoris tightness
Posterior superior iliac spine tenderness	Various possible implications, involving low back, gluteal and sacroiliac region
Lateral aspects of symphysis pubis	Adductors tight. Hip or sacroiliac dysfunction
Pain on coccyx	Gluteus maximus tightness, possibly piriformis or levator ani involvement
Crest of ilium – pain	Tight quadratus lumborum/gluteus medius and/or lumbodorsal dysfunction
Pain on greater trochanter	Tight abductors/hip dysfunction
Pain on lumbar spinous processes (especially L5)	Tight paraspinal muscles
Pain mid-dorsal spinous processes	Lower cervical dysfunction
Pain spinous process of C2	Levator scapular tight: C1–2, 2–3, dysfunction
Pain on xyphoid process	Rectus abdominus tight. 6–8 rib dysfunction
Pain on ribs, on mammary or axillary line	Pectoralis tightness. Visceral dysfunction referred to here
Pain at sternocostal junction upper ribs	Scalenus tightness
Pain on clavicle, medial aspect	Tight sternocleidomastoid
Pain transverse process of atlas	Tight sternocleidomastoid and/or recti capitis lateral. Atlanto-occipital dysfunction
Pain on occiput	Upper cervical or atlas dysfunction
Pain on styloid process of radius	Elbow dysfunction
Pain on epicondyles	Local muscular or elbow dysfunction
Pain at deltoid attachment	Scapulohumeral dysfunction
Mandibular condyles painful	Temporomandibular joint dysfunction. Tight masticators

Table 4.5 Periosteal acupuncture points and associations

Site	Associated with
1. Appropriate transverse cervical process	Headache, migraine, interscapular pain and cervical spondylosis
2. Area of sacroiliac joint	Low back pain, sciatica without neurological deficit, testicular pain
3. Coracoid process	Painful shoulder joint
4. Medial condyle tibia	Knee pain, without advanced pathology
5. Neck of femur	Hip pain, without major changes evident on radiography
6. Lateral aspect of posterior spine of lower lumbar vertebrae	If sacroiliac joint (2 above) does not yield benefit, these areas may be used

The various theories, methods and descriptive terminologies relating to the many point systems and classifications of 'points' are significant inasmuch as NMT offers the opportunity to access and use their potential. If we accept that there are many ways of looking at and interpreting the same phenomenon, then it will be an easy step to acknowledging that an acupuncture point and a trigger point and a Chapman's reflex point, for example, can all be the self-same point, but with different aspects of its reflex potential being considered in each classification.

NMT can (with other modalities) be used as an effective measure to detect and eliminate noxious trigger points and areas that generate or help to maintain dysfunction, or that influence reflexive activity. Such dysfunction can take the form of muscular weakness, muscular contraction, pain, vasodilatation, vasoconstriction, tissue degeneration, gastrointestinal disturbances, sympathetic nervous system abreactions, respiratory and a myriad other disorders including emotional and 'psychological' disorders such as anxiety.

Noxious (pain producing) points that are the end result of various forms of stress imposed on the tissues housing them may reside in either hypertonic or hypotonic muscle, or in ligamentous or fascial tissues, or in apparently normal tissues. When active, such points will always be sensitive to correctly applied pressure and can often be neutralised by manual pressure or a combination of chilling and manual pressure and stretching.

In the treatment sections there will be discussion of methods for locating and treating such points; however, what effects each therapist attempts to achieve by manipulating reflexively active points depends on the individual's professional training and beliefs.

REFERENCES

Arbuckle B 1977 The selected writings of Beryl Arbuckle. National Osteopathic Institute and Cerebral Palsy Foundation

Baldry P 1993 Acupuncture, trigger points and musculoskeletal pain. Churchill Livingstone, Edinburgh

Bischof I, Elmiger G 1960 Connective tissue massage. In: Licht E, ed. Massage, manipulation and traction. New Haven, Connecticut

Bosey J 1984 Acupuncture and Electro-Therapeutics Research 9(2):79–106

Botek S 1985 Acupuncture and Electro-Therapeutics Research 10(3):241

Chaitow L 1965 An introduction to Chapman's reflexes. British Journal of Naturopathy (Spring)

Chaitow L 1991 Acupuncture treatment of pain. Healing Arts Press, Vermont

Chaitow 2001 Positional release techniques. 2nd ed. Churchill Livingstone, Edinburgh

D'Ambrogio K, Roth G 1997 Positional release therapy. Mosby, St Louis, Missouri

Degenhardt B, Kuchera M 1996 Update on osteopathic medical concepts and the lymphatic system. Journal of the American Osteopathic Association 96(2):97–100

Deig D 2001 Positional release technique. Butterworth-Heinemann, Boston

DiGiovanna E 1991 An osteopathic approach to diagnosis and treatment. Lippincott, Philadelphia

Ebner M 1962 Connective tissue massage. Churchill Livingstone, Edinburgh

Ernst M 1983 Acupuncture and Electro-Therapeutics Research 8(3/4):343

Gray H 1973 Gray's anatomy. 35th edn. Longman, London

Jones L 1980 Strain and counterstrain. Academy of Applied Osteopathy, Boulder, Colorado.

JPR 1983 Anxiety states: preliminary report on the value of connective tissue massage. Journal of Psychosomatic Research 127(2):125–129

Kuchera W 1997 Lumbar and abdominal region. In: Ward R, ed. Foundations for osteopathic medicine. Williams & Wilkins, Baltimore

Lewit K 1992 Manipulative therapy in rehabilitation of the locomotor system. Butterworths, London

Lewith G, Kenyon J 1984 Social science and medicine. 19(12):1367–1376

Mann F 1963 The treatment of disease by acupuncture. William Heinemann Medical, London

Mann F 1983 International Conference of Acupuncture and Chronic Pain. September 1983

Mannino J 1979 The application of neurological reflexes to the treatment of hypertension. Journal of the American Osteopathic Association 79(4):225–230

Martin R, ed. 1977 Dynamics of correction of abnormal function. Ralph Martin, Sierra Madre

Melzack R, Stillwell D, Fox E 1977 Trigger points and acupuncture points of pain. Pain 3:3–23

Nimmo R, Vannerson J 1971 Receptor tonus technique. The Receptor 12(1):47

Northup G 1941 The role of the reflexes in manipulative therapy. Journal of the American Osteopathic Association 40:521–524

Oszeweski W, Engeset A 1979 Intrinsic contractility of leg lymphatics in man. Lymphology 21:81–84

Owens C 1980 An endocrine interpretation of Chapman's reflexes. American Academy of Osteopathy, Newark, Ohio

Patriquin D 1997 Chapman's reflexes. In: Ward R, ed. Foundations for osteopathic medicine. Williams & Wilkins, Baltimore

Serizawe K 1976 Tsubo: vital points for oriental therapy. Japan Publications, San Francisco

Simons D 2002 Understanding effective treatments of myofascial trigger points. Journal of Bodywork and Movement Therapies 6(2) (81–88).

Takeshige C 1985 Acupuncture and Electro-Therapeutics Research 10(3):195–203

Thie J 1973 Touch for health. DeVorss, California

Travell J, Simons D 1992 Myofascial pain and dysfunction. vol. 2. Williams & Wilkins, Baltimore

Vannerson J, Nimmo R 1971 Specificity and the law of facilitation in the nervous system. The Receptor 2(1)

Wall P, Melzack R 1989 Textbook of pain. Churchill Livingstone, Edinburgh

Walther D 1988 Applied kinesiology. SDC Systems, Pueblo

5

Diagnostic methods

In previous chapters we have dipped into the vast amount of information that exists relating to the neuromuscular component of the human body. A great many diagnostic aids exist for discovering just what is happening when aspects of this network of tissues malfunction. The great beauty of neuromuscular technique, as devised by Lief, is the way in which diagnostic and therapeutic processes are combined. The thumb, as it glides close to the spinal attachments of the paraspinal musculature, is assessing the tissue tone, density, temperature, etc., and at the same moment is capable of treating any tissues that display evidence of dysfunction (see discussion of STAR characteristics – sensitivity, tissue texture alteration, asymmetry, reduced range of motion – in Ch. 3). The response of the searching thumb or finger to whatever information the tissues impart can be immediate. The use of greater or lesser degrees of pressure, varying in direction and duration, allows the practitioner to judge and treat at the same time, and with great accuracy (Figs 5.1 & 5.2).

If treatment of musculoskeletal dysfunction is to be focused and meaningful, a diagnostic or assessment plan is required. Whilst local muscular changes will become more apparent as treatment progresses, an overall diagnostic picture is required to enable a coherent plan to emerge and for prognosis and progress to be judged.

NEUROMUSCULAR TECHNIQUE – ASSESSMENT AND DIAGNOSIS

If therapeutic intervention is to be structured and organised – and something other than hit

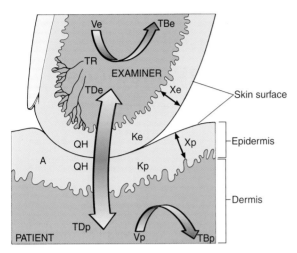

Figure 5.1 This diagram depicts some of the physical and physiological factors that affect the thermoreceptor (TR) discharge rate and consequently the temperature sensed in an examiner's skin in contact with a patient's skin. The temperature and rate of change of the examiner's thermoreceptors are functions of the net effects of the time that the tissues are in contact, their contact area (A), the temperatures (TBe and TBp) and volume flow rates (Ve and Vp) of blood perfusing the examiner's and patient's skin, epidermal thickness (Xe and Xp) and thermal conductivity (Ke and Kp) of both, dermal temperature (TDe and TDp) of both, as well as of the net heat exchange rate (QH) between the two tissues. QH is strongly affected by the heat transfer properties of material trapped between the two skin surfaces, for example air, water, oil, grease, hand lotion, dirt, tissue debris and fabric (Adams, Steinmetz, Heisey, Holmes & Greenman 1982).

and miss – there is a basic need for evaluation and assessment of the way in which the mechanical component of the body is adapting to its current situation, of the extent of changes from the norm, and of the ways in which patterns of pain, malcoordination and restriction are interacting. These changes might involve reflexively active structures such as myofascial trigger points, locally traumatised areas, fibrotic alterations, shortened and/or weakened muscles, joint restrictions and/or general or systemic factors (such as exist in arthritic conditions).

NMT provides a diagnostic/assessment tool and also offers, when it switches from assessment to actively therapeutic mode, a means whereby precisely focused and modulated degrees of force can be directed towards influencing restricted tissues. Myofascial release tech-

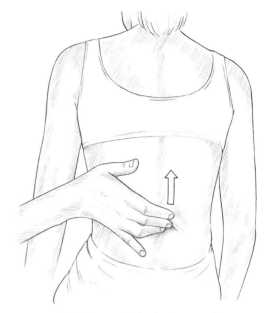

Figure 5.2 Light 'skin on skin' palpation can give indications of deeper dysfunction due to modification of sympathetic and circulatory activity.

niques, as well as ischaemic compression (osteopathic inhibitory technique), can be applied to precise targets via the contacting thumb or finger in NMT. Perhaps NMT's greatest usefulness in assessment relates to the opportunity it offers for the identification of local soft tissue dysfunction in a gentle non-invasive manner. In the USA, as well as in the UK, the focus of many therapists utilising NMT in recent years has been towards the identification and treatment of myofascial trigger points (and the often widespread musculoskeletal dysfunction that produces or is associated with them).

PALPATION

There is no valid substitute for skilful palpatory diagnosis in ascertaining the relatively minute structural changes – primary or reflex – that often have far-reaching effects on the body's economy.

It is generally agreed that the pads of the fingers are the most sensitive portion of the hand available for use in diagnosis. Indeed, the combination of the thumb and first two fingers is the finest mechanism, and can be adapted to conform with the variable areas under palpatory consideration.

Palpatory diagnosis
(Baldry 1993, Beal 1983, DiGiovanna 1991, Travell & Simons 1983, 1992)

Skin assessment before adding lubricant

One of the most successful methods of palpatory diagnosis is to run the pads of a finger or several fingers extremely lightly over the (unlubricated) area being assessed, feeling for changes in the skin texture, which may signify alterations in the tissues below. After localising any changes in this way, deeper periaxial structures can be evaluated by means of the application of greater pressure. There are a number of specific changes to be sought in light palpatory examination. This applies to both acute and chronic dysfunction.

Skin changes (Lewit 1992). Over an area of acute or chronic dysfunction, skin will feel tense and will be relatively difficult to move or glide over the underlying structures. The skin above reflexively active structures will therefore be more adherent to the underlying fascia, something that will be evident in any attempt to glide or roll it, compared with normal areas. By application of a series of bilateral 'pushes' of skin on fascia, comparison is possible for asymmetry of movement.

The skin overlying reflexively active areas such as trigger points (or active acupuncture points) tends to produce a sensation of 'drag' as it is lightly stroked, because of increased hydrosis. There is also an apparent – very slight – sensation of undulation, a rising and falling, palpable on a light stroke, described illustratively as 'hills and valleys'.

Over areas of reflexogenically induced dysfunction the skin will also lose its fully elastic quality, so that on light stretching (taking an area of skin to its easy resistance barrier on stretching) it will test as less elastic than neighbouring skin.

Methods for assessing these skin changes are described in more detail later in this chapter.

Assessment after adding lubricant

Dysfunctional patterns revealed by means of assessment of skin changes should become apparent in the application of neuromuscular palpation/assessment strokes, as described in detail in Chapters 6 & 7.

Induration. A slight increase in diagnostic pressure will ascertain whether or not the superficial musculature has an increased indurated feeling. When chronic dysfunction exists, the superficial musculature will demonstrate a tension and immobility indicating fibrotic changes within and below these structures. These changes are discussed further in the text dealing with the application of basic spinal and abdominal NMT (Chs 6 & 7).

Temperature changes. In acute dysfunction a localised increase in temperature may be evident. In chronic lesion conditions there may, because of relative ischaemia, be a reduced temperature of the tissues. This usually indicates that fibrotic alterations have occurred.

Tenderness. Tenderness of palpated tissues requires investigation. Is the tissue inflamed? Is the local area reflexively active? What is the nature and cause of the sensitivity?

Oedema. An impression of swelling, fullness and congestion can often be obtained in the overlying tissues in acute dysfunction. In chronic dysfunction this is usually absent, having been replaced by fibrotic changes.

Localised contractures. Local, sometimes very small, areas may display evidence of trigger point activity by the presence of taut bands, or minute contracture 'knots' which are exquisitely painful on application of pressure, and which may refer pain to distant areas.

The questions that need to be asked when palpation elicits the sort of changes briefly covered above include:

- What am I feeling?
- What significance does it have in relation to the patient's condition or symptoms?
- How does this relate to any other areas of dysfunction I have noted?

- Is this a local problem or part of a larger pattern of dysfunction?
- What does this mean?

In deeper NMT palpation, the pressure of the palpating fingers or thumb needs to increase sufficiently to make contact with deeper structures such as the periaxial (paravertebral) musculature, without provoking a defensive response. The changes that might be noted could include immobility/rigidity, tenderness, oedema, deep muscle tension, fibrotic and interosseous changes. Apart from the fibrotic changes, which are indicative of chronic dysfunction, all these changes can be found in either acute or chronic problems.

As Peter Lief (1963), son of the innovator of NMT, explains:

Palpation is the main method of detection. Gross lesions are easily palpable but sometimes they are so minute that their detection presents considerable difficulty, especially to the beginner. It sometimes takes many months of practice to develop the necessary sense of touch, which must be firm, yet at the same time sufficiently light, in order to discern the minute tissue changes which constitute the palpable neuromuscular lesion.

The presence of a lesion is always revealed by an area of hypersensitivity to pressure, an area which may be better described as being a painful spot. After these have been detected and noted, specific attention is given to them in the subsequent treatments.

Youngs (1964) has described what it is that the palpating fingers are seeking and finding and, as in NMT diagnosis and treatment often take place together, what they are achieving:

The changes which are palpable in muscles and soft tissues associated with reflex effects have been listed by Stanley Lief. They are essentially 'congestion'. This ambiguous word can be interpreted as a past hypertrophic fibrosis. Reflex cordant contraction of the muscle reduces the blood flow through the muscular tissue and in such relatively anoxic regions of low pH and low hormonal concentration, fibroblasts proliferate and increased fibrous tissue is formed. This results in an increase in the thickness of the existing connective tissue partitions – the epimysia and perimysia and also this condition probably infiltrates deeper between the muscle fibres to affect the normal endomysia. Thickening of the fascia and subdermal connective tissue will also occur if these structures are similarly affected by a reduced blood flow. Fat may be deposited, particularly in endomorphic types, but fibrosis is most pronounced in those with a strong mesomorphic component – a useful pointer for both prognosis and prophylaxis.

Fibrosis seems to occur automatically in areas of reduced blood flow, e.g., in a sprained ankle – where swelling is marked and prolonged, in the lower extremities where oedema of any origin has been constant over a period, in the gluteals where prolonged sitting is a postural factor, and in the neck and upper dorsal region where psychosomatic tension is frequent to a marked degree – depending upon the constitutional background. Where tension is the aetiological factor, fibrosis seems teleological.

Many devices have been developed to ease the strain on muscles which tend to be permanently contracted, e.g., locking of the kneejoint, or the exact balance of the head on the shoulders, where only gentle contraction is needed to maintain postural integrity. If postural integrity is lost through some cause or another then the strain on the muscle may be eased by structural alteration and the increase of fibrous tissue in the muscles acts to maintain normal position of the head. Fibrous tissue can then take the strain instead of the muscle fibres. It is this long-term homeostatic reflex which apparently operates in all cases of undue muscle contraction, whether due to strain or tension.

From this one can amplify Stanley Lief's beneficial effects of neuromuscular treatment as follows:

1. To restore muscular balance and tone.
2. To restore normal trophicity in muscular and connective tissues by altering the histological picture from a patho-histological to a physiologic–histological pattern with normal vascular and hormonal response.
3. To affect reflexly the related organs and viscera and to tonify them naturally.
4. To improve drainage of blood and lymph through the areas subject to gravitational or postural stasis, e.g., abdominal vessels not necessarily connected with viscera.
5. To reduce fatty deposits.

Thus the hyperaemia resulting from treatment automatically operates to reverse the original patho-histological picture and consequently normality will be approached.

In clinical terms it is safe to say that a chronic state of dysfunction exists if soft tissues have been consistently stressed for more than a few weeks, for after such a short period fibrotic adaptations begin to be palpable.

There is clinical evidence that trigger points have a consistent distribution, and their localisation can be predicted by studying the patterns of referred dysfunction and pain to which they give rise. Similarly patterns of referred pain are predictable if the trigger point can be located (Travell 1957).

A patient with unexplained pain, the examination of which reveals no local cause, may well have trigger points feeding pain messages into the target area. Thus the point at which the patient feels pain and the point at which the pain originates are often not the same, and knowledge of the reference patterns as illustrated in Chapter 3 (see Fig. 3.6) is therefore desirable.

Whether treatment of trigger points consists of anaesthetic injections, acupuncture, cryotherapy, or pressure and stretch techniques (NMT) or combinations such as INIT (see Ch. 9), the diagnostic aspect remains the same. Deep palpation and pressure on the located point must reproduce the symptoms in the target area in order to 'prove' the connection.

Zones of dysfunction: connective tissue changes

As well as trigger points there exist a number of palpable and often visible (Box 5.1) zones of soft tissue alteration, possibly involving viscerosomatic activity, in which diseased or stressed organs negatively influence soft tissues paraspinally and elsewhere (Bischof & Elmiger 1960). Viscerosomatic reflexes and the processes of facilitation (sensitisation) were discussed in Chapter 3. Some of these zones overlap and incorporate 'trigger' points, so a general awareness and knowledge of their existence is useful if an understanding of what can be achieved in NMT is to be more complete (Fig. 5.3).

As organs mainly receive their autonomic supply homolaterally, changes of a reflex nature will normally be found on the same side of the body surface:

- On the right side will be found the connective tissue reflex zones from the liver, gall bladder, duodenum, appendix, ascending colon, ilium, etc.

Box 5.1   Assessing the dominant eye

In making a visual diagnosis it is important for the operator to be sure of the information he or she is acquiring. American osteopathic physician Edward Stiles (1984) makes a valuable contribution to this area by pointing out that it is often for reasons of position, in observing structure, that a student or practitioner fails to see what is obvious:

By being so positioned as to bring into play the non-dominant eye this becomes far more likely. The orientation of the subject in the field of view is determined by the position of the dominant eye, and thus it is essential to initially ascertain which eye this is.

Hold your hands straight in front of you with the palms facing each other. Bring them together to make an aperture (gap) of about 1–2 inches across. Looking through this aperture, focus on an object across the room from you. Close first one eye and then the other. When the non-dominant eye is closed the image you see through the aperture will not change. When you close the dominant eye the image shifts out of the field of vision.

The dominant eye is not always on the same side as the dominant hand. If dominant hands and eyes are on different sides, this can lead to problems of accurately assessing palpatory findings, and the advice given is to palpate with eyes closed, where possible, in such cases.

When assessing visually, make sure that the dominant eye is lined up with the area or object being viewed. In an example where assessment of the chest is being made, Stiles suggests that, because most accurate visual information will be gained when the dominant eye is over the midline, the observation of the supine patient should be from the head of the table, and this should be approached from the side that brings the dominant eye closer to the patient.

- On the left side will be found the reflex zones from the heart, stomach, pancreas, spleen, jejunum, transverse colon, descending colon, rectum, etc.
- Central zones occur as a result of dysfunction in the bladder, uterus and head.
- Changes on the homolateral side of the body occur due to dysfunction of the lungs, suprarenal glands, ovaries, kidneys, blood vessels and nerves on that side.

According to Teiriche-Leube & Ebner (quoted in Teiriche-Laube 1960), these changes in the connective tissue and muscles can take the following forms:

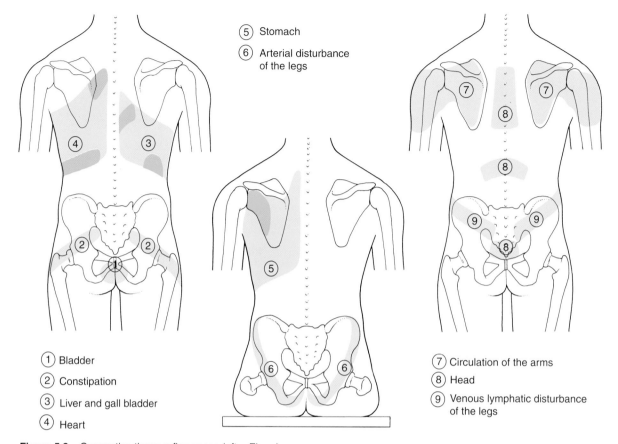

(5) Stomach

(6) Arterial disturbance of the legs

(1) Bladder

(2) Constipation

(3) Liver and gall bladder

(4) Heart

(7) Circulation of the arms

(8) Head

(9) Venous lymphatic disturbance of the legs

Figure 5.3   Connective tissue reflex zones (after Ebner).

- drawn-in bands of tissues
- flattened areas of tissue
- elevated areas, giving the impression of localised swelling
- muscle atrophy or hypertrophy
- osseous deformity of the spinal column.

For Teiriche-Leube & Ebner's description of some of these zones, see Box 5.2.

Using NMT in its assessment mode, as described in Chapters 6 & 7, or in specialised skin diagnosis (see below), these and other areas of soft tissue dysfunction can be readily located, identified and treated, even if no obvious symptoms of the associated conditions or diseases are present. It is clear that soft tissue changes often precede the appearance of symptoms of underlying pathology, and in this alone the diagnostic value of these zones is evident. Practitioners

using German connective tissue massage claim that it is often possible beneficially to influence symptoms of organ dysfunction, and to improve the function of these organs (liver, stomach, etc.), by treatment of the congested fibrotic reflex zone. This is not, however, to be considered an end in itself because it is clear that underlying causative factors and pathology (nutrition, infection, etc.) must also be dealt with. However, the value of the neuromuscular tool should not be minimised.

Mackenzie's abdominal reflex areas

Youngs (1964) points out that Sir James Mackenzie established a clear relationship between the abdominal wall and the internal abdominal organs (Mackenzie 1909). Mackenzie

Box 5.2 Altered connective tissue zones resulting from disturbed organs and functions

1. **Bladder**
   Small 'drawn in' area above anal cleft. Iliotibial tract may be drawn in. Swelling lateral aspect of ankles.
   Symptoms – Bladder dysfunction. Cold feet and legs (below the knee). Rheumatic diagnosis.

2. **Constipation**
   'Drawn in' band 2–3 inches (5–8 cm) wide, running from middle third of the sacrum downwards and laterally.
   Symptoms – Tendency to, or actual, constipation.

3. **Liver and gall bladder**
   Large 'drawn in' zone over right thoracic region and a band along lateral costal border on the right side. Small 'drawn in' area between lower vertebral border of scapula to spine at the 5th and 6th dorsal level. 7th cervical area appears swollen or congested.
   Symptoms – Liver and gall bladder dysfunction and anyone who has suffered from hepatitis.

4. **Heart**
   Tension over left thoracic region including lower costal margin. If hepatic circulation is involved, right costal margin will also be affected. The area between the left scapula and 2nd and 3rd dorsal vertebrae will be indurated. Posterior aspect of axilla appears thickened.
   Symptoms – Coronary and valvular diseases of the heart.

5. **Stomach**
   (a) Overlapping the heart zones (above).
   Symptoms – Stomach dysfunction.
   (b) Localised tension area below lateral aspect of the left scapular spine.
   Symptoms – Gastric ulcer and gastritis.

6. **Arterial disease of legs**
   A V-shaped configuration of the buttocks when sitting is noticed, rather than the normal rounded shape.
   Symptoms – Circulatory disturbance accompanied by angiospasm.

7. **Arms**
   'Drawn in' areas over scapula extending over posterior deltoid.
   Symptoms – Circulatory arm and hand problems. Neuritis paraesthesia.

8. **Head**
   (a) Thoracic area between scapulae.
   Symptoms – Insomnia and all types of headache.
   (b) Lower third of sacrum just above bladder zone.
   Symptoms – Headaches related to digestive dysfunction.
   (c) Just below origin of trapezius.
   Symptoms – Headaches due to tension.

9. **Venous lymphatic disturbance of the legs**
   A tight band from middle third of sacrum, parallel to iliac crest laterally and anteriorly over gluteus medius.
   Symptoms – Cramp. Swollen legs in summer, varicose veins and paraesthesia.

showed that organs that cannot react directly to painful stimuli (i.e. the majority) react by producing spasm and paraesthesia in the reflexly related muscle wall (the myotome), often augmented by hyperaesthesia of the overlying skin (dermatome).

The reflexes involved occur via the autonomic nervous system and may be viscerosomatic or – as has been shown by many researchers, including Lief – the origin may be somatic and the reflex, therefore, somaticovisceral.

Mackenzie's abdominal reflex areas are as illustrated in Fig. 5.4 and, although there is sometimes a degree of individualisation, it is reasonable to state that the presence in abdominal muscles and connective tissues of contracted or sensitive areas indicates (in the absence of recent trauma or strain) some underlying dysfunction that is causing or resulting from the soft tissue lesion. (See also discussion in Chapter 7 of Pain variables in somatic abdominal tissues.)

SKIN: REFLEX EFFECTS AND HYPERALGESIC SKIN ZONES

The work of Mackenzie early in the 20th century, as well as research into connective tissue zones evolving out of Bindegewebsmassage in Germany, demonstrates that the surface of the body offers evidence of internal dysfunction, and that it is possible to influence the interior by application of reflexively powerful stimuli from the surface.

Koizumi (1978) found that stimulation of the skin of the abdomen produced profound inhibition of intestinal movement. Stimulation of the skin produces an increase in sympathetic activity associated with the intestine, thereby inhibiting the mobility of the region. Koizumi noted that this was a strong effect, and that the intestine often became completely quiescent.

Stimulation of other skin areas, notably the neck, chest, forelimbs and hindlimbs, inhibited sympathetic activity, and therefore actually augmented intestinal motility. Vagal involvement in these changes was thought to be minimal, for when the vagi were sectioned the same responses were still noted. Reflexes disappeared,

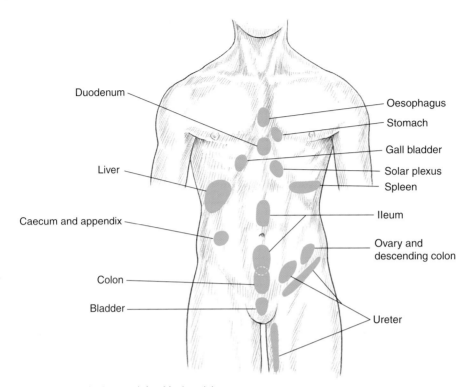

Duodenum

Oesophagus

Stomach

Gall bladder

Liver

Solar plexus

Spleen

Caecum and appendix

Ileum

Ovary and
descending colon

Colon

Bladder

Ureter

Figure 5.4 Reflex abdominal areas (after Mackenzie).

however, when the sympathetic nerve supply to the intestine (the splanchnic nerves) was sectioned. The somatic sympathetic reflex from the abdominal skin is a spinal reflex, whereas the reflexes originating from the other skin areas were thought to be a supraspinal reflex. Koizumi pointed out that, whereas the parasympathetic system plays little part in these reflexes, its involvement increases aspects of emotional reactions. If we consider the involvement of these mechanisms in affecting internal function, via stimulus applied to the skin, we may better appreciate the findings of Chapman (Owen 1980), Bennett (Arbuckle 1977) and others, in their work on the multitude of reflex areas, which they have so painstakingly charted, and which are available to us.

The sometimes dramatic effects obtained by the use of connective tissue massage methods can also be seen to relate to the patterns of therapeutic and diagnostic opportunities, which this knowledge opens.

For example, various techniques are available to us in diagnosing from, and treating, the cutaneous structures for reflex effect. These include skin rolling, as well as the delicate 'skin distraction' or stretching method, advocated by Lewit (1992). Lewit discusses hyperalgesic skin zones that are likely to be present in the skin overlying most areas of reflex activity. He points out a major advantage afforded by an awareness of hyperalgesic skin zones (HSZs): unlike the eliciting and mapping of areas, points or zones, which rely upon the subjective reporting of the patient, these areas are palpable to the operator.

A popular method of noting relative tension in skin is to 'roll' it. A fold of skin is formed, and this is rolled between the fingers (see Fig. 8.17). This method may produce some discomfort, or even transient pain, but is useful in that the increased tension and visibly thicker skin fold thus produced (compared with surrounding tissues) is diagnostic of a HSZ.

Lifting skin folds (assessment)

The assessment methods used in connective tissue massage are designed to obtain a picture of the mobility of the various layers of the connective tissue, as well as an idea of their consistency. One such method involves the lifting of skin folds, with the patient sitting. The skin is gripped between thumb and fingers, with care being taken not to pinch the fold (Fig. 5.5). The fold comprises sufficient tissue to allow it to be lifted away from the fascial layer. This is usually performed by starting at the lower costal margin and going up as far as the region of the shoulders. In some areas, especially overlying the mid-dorsal region, if there is any dysfunction involving the liver, gall bladder, stomach or heart, restriction of tissue elasticity will be noted. By lifting two folds simultaneously, right and left, it is possible to compare the relative freedom of these tissues.

 ## Stretching superficial tissue (assessment)

A second method may be used, in which relatively smaller areas are assessed with the patient prone or seated. With fingers lightly flexed, and using only enough pressure to produce adherence between the fingertips and the skin, a series of short pushing motions are made simultaneously with both hands, which stretches the tissues to their elastic barrier (Fig. 5.6). Usually the pattern of testing goes from inferior to superior, sometimes in an obliquely diagonal direction towards the spine. If the patient is seated and the operator works from behind, tissues from the buttocks to

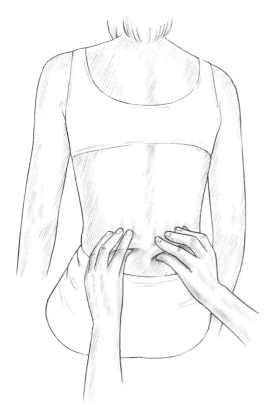

Figure 5.5 Skin folds can be lifted from the underlying fascial layer to test for restrictions, which may indicate local or reflexive dysfunction.

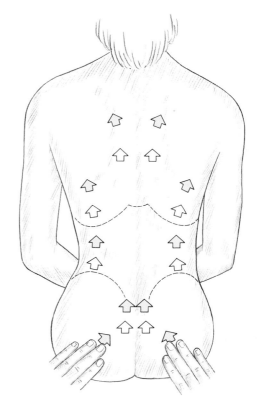

Figure 5.6 Testing and comparing skin and fascial mobility as bilateral areas are 'pushed' to their elastic barriers.

the shoulders may be tested, always comparing the sides for symmetry of range of movement to the elastic barrier. Two quite different evaluations can be performed simultaneously: (1) becoming aware of asymmetry and noting areas of interest for more refined assessment wherever skin does not slide as easily on the underlying tissue on one side, compared with the other, and (2) additionally and alternatively, the possible organ or system reflexes may be noted, if that is of interest to the therapist (see Box 5.1).

Areas investigated, direction of stretch of tissues, and possible implications of reduced elasticity include:

1. The buttocks – stretching tissue from the ischial region towards the lateral borders of the sacrum (arterial and constipation zone).

2. From the posterior aspect of the trochanters, towards the iliac crests (venous lymphatic and arterial disturbances of legs).

3. From the trochanters, towards sacroiliac joints (venous lymphatic zone).

4. Over the sacrum, working from the apex towards the upper sacral segments (bladder and headache zones).

5. Over the lumbar region, on either side of the spine, working upwards (kidney zone).

6. Bilaterally up the spine, from lower costal region to the mid-thoracic level (liver and gall bladder zone (right side), and heart, stomach (left) and pulmonary (bilateral)).

7. Between the scapulae (headache zone).

8. Over the scapulae, from inferior angle, towards spine of scapula (arm zone).

Normal variations will exist independent of reflex activity, and in individuals carrying increased adipose tissue a generally greater degree of tension or adherence will be noted, compared with a thinner individual. An older person's skin will feel looser, in comparison with that of a younger individual. The skin over the lumbar region is naturally less mobile than that in other regions.

Note that it is adherence ('tightness of tissues to each other') that is being assessed, and this may or may not be accompanied by sensitivity. In connective tissue massage an assessment of this sort is made regularly, as it is seen to be both diagnostic and prognostic, showing the rate of progress or lack of it, and providing a possible insight into visceral and functional status.

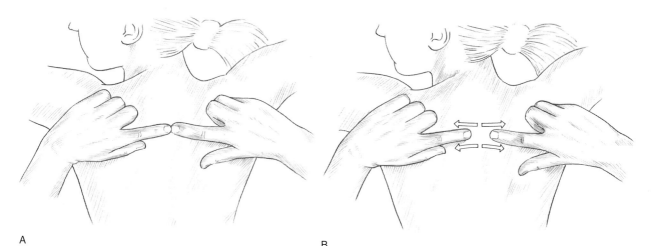

A   B

Figure 5.7A,B Hyperalgesic skin zones that lie above reflexive dysfunction (e.g. trigger points) are identified by means of the sequential stretching to their elastic barrier of local areas of skin. A series of such stretches indicates precisely those areas where elasticity is reduced in comparison to surrounding tissues. These are then tested for sensitivity and potential to cause referred pain by the application of ischaemic compression (inhibition).

Skin distraction (diagnostic and therapeutic)

Lewit (1992) describes a method that he finds reliable, painless and therapeutically very useful. Any area of skin may be assessed in this way, large or small, with fingertip or hand contact.

In a small area, the fingertips (both index fingers) or index and middle fingertips of both hands, are placed close together, resting on the tissues to be tested. By separating the fingers, the skin is pulled apart and stretched to its easy elastic barrier (Fig. 5.7).

A minimum of force is used, in order simply to take out the slack in the skin. The 'easy' end-position is noted, as is the degree of 'springing' available in the tissues. This is compared in several directions, over the area, and comparison is also made with the presumably healthy tissue on the contralateral side. If a HSZ is present, then a greater degree of resistance will be noted after the slack has been taken up. Where there is such resistance, if the end-position of stretch is held for between 10 and 20 seconds, the resistance will be felt to ease, and the normal physiological degree of springing will then be noted. This is a measurable phenomenon and, by marking the first stretch position with a skin pencil and marking the stretch position available after 'release of the tissue', a significant increase is usually noted.

The techniques may be used even for small areas (e.g. between the toes). These may be stretched by fingertip (light) pressure and separation. Larger areas, such as regions of the back, may be contacted by the ulnar border of the hands in order to introduce separation stretch. The hands are crossed and placed on the tissue to be tested or treated. Separation of the hands introduces stretch to take up the slack.

Having introduced this initial degree of stretch, resistance (end-feel) is then noted. If the tissues are resistant to stretch, and springiness is absent, the maintenance of the stretch (painless) achieves a release of the tissues over a period of less than half a minute as a rule.

All trigger points, tender points, connective tissue zones, Mackenzie's abdominal areas, etc. are characterised by the presence of such a HSZ in the overlying tissues. This very useful tool allows easy identification of reflex activity and is itself an ideal form of treatment of these reflexes in sensitive individuals, and further provides accurate evidence of the subsequent situation. Techniques for treating skin and superficial tissue are further discussed in Chapter 8.

Scar tissue often leads to the presence of HSZs around the scar, and these frequently become focal points of reflex activity. Specific release methods, as described in Chapter 8, may be used to alter the status of tissues affected by scar tissue. Acupuncture is a useful method of treating any very sensitive aspect of the scars themselves (Baldrey 1993).

CHAPMAN'S REFLEXES IN DIAGNOSIS AND TREATMENT

The reflexes described by Chapman are now commonly termed 'neurolymphatic' reflexes. These can be used in diagnosis and treatment, and as a guide to the effectiveness of treatment. See additional discussion of these reflexes in Chapter 4.

In 1965 I described the technique, for using these as follows (Chaitow 1965):

Treatment applied through these reflexes, as advocated by Chapman and Owens, consists of a firm but gentle rotary pressure imparted by the index or middle finger. The finger should not be allowed to slip. As these areas are acutely sensitive great care should be taken not to overtreat as the reflex will become fatigued and no benefit will be derived.

My current view coincides with the above method except that I now use a variable thumb pressure that fits in with the general neuro-muscular technique. Knowledge of the exact location of the reflexes is of primary importance.

By gentle palpation, the operator should first ascertain the presence of involved reflexes. The anterior reflexes should be tested first. If found to be present, the anterior reflex should be treated first, then the posterior counterpart of the involved anterior reflexes should be treated.

The anterior reflex has, therefore, a dual role: namely, for diagnosis and then to initiate the reflex treatment. The anterior reflex is later of value to ascertain the effectiveness of treatment (after both anterior and posterior reflexes have been treated).

If, on repalpating the reflexes, there is no change in the feel or tenderness, the treatment should be repeated. If there is again no change, this indicates either that the pathology is too great for rapid change, or that pathology is irreversible. It may also indicate that some musculoskeletal factor is maintaining the reflex. Primary treatment should then be directed at this factor rather than the reflex. The degree of treatment should be ascertained by palpation. Chapman and Owens described dosage of treatment in terms of seconds, but in practice I feel that anyone experienced in neuromuscular treatment would have the degree of sensory awareness required to 'feel' when sufficient treatment had been given.

I would stress that I have found the reflexes of Chapman useful in differential diagnosis, and in the treatment of various conditions from spastic constipation to migraine – but always as a part of a broader approach to the patient as a whole. That they can influence lymphatic drainage dramatically, I have no doubt. I am less sure of the effect on visceral conditions, but have found that the reflexes themselves provide an excellent guide to progress. If they are no longer present, then invariably the condition is progressing well. These personal observations are confirmed by Patriquin (1997).

Technique and charts for use of Chapman's reflexes (Fig. 5.8A–F)

Chapman (Owen 1980) suggested a vibratory treatment in stimulating the neurolymphatic reflexes, lasting 10–15 seconds. He used fingertip pressure to impart the required energy, although thumb pressure of varying intensity is just as effective. This can be applied as a gradually intensifying pressure building up over 5–8 seconds, easing for 2 or 3 seconds and then repeated. Altogether this should not take more

than half a minute. These points can be overtreated and the optimum time would seem to be from 15 to 30 seconds with the pressure (or squeeze) of a variable nature. If the patient is able to report a referred pain resulting from the pressure, then pressure/treatment can be continued for up to 1 minute, with fluctuations in the degree of pressure, until the patient indicates a diminution in the referred pain or until the time has elapsed.

It is important to realise that the objective 'feel' of these contractions is unlikely to change during such treatment. Any changes resulting from the treatment will occur later, when homeostatic forces have come into operation. The variation in pressure during the treatment is more desirable than a constantly held degree of pressure, which may irritate and exacerbate the condition. In the foreword to Owen's book *An Endocrine Interpretation of Chapman's Reflexes* (1980), in which Owen describes his and Chapman's research, noted osteopathic researcher Fred Mitchell recommends that pressure be applied by the pad of the middle finger. This should be maintained as a light direct pressure in an effort to decongest the fluid content of the palpable reflex point. Mitchell believes that the determining factor for the amount of treatment is whether a decrease in oedema takes place, or whether a dissolution of the gangliform contraction occurs, together with reduction in the sensitivity of the point over a period of between 20 and 120 seconds. The stimulation threshold is being raised in these points and inhibition of noxious impulses is being achieved. There is nothing to be gained from achieving local pressure anaesthesia (numbing) by exaggerated effort. Reflexes that are not painful should not be treated: only an active (and therefore sensitive) reflex point requires attention.

The reflexes may be treated as part of a general neuromuscular treatment or on their own in accordance with the recommendations of Chapman, Owen and Mitchell, which suggest the treating of the reflexes by light digital pressure of the anterior reflex followed by the corresponding posterior reflex. The anterior point should then be re-examined and, if there has

Table 5.1 Location of Chapman's neurolymphatic reflexes

No.	Symptoms/area	Anterior	Fig.	Posterior	Fig.
1.	Conjunctivitis and retinitis	Upper humerus	5.8A	Occipital area	5.8C
2.	Nasal problems	Anterior aspect of first rib close to sternum	5.8A	Posterior the angle of the jaw on the tip of the transverse process of the 1st cervical vertebra	5.8C
3.	Arms (circulation)	Muscular attachments pectoralis minor to 3rd, 4th & 5th ribs	5.8A	Superior angle of scapula and superior third of the medial margin of the scapula	5.8C
4.	Tonsillitis	Between 1st and 2nd ribs, close to sternum	5.8A	Midway between spinous process and tip of transverse process of 1st cervical vertebra	5.8E
5.	Thyroid	Second intercostal space close to sternum	5.8A	Midway between spinous process and tip of transverse process of 2nd thoracic vertebra	5.8C
6.	Bronchitis	Second intercostal space close to sternum	5.8A	Midway between spinous process and tip of transverse process of 2nd thoracic vertebra	5.8E
7.	Oesophagus	As no. 6	5.8A	As no. 6	5.8E
8.	Myocarditis	As no. 6	5.8A	Between the 2nd and 3rd thoracic transverse processes. Midway between the spinous process and the tip of the transverse process	5.8D
9.	Upper lung	3rd intercostal space close to sternum	5.8A	As no. 8	5.8D
10.	Neuritis of upper limb	As no. 9	5.8A	Between the 3rd and 4th transverse processes, midway between the spinous process and the tip of the transverse process	5.8D
11.	Lower lung	4th intercostal space, close to sternum	5.8A	Between 4th and 5th transverse processes. Midway between the spinous process and the tip of the transverse process	5.8D
12.	Small intestines	8th, 9th & 10th intercostal spaces, close to cartilage	5.8A	8th, 9th & 10th thoracic intertransverse spaces	5.8C
13.	Gastric hypercongestion	6th intercostal space to the left of the sternum	5.8A	6th thoracic intertransverse space, left side	5.8C
14.	Gastric hyperacidity	5th intercostal space to the left of the sternum	5.8A	5th thoracic intertransverse space, left side	5.8F
15.	Cystitis	Around the umbilicus and on the pubic symphysis, close to the midline	5.8A	Upper edge of the transverse processes of the 2nd lumbar vertebra	5.8F
16.	Kidneys	Slightly superior and lateral to the umbilicus	5.8A	In the intertransverse space between the 12th thoracic and the 1st lumbar vertebra	5.8F
17.	Atonic constipation	Between the anterior superior spine of the ilium and the trochanter	5.8A	11th costal–vertebral junction	5.8C
18.	Abdominal tension	Superior border of the pubic bone	5.8A	Tip of the transverse process of the 2nd lumbar vertebra	5.8D
19.	Urethra	Inner edge of pubic ramus near superior aspect of symphysis	5.8A	Superior aspect of transverse process of 2nd lumbar vertebra	5.8F
20.	Depuytren's contracture, and arm and shoulder pain	None		Anterior aspect of lateral margin of scapulae, inferior to the head of humerus	5.8F
21.	Cerebral congestion (related to paralysis or paresis)	(On the posterior aspect of the body). Lateral from the spines of the 3rd, 4th & 5th cervical vertebrae	5.8A	Between the transverse processes of the 1st and 2nd cervical vertebrae	5.8E

Table 5.1 (cont'd)

No.	Symptoms/area	Anterior	Fig.	Posterior	Fig.
22.	Clitoral irritation and vaginismus	Upper medial aspect of the thigh	5.8A	Lateral to the junction of the sacrum and coccyx	5.8D
23.	Prostate	Lateral aspect of the thigh from the trochanter to just above the knee. Also lateral to symphysis pubis as in uterine conditions (see no. 43)	5.8A	Between the posterior superior spine of the ilium and the spinous process of the 5th lumbar vertebra	5.8D
24.	Spastic constipation or colitis	Within an area of an inch or two wide extending from the trochanter to within an inch of the patella	5.8A	From the transverse processes of the 2nd, 3rd & 4th lumbar vertebrae to the crest of the ilium	5.8C
25.	Leucorrhoea	Lower medial aspect of thigh, slightly posteriorly (on the posterior aspect of the body)	5.8A & 5.8C	Between the posterior/superior spine of the ilium and the spinous process of the 5th lumbar vertebra	5.8D
26.	Sciatic neuritis	Anterior and posterior to the tibiofibular junction	5.8A	1. On the sacroiliac synchondrosis 2. Between the ischial tuberosity and the acetabulum 3. Lateral and posterior aspects of the thigh	5.8C
27.	Torpid liver (nausea, fullness malaise)	5th intercostal space, from the mid-mammillary line to the sternum	5.8B	5th thoracic intertransverse space on the right side	5.8C
28.	Cerebellar congestion (memory and concentration lapses)	Tip of coracoid process of scapula	5.8B	Just inferior to the base of the skull on the 1st cervical vertebra	5.8E
29.	Otitis media	Upper edge of clavicle where it crosses the 1st rib	5.8B	Superior aspect of 1st cervical transverse process (tip)	5.8C
30.	Pharyngitis	Anterior aspect of the 1st rib close to the sternum	5.8B	Midway between the spinous process and the tip of the transverse process of the 2nd cervical vertebra	5.8E
31.	Laryngitis	Upper surface of the 2nd rib, 2–3 inches (5–8 cm) from the sternum	5.8B	Midway between the spinous process and the tip of the 2nd cervical vertebra	5.8E
32.	Sinusitis	Lateral to the sternum on the superior edge of the 2nd rib in the first intercostal space	5.8B	As no. 31	5.8E
33.	Pyloric stenosis	On the sternum	5.8B	10th costovertebral junction on the right side	5.8F
34.	Neuraesthenia (chronic fatigue)	All the muscular attachments of pectoralis major on the humerus, clavicle, sternum, ribs (especially 4th rib)	5.8B	Below the superior medial edge of the scapula on the face of the 4th rib	5.8D
35.	Wry neck (torticollis)	Medial aspect of upper edge of the humerus	5.8B	Transverse processes of the 3rd, 4th, 6th & 7th cervical vertebrae	5.8E
36.	Splenitis	7th intercostal space close to the cartilaginous junction, on the left	5.8B	7th intertransverse space on the left	5.8C
37.	Adrenals (allergies, exhaustion)	Superior and lateral to umbilicus	5.8B	In the intertransverse space between the 11th and 12th thoracic vertebrae	5.8F
38.	Mesoappendix	Superior aspect of the 12th rib, close to the tip, on right	5.8B	Lateral aspect of the 11th intercostal space on the right	5.8C
39.	Pancreas	7th intercostal space on the right, close to the cartilage	5.8B	7th thoracic intertransverse space on the right	5.8F

Table 5.1 (cont'd)

No.	Symptoms/area	Anterior	Fig.	Posterior	Fig.
40.	Liver and gall bladder congestion	6th intercostal space, from the mid-mammillary line to the sternum (right side)	5.8A	6th thoracic intertransverse space, right side	5.8F
41.	Salpingitis or vesiculitis	Midway between the acetabulum and the sciatic notch (this is on the posterior aspect of the body)	5.8F	Between the posterior, superior spine of the ilium and the spinous process of the 5th lumbar vertebra	5.8D
42.	Ovaries	Round ligaments from the superior border of the pubic bone, inferiorly	5.8B	Between the 9th and 10th intertransverse space and the 10th and 11th intertransverse space	5.8D
43.	Uterus	Anterior aspect of the junction of the ramus of the pubis and the ischium	5.8B	Between the posterior superior spine of the ilium and the 5th lumbar spinous process	5.8D
44.	Uterine fibroma	Lateral to the symphysis, extending diagonally inferiorly	5.8B	Between the tip of the transverse process of the 5th lumbar vertebra and the crest of the ilium	5.8C
45.	Rectum	Just inferior to the lesser trochanter	5.8B	On the sacrum close to the ilium at the lower end of the iliosacral synchondrosis	5.8F
46.	Broad ligament (uterine involvement usual)	Lateral aspect of the thigh from the trochanter to just above the knee	5.8B	Between the posterior, superior spine of the ilium and the 5th lumbar spinous process	5.8D
47.	Groin glands (circulation and drainage of legs and pelvic organs)	Lower quarter of the sartorius muscle and its attachment to the tibia	5.8B	On the sacrum close to the ilium at the lower end of the iliosacral synchondrosis	5.8F
48.	Haemorrhoids	Just superior to the ischial tuberosity. (These areas are on the posterior surface of the body)	5.8D	On the sacrum close to the ilium, at the lower end of the iliosacral synchondrosis	5.8D
49.	Tongue	Anterior aspect of 2nd rib at the cartilaginous junction with the sternum	5.8A	Midway between the spinous process and the tip of the transverse process of the 2nd cervical vertebra	5.8E

been a palpable change or sensitivity has diminished, then no more action would be required. If no such change is found, the treatment to the anterior and then the posterior points is again carried out and, if still no change is noted, it is assumed that pathology is too great for a rapid change or is irreversible, or that there is a musculoskeletal factor maintaining the dysfunction.

If this approach is adopted, the grouping of reflexes into systems is a useful method. If one of a group is found to be active then all others in the group should be examined and, if active, treated; for example:

• The endocrine group comprises: prostate, gonads, broad ligaments, uterus, thyroid and adrenals.

• The gastrointestinal group comprises the colon, thyroid, pancreas, duodenum, small intestine and liver.

• The infections group comprises liver, spleen and the adrenals.

The advice, therefore, is to use reflexes intelligently, treating only what is palpable and sensitive. Some of the anterior reflexes (the ones that should, in theory, be treated first) lie on the posterior aspect of the body. These include those for:

• haemorrhoids (no. 48)
• cerebellar congestion (no. 21)
• leucorrhoea (no. 25)
• salpingitis (no. 41).

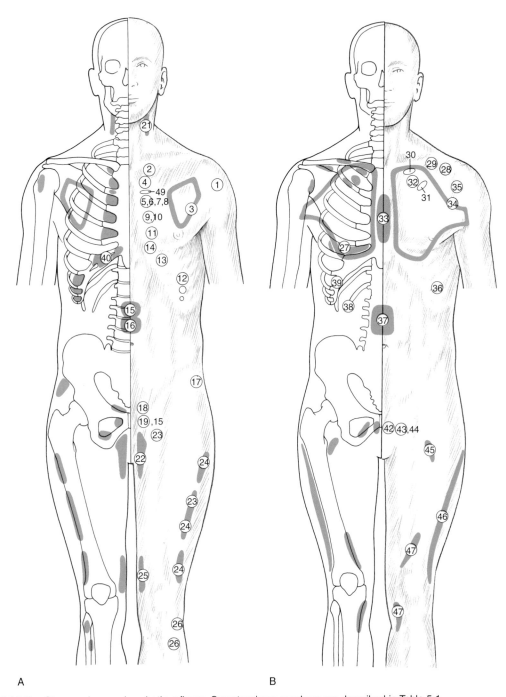

A   B

Figure 5.8A,B   Chapman's neurolymphatic reflexes. Symptom/area numbers are described in Table 5.1.

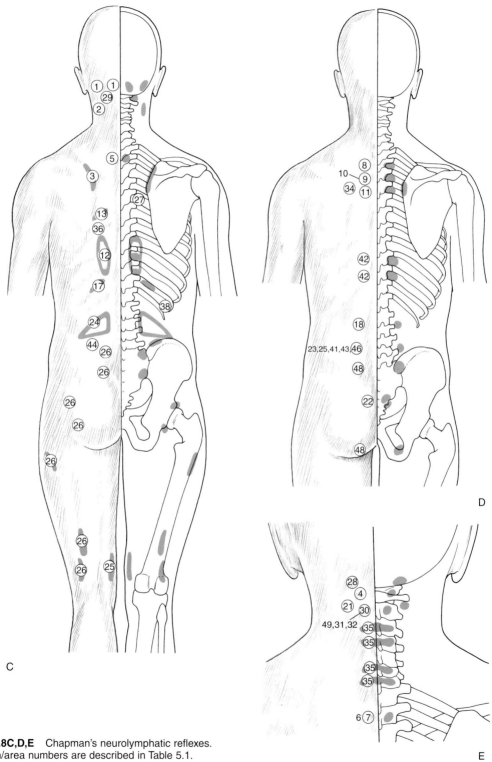

Figure 5.8C,D,E   Chapman's neurolymphatic reflexes.
Symptom/area numbers are described in Table 5.1.

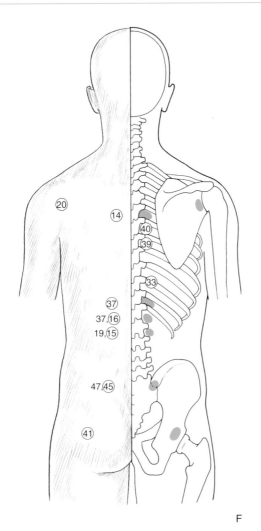

F

Figure 5.8F Chapman's neurolymphatic reflexes. Symptom/area numbers are described in Table 5.1.

It is suggested that reference be made to Owen (1980) for more detailed study. Table 5.1 gives the reflex by name, number and description of location, together with an indication of the figure on which it is indicated (it was not possible to incorporate all the drawings on to one picture without creating a confusing series of overlaps). It is suggested that the practitioner learns to search appropriate areas for the type of sensitive tissue changes that represent the superficial manifestation of these reflexes and to use Fig. 5.8A–F and Table 5.1 to become familiar with the patterns and groups of these important

aids to healing. The illustrations will aid the practitioner in locating these useful diagnostic and therapeutic areas.

BENNETT'S NEUROVASCULAR REFLEXES
(Note these will be sensitive to light pressure if active.) (See Figs 5.9A–C & Box 5.3.)

The way in which Bennett's neurovascular (NV) reflex points are used depends largely on the therapeutic objective: as diagnostic indicators; to influence specific muscle function; or to ease symptoms, particularly those deriving from emotional causes.

As with Chapman's neurolymphatic points, neurovascular points might be seen as useful additional sources of information regarding the organ, structure or function to which they appear to be linked. If the region of the point palpates as sensitive, further confirmation should be sought of the dysfunction indicated by the reflex.

Applied kinesiology methodology tends to use these neurovascular points as a means of modifying specific muscles with which they are purported to be reflexly linked. Walther (1988) explains: 'A specific muscle responds to only one [neurovascular] reflex, but most reflexes influence more than one muscle. Bennett's reflexes are primarily on the anterior surface of the trunk and on the head. The reflexes on the head are those used in applied kinesiology, with few exceptions.'

The way in which these reflexes are treated is as follows:

1. The point is located and a contact is made with the pad or tip of one finger.
2. The skin overlying the point is 'tugged' lightly and the finger contact is maintained until a pulsation is noted.
3. If the pulsation does not appear, the direction in which the skin 'tug' is made is varied until a pulsation is noted.
4. After the pulsation is noted, the finger contact is maintained for a further 15–20 seconds.

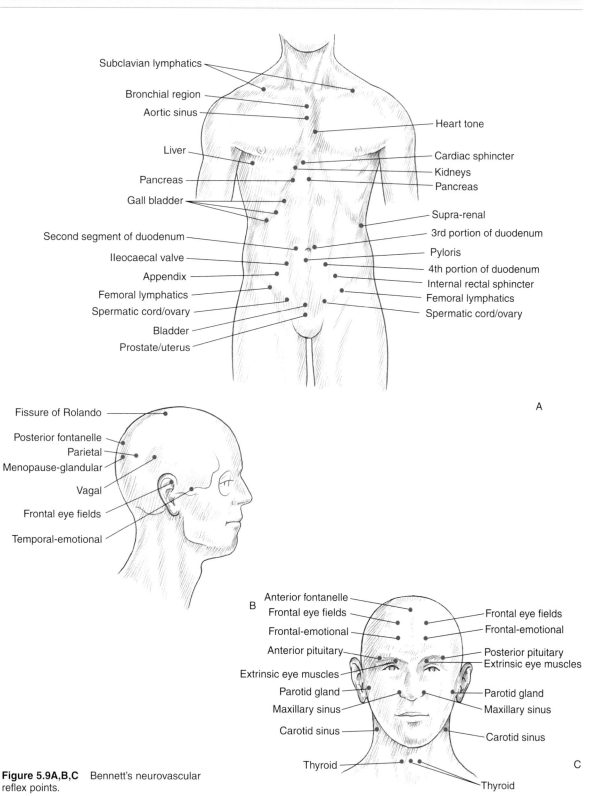

Subclavian lymphatics
Bronchial region
Aortic sinus
Heart tone
Liver
Cardiac sphincter
Pancreas
Kidneys
Gall bladder
Pancreas
Supra-renal
Second segment of duodenum
3rd portion of duodenum
Ileocaecal valve
Pyloris
Appendix
4th portion of duodenum
Femoral lymphatics
Internal rectal sphincter
Spermatic cord/ovary
Femoral lymphatics
Bladder
Spermatic cord/ovary
Prostate/uterus

A

Fissure of Rolando
Posterior fontanelle
Parietal
Menopause-glandular
Vagal
Frontal eye fields
Temporal-emotional

B

Anterior fontanelle
Frontal eye fields
Frontal eye fields
Frontal-emotional
Frontal-emotional
Anterior pituitary
Posterior pituitary
Extrinsic eye muscles
Extrinsic eye muscles
Parotid gland
Parotid gland
Maxillary sinus
Maxillary sinus
Carotid sinus
Carotid sinus
Thyroid
Thyroid

C

Figure 5.9A,B,C Bennett's neurovascular reflex points.

Box 5.3 Bennett's neurovascular reflexes

Reflex name	Site
1. **Parotid gland**	Raised area on masseter when jaw clenched *Diagnostic and treatment point*. Associated conditions: prostate problems, mumps, premenstrual problem, mastitis, lymphatic stasis.
2. **Cardiac sphincter**	Tip of xyphoid process *Diagnostic and treatment point*. If sensitive may relate to incompetent sphincter, heartburn.
3. **Liver**	Midclavicular line; right 5th intercostal *Diagnostic and treatment point*.
4. **Gall bladder**	Below costal cartilages right 9th, 10th, 11th ribs *Diagnostic and treatment point*. All points mentioned are treatment points; only 11th rib point is diagnostic. Pain may be noted as far lateral as mid-axillary line.
5. **Pancreas**	Medial to 6th and 7th rib heads. 1 inch below xyphoid process *Diagnostic point*. 5th and 6th costal cartilages right and left.
6. **Pyloris**	Lower border of umbilicus *Diagnostic and treatment point*.
7. **2nd segment of duodenum**	1 inch and 45° above umbilicus on right *Diagnostic and treatment point*. *Note*: Order of treatment in this region should follow sequence of pyloris–duodenum–pancreas–liver–gall bladder.
8. **3rd portion of duodenum**	1 inch and 45° above umbilicus on left *Diagnostic and treatment point*.
9. **4th portion of duodenum**	1 inch and 45° lateral and below umbilicus (left) *Diagnostic and treatment point*.
10. **Kidneys**	Tip of 8th rib. Bilateral *Diagnostic and treatment point*.
11. **Ileocaecal valve**	On right side midway between anterior–superior iliac spine and umbilicus *Diagnostic and treatment point*.
12. **Internal rectal sphincter**	On left midway between anterior/superior iliac spine and umbilicus *Diagnostic and treatment point*.
13. **Appendix**	Directly over the organ *Diagnostic and treatment point*.
14. **Bladder**	Just above pubic arch on midline *Diagnostic and treatment point*.
15. **Prostate/uterus**	Symphysis pubis *Diagnostic and treatment point*.
16. **Spermatic cord/ovary**	Approx. 1–1½ inches either side of bladder reflex (*Note*: thyroid to be treated when ovaries receiving attention) *Diagnostic and treatment point*.
17. **Supra-renal**	One finger-width below tip 12th rib. Diagnostic point is tip of 12th rib. *Diagnostic and treatment point*.
18. **Anterior pituitary**	Right, lateral aspect of eyebrow *Diagnostic and treatment point*.
19. **Posterior pituitary**	Left, lateral aspect of eyebrow *Diagnostic and treatment point*.
20. **Thyroid**	Over the organ *Diagnostic and treatment point*.
21. **Carotid sinus**	On carotid artery, below angle of jaw *Diagnostic and treatment point*.
22. **Aortic sinus**	Manubriosternal junction on ridge, or just inferior *Diagnostic and treatment point*.
23. **Heart tone**	Sternal end of 3rd rib. Contact on cartilage (left) *Diagnostic and treatment point*.
24. **Subclavian lymphatics**	Just inferior to and slightly medial to midpoint of clavicle *Diagnostic and treatment point*.
25. **Femoral lymphatics**	On Poupart's ligament. Midway between symphysis pubis and anterior superior iliac spine *Diagnostic and treatment point*.

Box 5.3 (cont'd)	
Reflex name	**Site**
26. **Maxillary sinus**	Lateral to nares; bilaterally *Diagnostic and treatment point.*
27. **Bronchial region**	Midway between manubrium sternum and epistemal notch *Diagnostic and treatment point.*
28. **Frontal-emotional**	Frontal eminences of forehead *Diagnostic and treatment point.*
29. **Vagal**	2 inches superior and 2 inches posterior to external auditory meatus *Diagnostic and treatment point.*
30. **Parletal**	2 inches superior and 3 inches posterior to external auditory meatus *Diagnostic and treatment point.*
31. **Temporal-emotional**	Midway between outer aspect of eye and external auditory meatus. Just superior to zygomatic bone *Diagnostic and treatment point.*
32. **Anterior fontanelle**	Over anatomical area *Diagnostic and treatment point.*
33. **Mid-sylvian**	1 inch superior to anterior aspect of external auditory meatus *Diagnostic and treatment point.*
34. **Fissure of Rolando**	Approx. $1\frac{1}{2}$ inches posterior to anterior fontanelle *Diagnostic and treatment point.*
35. **Frontal eye fields**	$1\frac{1}{2}$ inches superior to frontal eminences *Diagnostic and treatment point.*
36. **Extrinsic eye muscles**	Superior to eyelids with closed eyes *Diagnostic and treatment point.*
37. **Posterior fontanelle**	Over anatomical area *Diagnostic and treatment point.*
38. **Menopause-glandular**	$\frac{1}{2}$ inch inferior and lateral to posterior fontanelle *Diagnostic and treatment point.*

All the points on the cranium are useful for treating emotional and stress conditions. Those marked 'emotional' are the strongest. Light pressure only is suggested. Reference to these reflexes will be found in the chapter on treatment techniques (Ch. 6).

Walther (1988) describes how neurovascular points can be used to treat symptoms related to emotional causes:

Many of the emotional problems dealt with by this technique are those found in general examination to determine the reason for a recurring [problem]. It is not necessary . . . to know the precise emotional factor . . . Ask the person to think about the problem with the eyes closed, and watch for rapid eye movement (REM) which [may be] associated with the emotional experience . . . The NV reflex is located bilaterally on the frontal bone eminence [see point 28 (frontal-emotional) on Fig. 5.9C and description in Box 5.3] and is treated with a light tugging contact [see above] . . . until a maximum pulsation is felt. It may be necessary to hold the contact points for several minutes.

CONCLUSIONS

Speransky (1943) has stated that the nervous system contains a record of the past history of the organism. For the practitioner, the signs present in the musculoskeletal system constitute a map of past and present dysfunctions. It presents him or her with the opportunity to treat, alleviate and prevent further dysfunction.

Apart from palpation for tissue changes and reflex trigger areas, diagnosis should involve an evaluation of the gross stress patterns and postural factors. Each patient is an individual challenge, and indeed this challenge is renewed at each visit. Thus, whilst the mechanics of treatment are similar, the emphasis will probably be different at each visit. It is important that the patient understands this, and the nature of the problem as well as the goal desired. A cooperative patient will accept the time and effort required to achieve that goal.

Observation of the dynamic posture or body in motion gives an idea of balance, posture, gravitational stress, gross structural anomalies, etc. Observation of certain body areas in individual movement will then help the understanding of their stress patterns, restrictions, and so on. The practitioner must learn to appreciate the arrangement of the various body structures and their interrelationships. The myofascial tensions can then be visualised. When these gross and local postural patterns in active and passive modes have been observed, an overall impression can be added to the palpatory impressions, both superficial and deep, which the hands can evaluate with the patient standing, supine or prone. By lightly passing the hands over the various structures, alterations in tissue density and configuration can be felt. The deeper palpation to localise the dysfunction can then be performed or left to the neuromuscular treatment, where diagnosis coincides with treatment.

A history will have been taken before observation, palpation and mobility tests, and such history should be comprehensive, taking note of traumatic incidents, habits, occupational positions and postures, emotional state and history, congenital deformity and surgery, as well as general medical history and specific details of the presenting problems.

Mobility tests form part of the diagnostic procedures in soft tissue assessment and, because all manual therapists are concerned with joint mobility, these tests will also be part of any overall assessment. Active motion, movement of one part of the body in relation to another, powered by conscious muscular effort as well as passive motion in which an outside force acts on the body to induce movement, are both of diagnostic importance. Eventually it is possible to distinguish rapidly between healthy tissue and tissue in which there is dysfunction. This can be learned only by experience.

Observation, static and active; palpation, superficial and deep; a comprehensive and detailed history; mobility tests as required; localisation of trigger areas; re-evaluation during the course of treatment; and an intelligent cooperative understanding of the patient's problems, are the diagnostic tools with which to undertake the task in hand.

Finding 'points' using NMT

Knowledge of Chapman's neurolymphatic areas, Bennett's reflexes, Mackenzie's reflex areas, connective tissue zones and trigger points might appear a massive task for the memory – and so it is. However, the application of the general knowledge of their existence enables treatment to be effective even without precise knowledge of all the individual reflexes involved. The aim of this chapter has been to try to classify some of the more obvious diagnostic indicators, so that the practitioner's awareness of the range of diagnostic and therapeutic possibilities can be broadened.

REFERENCES

Arbuckle B 1977 Selected writings. National Osteopathic Institute
Baldry P 1993 Acupuncture, trigger points and musculoskeletal pain. Churchill Livingstone, London
Beal M 1983 Palpatory testing for somatic dysfunction in patients with cardiovascular disease. Journal of the American Osteopathic Association 82:822–831
Bischof I, Elmiger G 1960 Connective tissue massage. In: Licht E, ed. Massage, manipulation and traction. New Haven, Connecticut

Chaitow L 1965 An introduction to Chapman's reflexes. British Naturopathic Journal 6(4):111–113
DiGiovanna E, ed. 1991 An osteopathic approach to diagnosis and treatment. Lippincott, Philadelphia
Koizumi K 1978 Autonomic system reactions, caused by excitation of somatic afferents: study of cutaneo-intestinal reflex. In: Korr I, ed. The neurobiological mechanisms in manipulative therapy. Plenum Press, New York
Lewit K 1992 Manipulative therapy in rehabilitation of the locomotor system. Butterworths, London

Lief P 1963 British Naturopathic Journal 5(10):304–324

Mackenzie J 1909 Symptoms and their interpretations. London

Owen C 1980 An endocrine interpretation of Chapman's reflexes. American Academy of Osteopathy, Newark, Ohio

Patriquin D 1997 Chapman's reflexes. In: Ward R, ed. Foundations for osteopathic medicine. Williams & Wilkins, Baltimore

Speransky A 1943 A basis for the theory of medicine. International Publishers, New York

Stiles E 1984 Patient Care 15 May: 16–87;15 August: 117–164

Teiriche-Leube H 1960 Grundriss der Bindesgewebsmassage. Fisher, Stuttgart

Travell J 1957 Symposium on mechanisms and management of pain syndromes. Proceedings of the Rudolph Virchow Medical Society

Travell J, Simons D 1983 Myofascial pain and dysfunction. vol. 1. Williams & Wilkins, Baltimore

Travell J, Simons D 1992 Myofascial pain and dysfunction. vol. 2. Williams & Wilkins, Baltimore

Walther D 1988 Applied kinesiology. SDC Systems, Pueblo, Colorado

Youngs B 1964 NMT of lower thorax and low back. British Naturopathic Journal 5(11):176–190, 340–358

6

Basic spinal NMT

DEFINING NMT

NMT, as the term is used in this book, is summarised in Box 6.1.

In this text the 'European' version of NMT, as developed by Stanley Lief, based partly on traditional Ayurvedic massage, has been described

---

Box 6.1 Aims of NMT and allied approaches

- Neuromuscular technique, as the term is used in this book, refers to the manual application of specialised pressure and strokes, usually delivered by a finger or thumb contact, which have a diagnostic (assessment mode) or therapeutic (treatment mode) objective.
- Therapeutically, NMT aims to produce modifications in dysfunctional tissue, encouraging a restoration of normality, with a primary focus of deactivating focal points of reflexogenic activity such as myofascial trigger points.
- An alternative focus of NMT application is towards normalising imbalances in hypertonic and/or fibrotic tissues, either as an end in itself or as a precursor to joint mobilisation/rehabilitation.
- NMT utilises physiological responses involving neurological mechanoreceptors, Golgi tendon organs, muscle spindles and other proprioceptors, in order to achieve the desired responses.
- Insofar as they integrate with NMT, other means of influencing such neural reporting stations, including positional release (strain/counterstrain) and muscle energy methods (such as reciprocal inhibition and post-isometric relaxation induction) are seen to form a natural set of allied approaches.
- Traditional massage methods that encourage a reduction in retention of metabolic wastes and enhanced circulation to dysfunctional tissues are included in this category of allied approaches.

along with the subsequent evolution of American NMT methods, resulting from the work of Nimmo, St John and Walker, among others (see Ch. 10).

A confusing element relating to the term NMT emerges, because of its use by Dvorak et al (1988), when they describe what are, in effect, variations on the theme of the use of isometric contractions in order to encourage a reduction in hypertonicity. These methods, all of which form part of what is known as muscle energy technique (MET) in osteopathic medicine, are described briefly in Chapter 8, and form the focus of a further title in the series of which this book is part (Chaitow 2001).

Use of the terms NMT 1, 2 and 3 by Dvorak et al (1988), in order to describe these methods, succeeds in adding to, rather than reducing, semantic confusion, and it is hoped that this aberrant set of descriptions will not persist.

Dvorak et al (1988) have listed various MET methods (as NMT) as follows:

1. Methods that involve self-mobilisation by patient action, to encourage movement past a resistance barrier, are described as 'NMT 1'.
2. Isometric contraction and subsequent passive stretching of agonist muscles, involving postisometric relaxation, become 'NMT 2'.
3. Isometric contraction of antagonists, followed by stretching, involving reciprocal inhibition, are described as 'NMT 3'.

What is unique to NMT, as discussed in this book, is its concentration on the soft tissues, not just to give reflex benefit to the body, not just to prepare for other therapeutic methods such as exercise or manipulation, not just to relax and normalise tense fibrotic muscular tissue, and not just to enhance lymphatic and general circulation and drainage, but to do all these things and, at the same time, to be able to offer the practitioner diagnostic information via the palpating and treating instrument, which is usually the thumb.

NMT can usefully be integrated in treatment aimed at postural reintegration, tension release, pain relief, improvement of joint mobility, reflex stimulation/modulation or sedation. There are many variations of the basic technique as developed by Stanley Lief, the choice of which will depend upon particular presenting factors, or personal preference. Similarities between some aspects of NMT and other manual systems (see Ch. 8) should be anticipated, as techniques have been borrowed from other systems where appropriate. For example, in Chapter 11 Dennis Dowling has demonstrated the clinical value of using progressive inhibition of neuromuscular structures (PINS), a unique way of utilising NMT effects, in pain control. Use of PINS in pain control offers an example of the evolution of new applications of the basics, which NMT provides (Dowling 2000).

NMT can be applied generally, or locally, and in a variety of positions (with the patient seated, supine, prone, side-lying, etc.). The order in which body areas are dealt with is not regarded as critical in general treatment, but seems to be of some consequence in postural reintegration (Rolf 1977).

The basic spinal NMT treatment and the basic abdominal (and related areas) NMT treatment (see Ch. 7) are the most commonly used, and will be described in detail in this and the next chapter. The methods described are in essence those of Stanley Lief and Boris Chaitow, both of whom achieved a degree of skill in the application of NMT that is unsurpassed. The inclusion of data on reflex areas and effects, together with basic NMT methods, provides the practitioner with a useful therapeutic tool, the limitations of which will be determined largely by the degree of intelligence and understanding with which it is employed. As Boris Chaitow has written (personal communication, 1983):

The important thing to remember is that this unique manipulative formula is applicable to any part of the body for any physical and physiological dysfunction and for both articular and soft tissue lesions.

To apply NMT successfully it is necessary to develop the art of palpation and sensitivity of fingers by constantly feeling the appropriate areas and assessing any abnormality in tissue structure for tensions, contractions, adhesions, spasms.

It is important to acquire with practice an appreciation of the 'feel' of normal tissue so that one is better able to recognise abnormal tissue. Once some level of diagnostic sensitivity with fingers has been achieved, subsequent application of the technique will be much easier to develop. The whole secret is to be able to recognise the 'abnormalities' in the feel of tissue structures. Having become accustomed to understanding the texture and character of 'normal' tissue, the pressure applied by the thumb in general, especially in the spinal structures, should always be firm, but never hurtful or bruising. To this end the pressure should be applied with a 'variable' pressure, i.e. with an appreciation of the texture and character of the tissue structures and according to the feel that sensitive fingers should have developed. The level of the pressure applied should not be consistent because the character and texture of tissue is always variable. These variations can be detected by one's educated 'feel'. The pressure should, therefore, be so applied that the thumb is moved along its path of direction in a way which corresponds to the feel of the tissues.

This variable factor in finger pressure constitutes probably the most important quality any practitioner of NMT can learn, enabling him to maintain more effective control of pressure, develop a greater sense of diagnostic feel, and be far less likely to bruise the tissue.

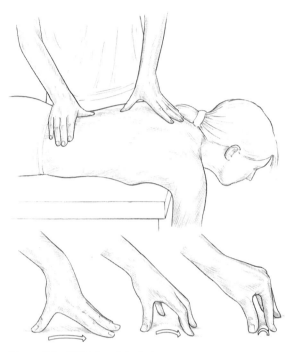

Figure 6.1 NMT thumb technique.

THUMB CONSIDERATIONS

NMT thumb technique (Fig. 6.1)

Thumb technique as employed in NMT, in either assessment or treatment modes, enables a wide variety of therapeutic effects to be produced. The tip of the thumb can deliver varying degrees of pressure via any of four facets; the very tip may be employed or the medial or lateral aspect of the tip can be used to make contact with angled surfaces. For more general (less localised and less specific) contact, of a diagnostic or therapeutic type, the broad surface of the distal phalange of the thumb is often used. It is usual for a light non-oily lubricant to be used to facilitate easy, non-dragging, passage of the palpating digit.

For balance and control, the hand should be spread, the tips of fingers providing a fulcrum or 'bridge' in which the palm is arched in order to allow free passage of the thumb towards one of the fingertips as the thumb moves in a direction that takes it away from the practitioner's body. During a single stroke, which covers between 2 and 3 inches (5–8 cm), the fingertips act as a

point of balance, while the chief force is imparted to the thumb tip via controlled application through the long axis of the extended arm of body weight. The thumb, therefore, never leads the hand but always trails behind the stable fingers, the tips of which rest just beyond the end of the stroke. Unlike many bodywork/massage strokes, the hand and arm remain still as the thumb, applying variable pressure (see below), moves through its pathway of tissue.

The extreme versatility of the thumb enables it to modify the direction of imparted force in accordance with the indications of the tissue being tested or treated. As the thumb glides across and through those tissues it becomes an extension of the practitioner's brain. In fact, for the clearest assessment of what is being palpated, the practitioner should have the eyes closed, in order that every minute change in the tissue can be felt and reacted to.

The thumb and hand seldom impart their own muscular force, except in dealing with small localised contractures or fibrotic 'nodules'.

In order that pressure/force be transmitted directly to its target, the weight being imparted should travel in as straight a line as possible, which is why the arm should not be flexed at the elbow or the wrist by more than a few degrees. The positioning of the practitioner's body in relation to the area being treated is also of the utmost importance in order to facilitate economy of effort and comfort.

The optimal height vis-à-vis the couch, and the most effective angle of approach to the body areas being addressed, must be considered and the descriptions and illustrations will help to make this clearer.

The degree of pressure imparted will depend on the nature of the tissue being treated, with a great variety of changes in pressure being possible during strokes across and through the tissues. When being treated, the patient should not feel strong pain, but a general degree of discomfort is usually acceptable as the seldom stationary thumb varies its penetration of dysfunctional tissues. A stroke or glide of 2–3 inches (5–8 cm) will usually take 4–5 seconds – seldom more unless a particularly obstructive indurated area is being dealt with. If reflex pressure techniques are being employed, a much longer stay on a point will be needed, but in normal diagnostic and therapeutic use the thumb continues to move as it probes, decongests and generally treats the tissues.

It is not possible to state the exact pressures necessary in NMT application because of the very nature of the objective, which in assessment mode attempts to meet and match the tissue resistance precisely, to vary the pressure constantly in response to what is being felt.

In subsequent or synchronous (with assessment) treatment of whatever is uncovered during evaluation, a greater degree of pressure is used and this too will vary, depending upon the objective – whether this is to inhibit, to produce localised stretching, to decongest and so on. Obviously, on areas with relatively thin muscular covering, the applied pressure would be lighter than in tense or thick, well covered areas such as the buttocks.

Attention should also be paid to the relative sensitivity of different areas and different patients. The thumb should not just mechanically stroke across or through tissue but should become an intelligent extension of the practitioner's diagnostic sensitivities so that the contact feels to the patient as though it is sequentially assessing every important nook and cranny of the soft tissues. Pain should be transient and no bruising should result if the above advice is followed.

The treating arm and thumb should be relatively straight because a 'hooked' thumb, in which all the work is done by the distal phalange, will become extremely tired and will not achieve the degree of penetration possible via a fairly rigid thumb.

Hypermobile thumbs

Some practitioners have hypermobile joints and it is difficult for them to maintain sustained pressure without the thumb giving way and bending back on itself. This is a problem that can be overcome only by attempting to build-up the muscular strength of the hand or by using a variation of the above technique; for example, a knuckle or even the elbow may be used to achieve deep pressure in very tense musculature. Alternatively, the finger stroke as described below can take over from a hypermobile thumb.

Alternatively an instrument such as the 'T'-bar (see Ch. 10, Fig. 10.1B,C) may be used to ease mechanical stress on the thumb joints.

 NMT finger technique (Fig. 6.2)

In certain localities, the width of the thumb prevents the degree of tissue penetration needed for successful assessment and/or treatment. In such regions the middle or index finger can usually be suitably employed. The most usual area for use of finger, rather than thumb, contact is in the intercostal musculature, and in attempting to penetrate beneath the scapula borders in tense fibrotic conditions.

The middle or index finger should be slightly flexed and, depending on the direction of the

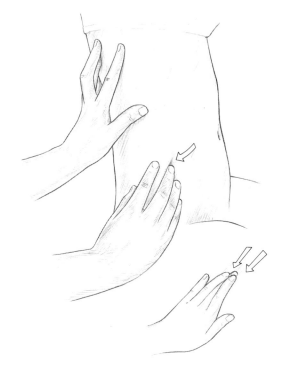

Figure 6.2   NMT finger technique.

stroke (most usually toward the practitioner) and density of the tissues, supported by one of its adjacent members. As the treating finger strokes with a firm contact, and usually a minimum of lubricant, a tensile strain is created between its tip and the tissue underlying it. This is stretched and lifted by the passage of the finger which, like the thumb, should continue moving unless or until dense, indurated tissue prevents its easy passage. When treating, these strokes can be repeated once or twice, as tissue changes dictate.

The angle of pressure to the skin surface is between 40° and 50°. The fingertip should never lead the stroke but should always follow the wrist, the palmar surface of which should lead, as the hand is drawn towards the practitioner. It is possible to impart a great degree of 'pull' on underlying tissues, and the patient's reactions must be taken into account in deciding on the degree of force to be used. Transient pain, or mild discomfort, is to be expected, but no more than that. All sensitive areas are indicative

of some degree of dysfunction, local or reflex, and are thus important, and their presence should be recorded. The patient should be told what to expect, so that a cooperative, unworried attitude evolves.

As mentioned above, unlike the thumb technique, in which force is largely directed away from the practitioner's body, in finger treatment the motive force is usually towards the practitioner. The arm position therefore alters, and a degree of flexion is necessary to ensure that the pull, or drag, of the finger across the lightly lubricated tissues is smooth. Unlike the thumb, which makes a sweep across the palm towards the fingertips, whilst the rest of the hand remains relatively stationary, the whole hand will move when finger technique is applied. Certainly some variation in the degree of angle between fingertip and skin is allowable during a stroke, and some slight variation in the degree of 'hooking' of the finger is sometimes also necessary. However, the main motive force is applied by pulling the slightly flexed, middle or index, finger towards the practitioner, with the possibility of some lateral emphasis if needed. The treating finger should always be supported by one of its neighbours.

Use of lubricant

The use of a lubricant to facilitate the smooth passage of, for example, the thumb over the surface is an essential aspect of NMT. The lubricant used should not allow too slippery a passage of the thumb or finger, and a suitable balance between lubrication and adherence is found by mixing 2 parts of rapeseed (or almond) oil to 1 part of lime or rose water. At times, the degree of stimulus imparted via this contact can be enhanced by increasing the tensile strain between the thumb or finger and the skin. If a cream is used, standard aqueous ointment, inexpensively available from any pharmacy, is hypoallergenic and offers an appropriate, nongreasy, medium.

If a stimulant effect is required (see notes on Connective tissue massage in Ch. 4), possibly to achieve a rapid vascular response, then no lubricant should be used. Clinical experience shows that similar reactions will be achieved (with lubricant) where NMT is applied along the intermuscular septa, or at the origins and insertions of muscles.

It should be clear to the practitioner that whatever underlying tissues are being treated should be visualised. Depending upon the presenting symptoms, and the area involved, any of a number of procedures may be undertaken as the hand moves from one site to another:

- superficial stroking in the direction of lymphatic flow
- direct pressure along the line of axis of stress fibres
- cross-fibre strokes
- deeper alternating 'make and break' stretching and pressure efforts
- subtle weaving, insinuating, movements that attempt to melt into the tissues to obtain information or greater access
- traction on fascial tissue
- crowding of bunched tissues toward the direction in which they are shortening.

As variable pressure is being applied, the practitioner needs to be constantly aware of diagnostic information that is being received via the contact hands, as this is what should determine the variations in pressure and the direction of force being applied.

Any changes in direction, or degree, of applied pressure should ideally take place without any sudden release, or application, of force, which might irritate the tissues and produce pain or a defensive contraction.

Lief's basic spinal treatment followed the pattern as set out below. The fact that the same pattern is followed at each treatment does not mean that the treatment is necessarily the same each time. The pattern gives a framework and a useful starting and ending point, but the degree of emphasis applied to the various areas of dysfunction that manifest themselves is a variable factor based always on what information the palpating hands are picking up: this is what makes each treatment different.

The areas of dysfunction noted during NMT application should be recorded on a case card, together with all relevant material and assessment and diagnostic findings relating to myofascial tissue changes, trigger points and reference zones, areas of sensitivity, restricted motion, fibrotic changes, areas of sensitivity, asymmetrical features, and so on.

LIEF'S BASIC SPINAL TREATMENT

Lief's basic spinal NMT treatment follows a pattern in which the patient is prone, with a pillow of medium thickness under the chest, forehead supported by the patient's hands or, ideally, resting in a split head-piece or face-hole. Alternatively – and more appropriately – a contoured cushion, which supports the entire body, should be used.

1. The whole spine from occiput to sacrum, including the gluteal area, should be lightly oiled or creamed.

2. The practitioner should begin by standing half-facing the head of the couch on the left of the patient, with the hips level with the mid-thoracic area.

3. To facilitate the intermittent application of pressure and the transfer of weight via the arm to the exploring and treating thumb, the practitioner should stand with the left foot forward of the right by 12–18 inches (30–45 cm), weight evenly distributed between them, knees slightly flexed.

4. The first contact, to the left side of the patient's head, is a gliding, light-pressured movement of the medial tip of the right thumb, from the mastoid process along the nuchal line to the external occipital protuberance. This same stroke, or glide, is then repeated with deeper pressure (see Fig. 6.4A,B).

The non-treating hand's role

- The practitioner's left hand should at this time rest on the upper thoracic or shoulder area to act as a stabilising contact.
- Whichever hand is operating at any given time, the other hand can give assistance by

means of gently rocking or stretching tissues to complement the efforts of the treating hand, or it can be useful in distracting tissues that are 'mounding' as the treating hand works on them.

• Whenever the practitioner changes to the other side of the table, it is suggested that one hand always maintains light contact with the patient. Indeed, it is suggested that, once treatment has commenced, no breaks in contact be allowed. There is often a noticeable increase in tension in the tissues if the series of strokes, stretching movements and pressure techniques that make up NMT are interrupted by even a few seconds because of a break in contact. Continuity would seem, in itself, to be of therapeutic value, simply as a reassuring and calming feature.

What the treating thumb feels

The movement of the right thumb through the tissue is slow – not uniformly slow, but deliberately seeking and feeling for 'contractions' and 'congestions' (to use two words that will be meaningful to any manual therapist). If and when such localised areas are felt, the degree of pressure can be increased and, in a variably applied manner, this pressure carries the thumb tip across, or through, the restricting tissues, decongesting, stretching and easing them.

The patient will often report a degree of pain but may say that it 'feels good'. This is a contradiction in terms, but constructive pain is usually felt as a 'nice hurt'.

 ## Practitioner's posture (Fig. 6.3)

• When applying thumb strokes, whether facing the head or the foot of the table, the treating arm should not be flexed, because the optimum transmission of weight from the practitioner's shoulder, through the arm to the thumb tip, is best achieved with a relatively straight arm.

• This demands that the practitioner ensures the table height is suitable for his or her own

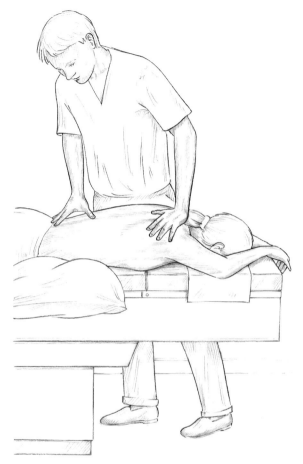

Figure 6.3   NMT – practitioner's posture should ensure a straight treating arm for ease of transmission of body weight, as well as leg positions that allow for the easy transfer of weight and centre of gravity. These postures assist in reducing energy expenditure and ease spinal stress.

height. The practitioner should not be forced to stand on tiptoe to treat the patient, nor should an unhealthy bent posture have to be adopted.

• The practitioner's weight should be evenly spread between the separated feet, both of which are forward facing at this stage.

• In this way, by slightly altering the weight distribution from the front to the back foot, and vice versa, an accurate, controlled degree of pressure can be exerted with minimal arm or hand effort.

The mechanics of NMT – achieving economy of effort

- The hand itself should not be rigid but in a relaxed state, moulding itself to the contours of the neck or back tissues.
- To some extent the fingertips stabilise the hand.
- The thumb's glide is controlled by this, so that the actual stroke is achieved by the tip of the extended thumb being brought slowly across the palm towards the fingertips.
- The fingers, during this phase of cervical treatment, would be placed on the opposite side of the neck to that being treated.
- The fingers maintain their position as the thumb performs its diagnostic/therapeutic glide. Figure 6.4A,B will aid the reader to a better understanding of this description.

However, were all the effort to be on the part of the thumb, it would soon tire. Consider which parts of the practitioner's arm/hand are involved with the various aspects of the glide/stroke as delivered by the thumb (finger strokes involve completely different mechanics):

1. The transverse movement of the thumb is a hand or forearm effort.
2. The relative straightness, or rigidity, of the last two thumb segments is also a local muscular responsibility.
3. The vast majority of the energy imparted via the thumb results from transmission of body weight, through the straight arm and into the thumb.
4. Any increase in pressure can be speedily achieved by simple weight transfer from back towards front foot, and a slight 'lean' on to the thumb from the shoulders.
5. A lessening of imparted pressure is achieved by reversing this body movement.

Treatment continues

The first two strokes of the right thumb having been completed – one shallow and almost totally diagnostic, and the second, deeper, imparting

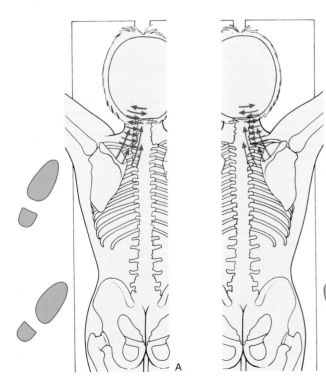

A B

Figure 6.4A, B First positions of suggested sequence of applications of NMT, to ensure optimal thumb and/or finger contact with primary trigger point sites and with the origins and insertions of most muscles. Note foot positions.

therapeutic effort – the next stroke is half a thumb-width caudal to the first. Thus a degree of overlap occurs as these strokes, starting on the belly of the sternocleidomastoid, glide across and through the trapezius, splenius capitus and posterior cervical muscles. A progressive series of strokes is applied in this way until the level of the cervicothoracic junction is reached. Unless serious underlying dysfunction is found, it is seldom necessary to repeat the two superimposed strokes at each level of the cervical region.

 ## Variable pressure – the key to painless pressure

- If underlying fibrotic tissue appears unyielding, a third, or fourth, slow deep glide may be necessary.
- The degree of discomfort felt by the patient is of some importance. The sensitivity of this region is well known and if pressure is too deep, or sustained for too long, the defensive resistance that may be created can make the treatment counterproductive.
- It is possible to achieve deep, penetrating pressure if it is variable in nature and not held for long, without undue pain or discomfort.
- Thus a thinking, intuitive feel for the work is a prerequisite of successful application.

Deactivating trigger points

Should trigger points be located during the NMT assessment/treatment strokes – as indicated by the reproduction, in a target area, of an existing, familiar, pain pattern – then a number of choices are open:

1. The point can be marked and noted (on a chart and if necessary on the body with a skin pencil) for later attention, or treatment can be offered immediately.
2. Sustained pressure, or 'make and break' pressure, can be used (see Chs 8 & 9 for details and choices).
3. Application of a positional release approach (strain/counterstain) will reduce activity in the hyperreactive tissue, as outlined in Chapter 8 (Simons 2002).
4. Initiation of an isometric contraction followed by local and whole muscle stretching should be used (Lewit 1999).
5. A combination of pressure, positional release and muscle energy technique (MET) (integrated neuromuscular inhibition technique (INIT), as described in Ch 9) can be introduced (Chaitow 1994).
6. Alternatively, spray and stretch methods can be used (vapocoolant technique, as discussed in Ch. 8) (Travell & Simons 1992).
7. An acupuncture needle or procaine injection can be used (as, it is suggested, can laser or microcurrent application) (Baldry 2001 McMakin 1998).
8. Sustained pressure, if applied, should be variable: deep pressure for 5–7 seconds, followed by a slight easing for a further few seconds, and so on, repeated until the local or reference pain changes (usually diminishing, but sometimes increasing), or until 2 minutes has elapsed. It is suggested that no more than this amount of manual pressure should be applied to a trigger point at any one session.
9. Further ease of the hyperreactive patterns in a trigger point can be achieved by applying ultrasound (pulsed), or by the application of a hot towel to the area, followed by effleurage (Lowe & Honeyman-Lowe 1999).
10. Whichever approach is used, a trigger point will only be permanently deactivated if the muscle in which it lies is restored to its normal resting length, and MET can assist in achieving this (Travell & Simons 1992).

The neck treatment continues

- Once the right thumb has completed its series of transverse strokes across the long axis of the cervical musculature, the left hand, which has been resting on the patient's left shoulder, now comes into play.
- A series of strokes is applied by the left thumb, upward from the left of the upper thoracic area towards the base of the skull.

- The fingers of the left hand rest (and act as a fulcrum) on the front of the shoulder area at the level of the medial aspect of the clavicle.
- The thumb tip should be angled to allow direct pressure to be exerted against the left lateral aspects of the upper thoracic and the lower cervical spinous processes as the thumb glides cephalad.
- The subsequent strokes of the thumb should be in the same direction but placed slightly more laterally.
- The fingers should then be placed on the patient's head at about the temporo-occipital articulation. The left thumb then deals in the same way with the mid and upper cervical soft tissues, finishing with a lateral stroke or two across the insertions on the occiput itself.

In travelling from the nuchal line to the level of the cervicothoracic junction, and back again, in a series of overlapping gliding movements, common sites of a number of possible trigger points will have been evaluated.

The midpoint of the sternomastoid, at the level of the posterior angle of the jaw, can be the source of an intensely painful trigger point, which refers its influence from the area above the temple in the ear region to below the angle of the jaw. Similar triggers exist in the splenius capitus, upper trapezius, posterior cervical and other muscles of the area, all with different target areas. (See Fig. 3.6 for these and other examples of trigger point distribution patterns.)

Posterior reflex centres

Also in this area there occur the posterior reflex centres of the neurolymphatic type (Chapman's reflexes), notably those connected with conjunctivitis, cerebellar congestion, and ear, nose and throat problems of an inflammatory or congested type, from sinusitis to tonsillitis. It is suggested that due study is made of the illustrations of neurolymphatic reflex positions (see Ch. 5). Treatment of these points is via lightly sustained pressure, as described in Chapter 4.

Recall at this point that Gutstein (see Ch. 3) found trigger areas in the cervical and upper

thoracic region that profoundly affected such diverse conditions as menopausal symptoms, imbalance in skin secretions and excessive perspiration. He stressed the importance of the cervical region and the interscapular area. Among the more important *tsubo* or acupressure points in the upper cervical area are:

- Gall bladder 20, which lies bilaterally in a depression midway between the occipital protuberance and the mastoid at the base of the skull.
- Bladder 10, which lies bilaterally just lateral to the large bundle of muscular insertions at the occiput.
- Triple heater 17, which lies bilaterally in the depression between the lobe of ear and the mastoid process.

These points, if sensitive, should receive a sustained or variable pressure, as for the other trigger points. Their influence is felt in a variety of conditions relating to the head, such as migraine, neuralgia, cold symptoms, hypertension and hypotension, and liver dysfunction.

Goodheart (1987) mentions levator scapulae 'weakness' as indicating digestive problems and recommends pressure techniques in the cervicothoracic area and on the medial border of the scapula to help normalise this.

Following treatment of the left side of the cervical area, the same procedures are repeated on the right. A tall practitioner can probably adapt to treat both sides of the area from one standing position; however, a move to the opposite side makes for a more controlled delivery of the appropriate strokes.

Origins and insertions

During NMT, special notice should be given to the origins and insertions of the muscles of the area. Where these bony landmarks are palpable by the thumb tip, they should be treated by the slow, variably applied, pressure technique. Indeed, all bony surfaces within reach of the probing digit should be searched for undue sensitivity and dysfunction of their attachments – described by Lewit (1999) as 'periosteal pain points' – which are amongst the commonest sites of trigger points, according to Travell & Simons (1992).

Duration of treatment

Treatment of the left cervical area should take no more than 2–3 minutes and, in the absence of dysfunction, can be comfortably and successfully dealt with in 90 seconds, or less. Indeed, in its assessment mode, the entire basic spinal NMT treatment can usually be completed in 15 minutes.

 ## Adopting a new position

Once both left and right cervical areas have been treated, the practitioner moves to the head of the table (Fig. 6.5).

- Resting the tips of the fingers on the lower, lateral aspect of the patient's neck, the thumb tips are placed just lateral to the first thoracic–spinal process.
- A degree of downward (toward the floor) pressure is applied via the thumbs, which are then drawn cephalad, alongside the lateral margins of the cervical spinous processes.
- This bilateral stroke culminates at the occiput, where a lateral stretch, or pull, is introduced across the bunched fibres of the muscles inserting into the base of the skull.
- The upward stroke should contain an element of pressure medially towards the spinous process, so that the pad of the thumb is pressing downward (towards the floor), whilst the lateral thumb tip is directed towards the centre, attempting to contact the bony contours of the spine, all the time being drawn slowly cephalad to end at the occiput.
- This combination stroke is repeated two or three times.
- The fingertips, which have been resting on the sternomastoid, may also be employed at this stage, to lift and stretch it posteriorly and laterally.
- The lateral stretch across the occipital protuberance may be likened to trying to break open a melon.

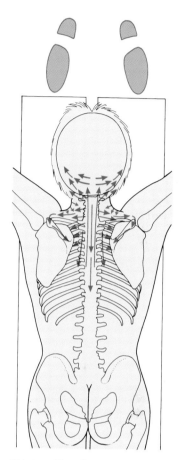

Figure 6.5 Third position of suggested sequence of application of NMT.

- The thumb tips dig deep into the medial fibres of the paraoccipital bundle and an outward stretch is instituted, using the leverage of the arms, as though attempting to open out the occiput.
- The thumbs are then drawn laterally across the fibres of muscular insertion into the skull, in a series of strokes culminating at the occipitoparietal junction.
- The fingertips, which act as a fulcrum to these movements, rest on the mastoid area of the temporal bone.
- Several strokes are then performed by one thumb or the other running caudad directly over the spinous process from the base of the skull to the upper thoracic area. Pressure should be moderate and slow.

• Standing in the same position, the left thumb will now be placed on the right lateral aspect of the first thoracic vertebra, and a series of strokes is performed caudad and laterally as well as diagonally towards the scapula.

• The fingers should be splayed out ahead of the thumb in whichever direction it is travelling, so that the force transmitted via the extended arm can be controlled.

• The fingers act as a fulcrum, with the thumb tip being drawn across the palm towards the diagonally opposite point – the tip of the middle or little finger.

• The thumb should never lead the hand nor be solely 'digging' or pressing, without the stabilising and controlling action of the hand or fingertips also being in operation.

• A series of strokes, shallow and then deep, is therefore applied from T1 to about T4 or T5, and outwards towards the scapula and along and across the upper trapezius fibres and the rhomboids.

• The left hand treats the right side, and vice versa, with the non-operative hand resting on the neck or head, stabilising it.

• Weight transfer to the thumb is achieved as described previously, by leaning forward.

Trapezius and sternomastoid muscles

Standing at the head of the table facing caudad allows the practitioner to access the region of the upper trapezius from above, so to speak. By lowering the angle at which the hand contacts the muscle, perhaps by kneeling or at least by lowering the centre of gravity significantly, and by standing a little to one side of the centre, it is possible to apply a series of sensitively searching contacts into the area of the thoracic outlet (see Fig. 6.5).

• Strokes that start in this triangular depression would move towards the trapezius fibres and through them towards the upper margins of the scapula. A treasure-house of trigger points awaits this searching digit.

• As it is often difficult to apply pressure to the trapezius or sternocleidomastoid muscles in such a way as to involve underlying bony structures, it may be necessary lightly to pinch, or squeeze, the more sensitive areas of dysfunction to assess trigger points and their related target areas of pain.

• Several strokes should also be applied directly over the spinous processes caudad as far down as the mid-thoracic area. Triggers sometimes lie on the attachments to the spinous processes, or between them.

By referring to the illustrations of trigger points (see Ch. 3, Fig. 3.6), the location of some of the commonest trigger points can be predicted, and their presence rapidly established.

When it is not possible to apply thumb pressure to such a point, a squeezing of the involved muscle area instead of direct pressure into it, again using varying pressure as described earlier in this chapter, will usually induce a reduction of the referred pain. Once pain reduces, the pressure should be released. If no success is achieved by these means, one of the other approaches, as previously outlined, can be used.

Left-side trunk treatment

The practitioner then moves to the patient's left side and stands in the same manner as at the commencement of the treatment, but at the level of the patient's waist.

• With the right hand now resting at the level of the lower thoracic spine, the left thumb commences a series of strokes cephalad from the mid-thoracic area.

• Each stroke covers two or three spinal segments and runs immediately lateral to the spinous process so that the angle of pressure imparted via the medial tip of the thumb is roughly towards the contralateral nipple.

• Again, light assessment and deep therapeutic strokes are employed and a degree of overlap is allowed on successive strokes.

• In this way the first two strokes might run from T8 to T5, followed by two strokes (one light, one deeper) from T6 to T3, and finally two strokes from T4 to T1.

● Deeper and more sustained pressure can be exerted upon discovering marked congestion or resistance to the gliding, probing thumb.

● In the thoracic area a second line of cephalad strokes may be employed, to include the spinal border of the scapula as well as one or two searching lateral probes along the inferior spine of the scapula, and across the musculature inferior to and inserting into the scapula (see Fig. 6.6A).

Right-side treatment

Treatment of the right side of the mid and upper thoracic region may be carried out without necessarily changing position, other than to lean across the patient. However, the shorter practitioner should change sides so that, standing half-facing the head of the patient, the right thumb can perform the strokes discussed above.

● Apart from trigger points in the lower trapezius fibres, others may be sought in levator scapulae, supraspinatus and infraspinatus, and subscapularis (by accessing via the axilla).

● The connective tissue zones affecting the arm, stomach, heart, liver and gall bladder are apparent in this region, and neurolymphatic reflexes relating to the arm, thyroid, lungs, throat and heart occur in the upper thoracic spine, including the scapular area (see Ch. 5).

● The intercostal spaces are a rich site of soft tissue dysfunction. The thumb tip, or a fingertip, should be run along both surfaces of the rib margin, as well as in the intercostal space itself.

● In this way the fibres of the small muscles involved will be treated adequately.

● If there is over-approximation of the ribs, a simple stroke along the space may be all that is possible until a degree of normalisation has taken place. These intercostal areas are extremely sensitive and care must be taken not to distress the patient. In most instances the intercostal spaces on the side opposite that on

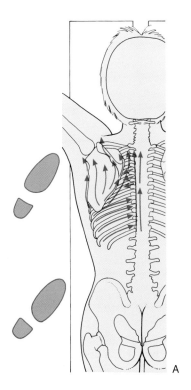
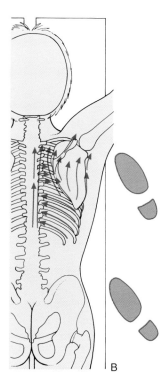

Figure 6.6A, B   Fourth (A) and fifth (B) positions of suggested sequence of applications of NMT.

which the practitioner is standing will be treated using the finger stroke, as illustrated (see Figs 6.2 & 6.6A, B).

● The tip of a finger is placed in the intercostal space and gently but firmly brought upwards and around the curve of the trunk towards the spine, feeling for contracted or congested tissues in which trigger points might be located.

 Change of position

● The practitioner now half turns so that, instead of facing the patient's head, he or she faces the patient's feet. The pattern of strokes is now carried out on the patient's left side by the practitioner's right hand (see Fig. 6.7).

● A series, starting from T8 to T11, followed by T11 to L1 and then L1 to L4, is carried out as before.

● Two or more gliding strokes with the pressure downwards but angled so that the medial aspect of the thumb is in contact with the lateral margin of the spinous process, are performed at each level.

● The lower intercostal areas are treated in much the same way as described above.

● The practitioner then steps back from the table and glides the thumb to allow access to a stroke that runs along the superior iliac crest from just above the hip to the sacroiliac joint.

● Several such strokes may be applied into the heavy musculature above the crest of ilium.

● To treat the opposite side, the practitioner changes sides so that he or she is facing the patient's waist and half-turned towards the feet; the left hand can deal with the lower thoracic and upper lumbar area, and the iliac crest, in the manner described above.

● One or two strokes should then be applied running caudad over the tips of the spinous processes from the mid-thoracic area to the sacrum, searching for attachment trigger points.

The area we have been describing contains a network of reflex areas and points:

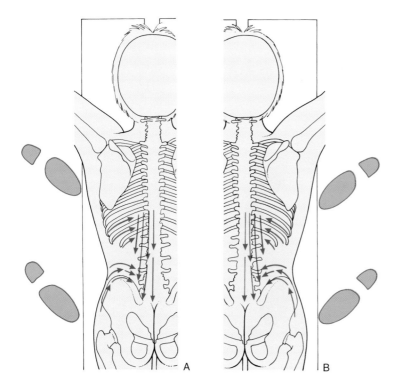

Figure 6.7A, B Sixth positions of suggested sequence of applications of NMT.

1. The *tsubo* or acupressure points lying symmetrically on either side of the spine and along the midline have great reflex importance. Associated points (see Fig. 4.3) are located alongside the spine.

2. The so-called 'Bladder meridian' points lie in two lines running parallel with the spine, one level with the medial border of the scapula and the other midway between it and the lateral border of the spinous processes.

3. Goodheart's work (1987) suggests that rhomboid weakness indicates liver problems and that pressure on C7 spinous process and a point on the right of the interspace between the 5th and 6th thoracic spinous process assists its normalisation. Latissimus dorsi weakness apparently indicates pancreatic dysfunction. Lateral to 7th and 8th thoracic interspace is the posterior pressure reflex to normalise this. These and other reflexes would appear to derive from Chapman's reflex theories and are deserving of further study.

4. In general terms, dysfunction of the erector spinae group of muscles, between 6th and 12th thoracic, indicates liver involvement. Similarly 4th, 5th and 6th thoracic area congestion or sensitivity usually involves stomach reflexes and gastric disturbance, whereas T12 and L2 indicate possible kidney dysfunction.

5. Connective tissue zones (see Ch. 5) relating to the stomach, head and lower limb circulation, are located in this region.

6. Jones' tender points (see Ch. 4, Fig. 4.5B in particular) in this region may relate to extension strains

 Left hip position

The next treatment position requires the practitioner to stand at the level of the patient's left hip, half-facing the head of the couch:

● The left hand and thumb describe a series of cephalad strokes from the sacral apex towards

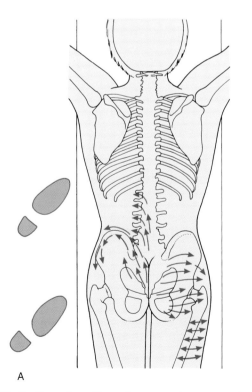
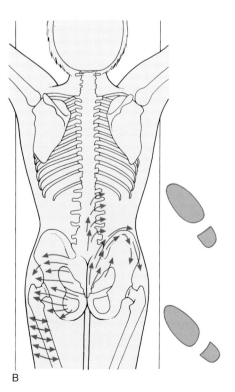

A   B

Figure 6.8A, B Seventh positions of suggested sequence of applications of NMT.

the sacroiliac area, and then laterally along the superior and inferior margins of the iliac crest to the insertion of the tensor fascia lata at the anterior, superior iliac spine (see Fig. 6.8).

● A further series of short strokes of the thumb upwards and laterally in the lumbar area may be described as attempting to stretch the paraspinal muscles away from the spine, notably the sacrospinal group.

● Having treated both left and right sides of the lumbar spine, as above, the practitioner uses a series of two-handed gliding manoeuvres in which the hands are spread over the upper gluteal area laterally, the thumb tips are placed at the level of the second sacral foramen with a downward (towards the floor) pressure; they glide cephalad and slowly laterally to pass over and through the fibres of the sacroiliac joint. This gliding stroke is repeated several times. (*Note*: the arrow directions on the figures are not meant to be definitive; for example, these strokes could be performed with the thumbs moving caudad, rather than cephalad, as illustrated).

● Still standing on the left, the practitioner leans across the patient's upper thigh and engages the right thumb on to the ischial tuberosity.

● A series of gliding movements is carried out from that point, laterally to the hip and caudad towards the gluteal fold.

● A further series of strokes, always applying deep, probing but variable pressure, is then carried out from the sacral border across the gluteal area to the hip margins. The fingertips during these strokes are splayed out so that they can guide and balance the hand and thumb movement.

● In these deep muscles the line of the thumb's direction is more towards the tip of the index finger, or middle finger, rather than to the little fingertip, as it was in the cervical area.

● In deep, tense gluteal muscle, the thumb may be inadequate to the task of prolonged pressure techniques, and the elbow may be used to sustain deep pressure for minutes at a time (see notes on the use of elbow in Ch. 8). Care should be taken, however, as the degree of pressure possible by this means is very great, and

> **Box 6.2** Trigger points, connective tissue zones and neurolymphatic reflexes of the lower lumbar, gluteal and lateral thigh areas
>
> ● The trigger points that may be found in the lower lumbar and gluteal areas include those in the following muscle groups: iliocostal, multifidus, longissimus, gluteus medius and gluteus minimus (see Fig. 3.6 for illustrations of many of these).
> ● The connective tissue zones that may be involved include those that involve arterial and venous disturbance to the legs, constipation, liver, gall bladder, heart and bladder (see Fig. 5.3).
> ● The neurolymphatic reflexes include those involving the following areas and conditions: the appendix, haemorrhoids, female generative organs, vasculitis, sciatic nerve, abdominal tension and constipation, prostate, colitis, kidneys, adrenal glands, digestive system, pancreas, liver, spleen and gall bladder. TFL contains neurolymphatic reflexes to the groin glands, the broad ligaments, spastic constipation and colitis, and the prostate (see Ch. 5).

tissue damage and bruising can result from its careless employment.

The practitioner may then move to the right side, repeating the strokes as described. Alternatively, rather than changing sides, the practitioner may lean across the patient, using hooked finger strokes to access the tissues above the hip and around the curve of the iliac crest effectively.

Trigger points, connective tissue zones and neurolymphatic reflexes that may be involved in the lower lumbar and gluteal areas are shown in Box 6.2.

Lateral thigh and gluteal structures

Having treated the low lumbar area and the gluteals, the practitioner might usefully include a series of strokes across the fibres of the tensor fascia lata (TFL) from the hip area to the lateral knee area. The tensor fascia lata contains neurolymphatic reflexes to the groin glands, the broad ligaments, spastic constipation and colitis, prostate, etc., and is itself a major contributor to knee, pelvic and low back problems via its influence on the mechanics of the region. It is commonly extremely sensitive to pressure, and care is needed to prevent patient distress in treating it. (See also Alternative methods for treating TFL in Ch. 8.)

Completion of treatment

This completes the basic spinal NMT treatment, apart from any manipulative procedures that might be indicated or thought desirable.

- Boris Chaitow completes the spinal treatment by standing at the head of the table, leaning over the patient's upper thoracic area, the palms of both hands totally in contact with the upper lumbar region so that the thenar eminence is resting on the paraspinal musculature and the fingers are pointing laterally.
- The heel of the hand imparts the main contact laterally.
- A series of gliding strokes is performed with the hands rhythmically alternating with each other so that, as the right hand strokes downwards to end its movement on the gluteals, the left is being brought back to the lower thoracic area.
- After it descends, the right hand comes back to the start.
- In this way a series of 10 to 20 deep rhythmic strokes is carried out in order to stimulate local circulation and drainage as well as to help relax the patient, who may well have tensed during the treatment of the lumbar and gluteal areas.

- As stated previously, the basic 'assessment' treatment should take no more than 15–20 minutes; however, far longer may be needed if whatever is found of a dysfunctional nature is treated.

The patient should have a sense of release from tension, and a sense of well-being that may last for some days. Many feel a sense of tiredness and a great desire to sleep; this should be encouraged. Pain may result in those areas that have borne the brunt of the pressure techniques, and this should be explained to the patient, who should be encouraged to note any changes in his or her condition and to report these at the subsequent visit.

The frequency of application of NMT will vary with the condition. In chronic conditions, one or two treatments weekly are as much as is ever required. This can be maintained until progress dictates that the interval be lengthened. In acute conditions, treatment may be much more frequent (but almost always less invasive): daily if possible until ease is achieved. Of necessity, this must depend upon what other modalities are employed.

REFERENCES

Baldry P 2001 Myofascial pain and fibromyalgia syndromes. Churchill Livingstone, Edinburgh

Chaitow L 1994 Integrated neuromuscular inhibition technique. British Journal of Osteopathy 13:17–20

Chaitow L 2001 Muscle energy techniques. 2nd edn. Churchill Livingstone, Edinburgh

Dowling D 2000 Progressive neuromuscular inhibition technique (PINS). Journal of the American Osteopathic Association 100(5):285–298

Dvorak J, Dvorak V, Schneider W 1988 Manual medicine therapy. Georg Thieme, Stuttgart

Goodheart G 1987 Applied kinesiology workshop procedure manuals 1976–1987. Published privately, Detroit

Lewit K 1999 Manipulation in rehabilitation of the motor system. 3rd edn. Butterworths, London

Lowe J-C, Honeyman-Lowe G 1999 Ultrasound treatment of trigger points: differences in technique for myofascial pain syndrome and fibromyalgia patients. Medecine du Sud-est April–May–June, no. 2:12–15

McMakin C 1998 Microcurrent treatment of myofascial pain in head, neck and face. Topics in Clinical Chiropractic 5(1):29–35

Rolf I 1977 Rolfing – integration of human structures. Harper & Row, New York

Simons D 2002 Understanding effective treatments of myofascial trigger points. Journal of Bodywork and Movement Therapies 6(2):81–88.

Travell J, Simons D 1992 Myofascial pain and dysfunction: the trigger point manual. Vol. 2: the lower extremities. Williams & Wilkins, Baltimore

7

Basic abdominopelvic NMT application

OBJECTIVES

The objectives for the use of NMT – and associated methods – in the treatment of abdominopelvic tissues vary considerably and may include:

1. To attempt to normalise local soft tissue dysfunction and pain (including symptoms produced by myofascial trigger points) resulting from postural or overuse strain (occupational or leisure activities, patterns of use, overload, repetition of movement, lifting, etc.), breathing pattern disorders, obesity, visceroptosis (causing drag of supporting structures, and associated congestion).

2. To enhance relaxation and reduction in symptoms relating to emotional or stress influences, particularly long-held psychological distress.

3. To improve function when the area has been traumatised (accidents, blows, surgery, etc.).

4. To influence internal organ function via reflex stimulation, for example using neurolymphatic (Chapman) reflexes and/or acupuncture points (see Ch. 4).

5. To modify painful and distressing symptoms such as those associated with interstitial cystitis and urgency (Weiss 2001). See Box 7.1 for details of research into such influences.

6. To attempt to improve function of the abdominopelvic organs by directly influencing circulatory and drainage functions (including lymphatic function) of the region (Wallace et al 1997).

7. To modify the negative local effects of viscerosomatic influences (see Ch. 3).

8. To improve diaphragmatic and respiratory function.

SOMATICOVISCERAL SYMPTOMS

In Chapter 3 there was discussion of the phenomenon in which organ dysfunction reflects reflexogenically to the soma, particularly as areas of segmental facilitation in the spinal region. These are, of course, the viscerosomatic reflexes. Later in this chapter possible variations on causes of viscerosomatic reflex pain will be outlined.

Simons et al (1999) reverse the consideration when they report details of somatovisceral responses, particularly arising from abdominal musculature, influencing internal visceral organs and functions. They note that injection of the trigger affecting an organ may offer symptomatic relief. This is not meant to suggest that local changes (such as trigger points) in the soma, muscles, etc. are necessarily the cause of such dysfunctions and diseases (see list below), but that there exists a strong possibility, in any given case, that the conditions/disease processes may be aggravated and/or maintained by reflexogenic activity associated with myofascial trigger points.

- projectile vomiting
- anorexia
- nausea
- intestinal colic
- diarrhoea
- urinary bladder and sphincter spasm
- dysmenorrhoea
- pain symptoms mimicking those of appendicitis and cholelithiasis
- symptoms of burning, fullness, bloating, swelling or gas (Gutstein 1944)
- heartburn and other symptoms of hiatal hernia
- urinary frequency
- groin pain
- chronic diarrhoea
- pain when coughing
- belching
- chest pain that is not cardiac in origin
- abdominal cramping
- colic in infants as well as adults.

JUNCTIONAL TISSUES

Simons et al (1999) have discussed the sites of trigger points as falling largly into two categories: (1) close to attachments and (2) close to motor end-points near the bellies of muscles. These guidelines also apply when treating abdominopelvic and related areas, where, in addition, the author's clinical experience suggests that particular attention should be given to specific junctional tissues, such as:

- the central tendon
- lateral aspect of the rectal muscle sheaths
- attachment of the recti muscles and external oblique muscles to the ribs
- the xiphisternal ligament, as well as the lower insertions of the internal and external oblique muscles
- intercostal areas from 5th to 12th ribs are equally important
- scars from previous operations may be the site of formation of connective tissue trigger points (Simons et al 1999). After sufficient healing has taken place, these incision sites can be examined by gently pinching, com-

pressing and rolling the scar tissue between the thumb and finger to examine for evidence of trigger points (Chaitow & DeLany 2000).

ASSISTING ORGAN DYSFUNCTION

Specific general areas are worthy of consideration in treating conditions that affect particular organs or functions, based on the evidence of the different reflex systems described in Chapter 4 (see also notes on percussive methods, such as spondylotherapy, in Ch. 8) (Baldry 1993, Chaitow & DeLany 2000, Kuchera & Kuchera 1994, Wallace et al 1997, Zhao-Pu 1991):

● Liver dysfunction and portal circulatory dysfunction calls for special attention to the right-side intercostal musculature, from the 5th to the 12th ribs. Especially important are the various muscular insertions into all these ribs.
● Gall bladder dysfunction involves similar areas, with extra attention to the area on the costal margin, roughly midway between the xiphisternal notch and the lateral rib margins.
● Spleen function may be stimulated by attention to the intercostal spaces between the 7th and 12th ribs on the left side.
● Digestive disorders in general may benefit from NMT applied to the central tendon between the recti and directly to the rectal sheaths.
● Stomach pain is treated via its reflex area to the left of the xiphisternal notch and to the tendon and rectal sheaths.
● Colonic problems and ovarian dysfunction may benefit from reflex NMT application to both iliac fossae as well as to the midline structures.
● Dysfunction of the kidneys, ureters and bladder requires attention to the inguinal borders of the internal and external oblique insertions, the suprapubic insertions of the recti, the overlying muscles and sheaths of the area, and the internal aspects of the upper thigh.
● In pelvic congestion relating to gynaecological dysfunction, NMT should be applied to the hypogastrium and both iliac fossae. This appears to relieve congestion and stimulates pelvic circulation.

● Ileitis and other functional disturbances of the transverse colon and small intestine may benefit from NMT applied to the umbilical area.
● Prostatic dysfunction may benefit from NMT to the central hypogastric region. Internal drainage massage of the prostate should also be considered.

The above brief indications should be considered in conjunction with other reflex systems and points (see below), as well as attention to the appropriate spinal areas (see notes on facilitation in Ch. 3), which may also benefit from NMT.

MORE ON ABDOMINAL REFLEX AREAS

Gutstein (1944) has noted trigger areas in the sternal, parasternal and epigastric regions and in the upper portions of the rectus, all relating to varying degrees of retroperistalsis. He also noted that colonic dysfunction related to triggers in the mid and lower rectus muscle. These were all predominantly left-sided. Other symptoms that improved or disappeared with the obliteration of these triggers include excessive appetite, poor appetite, flatulence, nervous vomiting, nervous diarrhoea, etc. The triggers were always tender spots, easily found by the palpation and situated mainly in the upper, mid and lower portions of the recti muscles, over the lower portion of the sternum and the epigastrium, including the xyphoid process and the parasternal region. The parasternal region corresponds to the insertions of the rectus muscle into the 5th, 6th and 7th ribs.

Fielder & Pyott (1955) described a number of reflexes occurring on the large bowel itself. These could be localised by deep palpation and treated by specific release techniques. These reflexes palpate as areas of tenderness and may include a degree of swelling and congestion resulting from adhesions, spasticity, diverticuli, chemical or bacterial irritation, etc.

In considering the reflexes available in the thoracic and abdominal regions, the neurolymphatic points of Chapman are also worthy of close attention (see Ch. 4 for more detail). When applying NMT in its evaluative mode to the anterior thorax and abdomen (as described later in this chapter), an awareness of the reflexes described by Chapman (Owen 1980) is a distinct advantage if there is a need to take account of visceral or thoracic organ dysfunction. Kuchera (1997) notes:

Palpate for tender anterior Chapman's [neurolymphatic] points as an indication to specific visceral irritation . . . Abdominal viscera, because of their innervations, have their first Chapman's [neurolymphatic] points at the level of the fifth intercostal spaces. If an anterior Chapman's [neurolymphatic] point is tender, ask the patient questions relating to dysfunction of the organ most likely to produce the tender point.

Anterior neurolymphatic reflexes for the upper lungs are found between the 3rd and 4th ribs, and between the 4th and 5th ribs (lower lung) close to the costal cartilage and the sternum. See Fig. 7.1 for the location of common abdominally related reflexes noted in this region (and also Fig. 5.8A,B).

Discussion

To what extent Gutstein's myodysneuric points are interchangeable with Chapman's or Fielder's reflexes, or other systems of reflex study (e.g. acupuncture or *tsubo* points and Travell's triggers), and to what extent these involve Mackenzie's work (Mackenzie 1909), is a matter for further research.

What is certain is that, within the soft tissues of this region, there abound palpable, sensitive, discrete areas of dysfunction that, on a local basis, interfere with or modify functional integrity to a greater or lesser degree, and reflexively are capable of massive interference with normal physiological function on a neural, circulatory and lymphatic level, to the extent of producing or mimicking serious pathological conditions. As these areas of dysfunction often yield to the simple, soft tissue manipulative techniques that are incorporated into Lief's NMT, the value of these techniques becomes apparent.

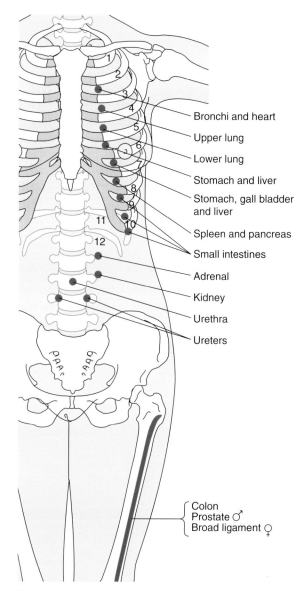

Bronchi and heart
Upper lung
Lower lung
Stomach and liver
Stomach, gall bladder and liver
Spleen and pancreas
Small intestines
Adrenal
Kidney
Urethra
Ureters

Colon
Prostate ♂
Broad ligament ♀

Figure 7.1 Common neurolymphatic points. From Ward (1997), with permission.

Many of Jones' (positional release/strain/counterstrain) tender points are found in the abdominal regions specifically relating to those strains that occur in a flexed position (Jones 1981).

Bennett's neurovascular points (see Ch. 4) are located mainly on the anterior aspect of the body and may be located during abdominal NMT work. This may be a link with the work of Mackenzie and others, who have demonstrated a clear relationship between the abdominal wall and the viscera. This and other reflex patterns provide the rationale for NMT application to the abdominal and sternal regions. These reflex patterns vary in individual cases, but it is clear that the majority of the organs are able to protect themselves by producing contraction, spasm and hyperaesthesia of the overlying, reflexively related, muscle wall – the myotome – which is also often augmented by hyperaesthesia of the overlying skin – the dermatome.

Baldry (1993) details a huge amount of research that validates the link (a somatovisceral reflex) between abdominal trigger points and symptoms as diverse as anorexia, flatulence, nausea, vomiting, diarrhoea, colic, dysmenorrhoea and dysuria. Pain of a deep aching nature, or sometimes of a sharp or burning type, is reported as being associated with this range of symptoms, which mimic organ disease or dysfunction (Hoyt 1953, Melnick 1954, Ranger et al 1971, Theobald, 1949, Travell & Simons 1983). Baldry (1993) has further summarised the importance of this region as a source of considerable pain and distress involving pelvic, abdominal and gynaecological symptoms. He says:

Pain in the abdomen and pelvis most likely to be helped by acupuncture is that which occurs as a result of activation of trigger points in the muscles, fascia, tendons and ligaments of the anterior and lateral abdominal wall, the lower back, the floor of the pelvis and the upper anterior part of the thigh. Such pain, however, is all too often erroneously assumed to be due to some intra-abdominal lesion, and as a consequence of being inappropriately treated is often allowed to persist for much longer than is necessary.

If we replace the word acupuncture with the term 'appropriate manual methods', we can come to appreciate that a large amount of abdominal and pelvic distress is remediable via the methods outlined in this book.

What activates these triggers? – similar factors that produce 'stress' anywhere else in the musculoskeletal system: postural faults, trauma, environmental stressors such as cold and damp,

surgery (another form of trauma) and so on. Differential diagnosis is obviously important in a region housing so many vital organs, and attention to the overall pattern of symptom presentation is critical. If in doubt, obtain expert opinion.

 Is the pain in the muscle or an organ?

As there is no underlying osseous structure available to allow compression of the musculature of many of the soft tissues of the abdomen, there is a need for a particular strategy that helps to screen palpated pain occurring at depth from that being produced in surface tissues.

When a local area of pain is noted using NMT or any other palpation method, it should be firmly compressed by the palpating digit, sufficient to produce pain/referred pain (if a trigger is involved) but not enough to cause distress. The supine patient is then asked to raise both (straight) legs from the table (heels must be raised by several inches). As this happens there will be a contraction of the abdominal muscles, which produces a compression of the trigger point between the muscle and the finger/thumb, and pain should increase. If pain decreases on the raising of the legs, the site of the pain is beneath the muscle and probably involves a visceral problem (Thomson & Francis 1977).

It is, of course, possible for there to be a problem in the viscera and also in the abdominal wall (see item 3 in the discussion immediately below), in which case this test would be in error in ascribing all symptoms of pain to a muscle wall lesion. The superficial musculature may be receiving distress sensations from an inflamed or irritated organ. The test described above therefore gives a clue, but not an absolute finding, as to the locality of the problem causing the pain.

Pain variables in abdominal somatic tissues

Kuchera (1997) points to three different manifestations of pain and discomfort arising from irritation or inflammation in the pelvic and abdominal viscera:

1. A 'vague, gnawing, deep, poorly localised, and midabdominal' pain, derives from afferent impulses from the organs of the region travelling towards the spinal cord.

2. Organs are supplied with their sympathetic input from specific spinal levels. Afferent messages also travel towards the spine, from the organs, along the same pathways, and when the organ is dysfunctional (inflamed, irritated, etc.) paraspinal changes (including tenderness, asymmetry, tissue changes and altered range of movement) will be noted at the level from which sympathetic innervation emerges for particular organs. (See notes on facilitation and viscerosomatic reflexes in Ch. 3, connective tissue massage in Ch. 4 and also zones of dysfunction in Ch. 5). Beal (1985) has summarised the levels as: T1–T5 = heart and lungs; T5–T10 = oesophagus, stomach, small intestine, liver, gall bladder, spleen, pancreas and adrenal cortex; T10–L2 = large bowel, appendix, kidney, ureter, adrenal medulla, testes, ovaries, urinary bladder, prostate gland and uterus. (See also notes under heading 'Assisting organ dysfunction' above).

3. Pain may be noted in the soft tissues superficial to the organ. Kuchera (1997) describes these as being due to irritation of contiguous peritoneal tissues and the abdominal wall, and as being 'responsible for rebound tenderness and abdominal guarding associated with severe abdominal pain.' (See also Fig. 5.4 showing abdominal reflexes, as described by Mackenzie in 1909).

 Treatment of attachment stress in the mesentery (e.g. visceroptosis effects)

The mesentery (literally 'the middle intestine') is the name given to the double layer of peritoneal membrane that supports the small intestine. It is shaped like a fan, with its shorter edge attaching to the back of the abdomen and the longer edge attaching to the small intestine for a length of around 20 feet (6 metres). The main mesenteric attachment is located in a line running from approximately 1 inch (2.5 cm) above and 1 inch (2.5 cm) to the left of the umbilicus, downward and to the right lower quadrant of the abdomen, just anterior to the sacroiliac joint (see Fig. 7.2).

If the organs of the abdomen sag, as occurs in obesity and visceroptosis, enormous degrees of drag occur on the mesenteric attachment tissues,

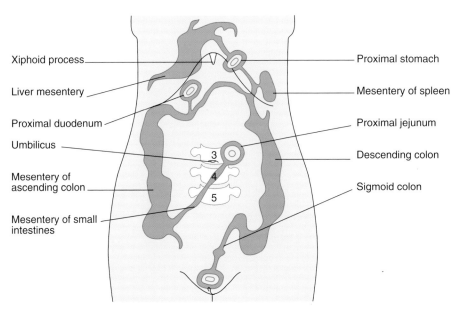

Figure 7.2 Mesenteric attachments as described by Kuchera. From Ward (1997), with permission.

with resulting congestion. Kuchera (1997) reports: '[Appropriate] treatment improves organ function, and can decrease many functional visceral symptoms, including bloating, constipation, and pelvic or abdominal pain.

Kuchera acknowledges the clinical research and teachings of the French osteopath Barral, whose work in visceral manipulation has opened this area to improved therapeutic intervention (Barral & Mercier 1988).

The mesenteric structures carry the sympathetic and parasympathetic fibres (as well as arteries) to the viscera, and also afferent fibres, lymphatic and venous vessels, away from the viscera.

Kuchera (1997) suggests that tenderness and tension in the mesentery can be palpated for tension and treated as follows:

By placing the extended fingers flat over the lateral margin of the ascending or descending colon and moving the viscera toward the midline of the body. The [practitioner] monitors continuously for changes in resistance to this movement.

- The mesentery of the sigmoid colon is moved toward the umbilicus. [See Fig. 7.3A,B].

- The 6-inch [15 cm] mesentery, along with the 30 feet [9 metres] of small intestines, is palpated by placing the extended fingers carefully into the lower left abdominal quadrant to obtain as much of the small intestines as possible, and moving this toward the upper right quadrant of the abdomen. [See Fig. 7.4]

To treat restrictions noted in such palpation:

- The patient lies supine, with knees flexed and feet flat on the table.
- The fingers are extended and placed flat over the lateral margin of the mesentery (to be treated).
- Medial pressure is then placed over the section of bowel, at right angles to its posterior, mesenteric, abdominal wall attachment.
- The tension is held as the patient takes a half-breath and holds it.

Wallace et al (1997) caution against causing any pain during these procedures, and further suggest that the tissues being held should be gently 'turned' clockwise and anticlockwise, to sense their position of greatest tissue freedom.

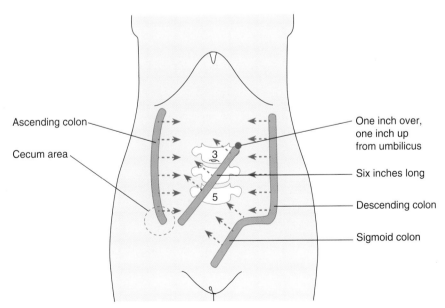

Figure 7.3A Suggested directions of movement in treating intestinal mesentery (after Kuchera). From Ward (1997), with permission.

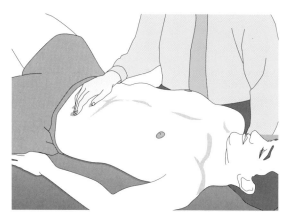

Figure 7.3B Lifting the small intestine/sigmoid colon to ease mesenteric drag (after Wallace et al). From Ward (1997), with permission.

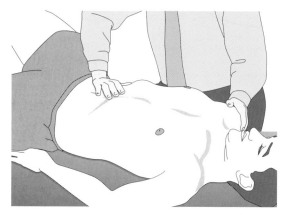

Figure 7.4 Lifting the caecum to ease mesenteric drag (after Wallace et al). From Ward (1997), with permission.

Box 7.2 Caution: pulsations

If, during palpation or treatment, any large pulsating mass is noted in the midline between the xyphoid and the umbilicus, caution should be exercised.

Kuchera (1997) notes: 'A normal abdominal aorta in an adult should not be wider than an inch (2.5 cm). Pulsations occurring anteriorly are normal, but lateral pulsations from the aorta suggest a weak vessel wall or aneurysm. Palpate [also] the inguinal area for a good pulse and compare the right and left sides. If a decreased pulse is found on one or both sides, ask the patient about claudication and then palpate and evaluate the pulse at the popliteal, posterior tibial, and dorsal pedis arteries in that leg, and compare to pulses in the opposite leg.'

The tissues are then held for not less than 90 seconds, or until a sense of relaxation is noted.

When breathing resumes, after this positional release approach, the tissues should be repalpated.

ABDOMINAL NMT APPLICATION
(Boxes 7.2 & 7.3)

In treating the abdominal and thoracic regions, the patient should be supine with the head

---

Box 7.3 Differential abdominal symptoms (Grieve 1994)

Most abdominal disorders can produce pain in the back (e.g. peptic ulcer, colonic cancer, abdominal arterial disease). Therefore, all other symptoms should be evaluated alongside the musculoskeletal assessment.

A hiatus hernia is usually associated with bilateral thoracic and shoulder pain. Anginal pain classically presents with chest, anterior cervical and (usually left) arm pain.

Thoracic facet or disc conditions can mimic angina, as can active trigger point activity. Aggravating and ameliorating factors usually offer clues as to whether the condition is cardiac related, or whether it is aggravated or eased by biomechanical influences.

A dysfunctional gall bladder commonly refers pain to the mid-thoracic area, unilaterally or bilaterally. Aggravating and ameliorating factors can usually offer clues as to whether the condition is related to digestive function or is biomechanically influenced.

Sacroiliac and right buttock pain may be produced by perforation of the ileum in regional ileitis (Crohn's disease).

Pronounced low back pain (possibly referring to the testicles in men) may be associated with an aneurysm that is about to rupture. Grieve (1994) reports that 'the onset of dissection of the ascending aorta or aortic arch is characterized by a sudden, tearing chest pain', which may radiate to the neck, thorax, abdomen and legs. The distinction between such symptoms and an acute musculoskeletal problem may be discerned by the 'suddenness, severity and spread' of the pain.

If a patient has a background of coronary, pulmonary or bronchial disease, the vertebral veins may have become varicosed, leading to an ill-defined backache. Grieve (1994) discusses the widespread nature of venous drainage from the vertebral column. These veins, as well as associated arteries and arterioles, are 'supplied with a dense plexiform arrangement of unmyelinated nerve fibers which constitute an important part of the vertebral column, and which may be irritated in a variety of ways to give rise to pain.'

supported by a medium-sized pillow and the knees flexed, either with a bolster under them or drawn right up so that the feet approximate the buttocks. Generous application of lubricant should be made to the area being treated.

Intercostal treatment

Abdominal and anterior intercostal NMT

The initial objective of the treatment strokes described below is to evaluate for soft tissue changes (active or latent trigger points, tissue texture changes, asymmetry, tenderness, etc.) with a contact that 'meets and matches' tissue tension. Only when a decision has been made to use subsequent strokes to attempt to alter the status of the tissues should pressure be increased to overcome tension, fibrotic resistance, etc., so stretching, inhibiting, draining and in other ways modifying structural features. (See Ch. 3, particularly Box 3.5, for notes on the effects of compressive force.)

The practitioner should be facing the patient and be half-turned towards the head, with legs apart for an even distribution of weight, and with knees flexed to facilitate the transfer of pressure through the arms. As many of the manoeuvres in the intercostal area, and on the abdomen itself, involve finger and thumb movements of a lighter nature than those applied through the heavy spinal musculature, the elbows need not be kept as straight as is necessary for spinal NMT (see Ch. 6).

However, when deep pressure is called for, and especially when this is applied via the thumb, the same criterion of weight transference, from the shoulder through the thumb, applies, and the straight arm is then an advantage for the economic and efficient use of energy.

The practitioner should be positioned to be level with the patient's waist and a series of strokes applied with the tip of the thumb, along the course of the intercostal spaces from the sternum, laterally. It is important that the insertions of the internal and external muscles receive attention. The margins of the ribs, both inferior and superior aspects, should receive firm gliding

pressure from the distal phalanx of the thumb or middle finger (see Box 7.5).

If there is too little space to allow such a degree of differentiated pressure, then a simple stroke along the available intercostal space has to suffice.

If the thumb cannot be insinuated between the ribs, a finger (side of finger) contact can be used (see description of NMT finger technique in Ch. 6), in which this is drawn towards the practitioner from the side, contralateral to that being treated, towards the sternum.

The intercostals, from the 5th rib to the costal margin below the 12th rib, should receive a series of two or three deep, slow-moving, gliding, sensitive strokes on each side, with special reference to points of particular congestion or sensitivity. These areas may also benefit from sustained or variable pressure techniques, depending on the objective. It is useful to note the possible presence, in the intercostal spaces, close to the sternum of neurolymphatic (Chapman) reflex points.

These points require only light circular pressure when being treated (see Ch. 5 for more detail). The practitioner should bear in mind other reflex patterns in the region, including those related to acupuncture alarm points and neurovascular points.

If a localised area of dysfunction is located, which refers pain or other symptoms that are familiar to the patient, an active trigger point will have been located (see Ch. 3).

Gentle probing on the sternum itself may elicit sensitivity in the rudimentary sternalis muscle, which has been found to house trigger points. If this is found to be sensitive, any of the various trigger point treatments recommended in Chapter 8 may be used.

It is not necessary for the practitioner to change sides during treatment of the intercostals, unless it is found to be more comfortable to do so.

Having treated the intercostal musculature and connective tissue, and having charted and/or treated any trigger points located during assessment, the practitioner, using either a deep thumb pressure or a contact with the pads of the fingertips, applies a series of short strokes in a combination of oblique lateral and inferior directions from the xyphoid process.

Rectal sheath

Thumbs or fingers may then be used to apply a series of deep slow strokes, along and under the costal margins. Whether diaphragmatic attachments can be located is questionable; however, sustained, firm (but not invasively aggressive) pressure allows for gradual access to an area that may reveal trigger points of exquisite sensitivity, with often surprising areas of referral. Many seem to produce sensations internally, while others create sensations in the lower extremities or in the throat, upper chest and shoulders. Deactivation of such triggers needs to be carried out slowly, carefully and with sensitivity.

A series of short strokes using fairly deep, but not painful, pressure is then applied by the thumb, from the midline up to the lateral rectal sheath. This series of strokes starts just inferior to the xyphoid and concludes at the pubic promontory. The series may be repeated on each side several times, depending on the degree of tension, congestion and sensitivity noted. It is useful during these applications to be aware of the mesenteric attachments as described by Wallace et al (1997) and Kuchera (1997) (see Figs 7.2 & 7.3).

A similar pattern of assessment/treatment is followed (using the thumb if working ipsilaterally, and the fingers if working contralaterally) across the lateral border of the rectal sheath, a series of short, deep, slow-moving (usually thumb) strokes being applied from just inferior to the costal margin of the rectal sheath, until the inguinal ligament is reached. Both sides are treated in this way (Fig. 7.5).

A series of similar strokes is then applied on one side and then the other laterally, from the lateral border of the rectal sheath (see Fig. 7.5). These strokes follow the contour of the trunk, so that the upper strokes travel in a slightly inferior curve whilst moving laterally (following the curve of the lower ribs), and the lower strokes have a superior inclination (following the curve

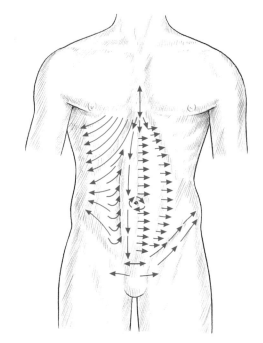

Figure 7.5 Neuromuscular abdominal technique. Suggested lines of application to access primary trigger point and attachment sites, and interfaces between different muscle groups. Note that the lines of application on this chart show one side only, and a full assessment/treatment involves these thumb or finger strokes being applied on each side of the body.

of the crest of the pelvis) as the hand moves laterally. A total of five or six strokes should be adequate to complete these movements, and this could be repeated, before performing the same strokes on the opposite side. Evidence is being sought of local soft tissue changes, as well as any underlying sense of tension or 'drag' on supporting tissues.

In treating the side on which the practitioner is standing, it may be more comfortable to apply the therapeutic stroke via the flexed fingertips, which are drawn towards the practitioner, or the usual thumb stroke may be used (see Ch. 6). In treating the opposite side, thumb pressure can be applied more easily, as in spinal technique, with the fingers acting as a fulcrum and the thumb gliding towards them in a series of 2–3-inch-long strokes. The sensing of contracted gangliform areas of dysfunction is more difficult in abdominal work, and requires great sensitivity of touch and great concentration on the part of the practitioner.

Symphysis pubis

The sheaths of the rectus abdominis muscles, from the costal margins downwards to the pubic bones, are evaluated by finger or thumb strokes. Attention should be given to the soft tissue component of, as well as the insertions into, the iliac fossa, the pubic bones and the symphysis pubis, including the inguinal ligaments (see Fig. 7.5).

Strokes should be made, commencing at the anterior superior iliac spine (ASIS), which attempt to evaluate the attachments of internal, external obliques and transversus abdominis, which can be contacted.

A deep but not painful stroke, employing the pad of the thumb, should be applied to the superior aspect of the pubic crest. This should start at the symphysis pubis and move laterally, first in one direction and, then after repeating it once or twice, in the other.

A similar series, starting at the centre and moving laterally, should then be applied over the anterior aspect of the pubic bone. Great care should be taken not to use undue pressure as the area is sensitive at the best of times, and may be acutely so if there is dysfunction associated with the insertions into these structures (as well as in relation to sacral torsions and sacroiliac dysfunction).

A series of deep slow movements is then performed, via the thumb, along the superior and inferior aspects of the inguinal ligament, starting at the pubic bone and running up to and beyond the iliac crest.

Positional release implications of abdominal tender points

In this lower abdominal area, close to the ASIS and towards the umbilicus, many of the tender points (see Ch. 4 on Jones' points, and Fig. 4.5A) associated with flexion strains of the lumbar and lower thoracic spine may be located. Positional release methods should be employed to relieve

---

Box 7.4   Positional release technique for abdominal muscles

Tender points (which may or may not also be trigger points) located in the abdominal musculature often represent dysfunction of the lumbothoracic region; they result from strain or stress, and occurred in flexion.

Tender points are almost always located in tissues shortened at the time of strain. For a greater understanding of the strain/counterstrain theory, which supports this assertion, see Chaitow 2002, Chaitow & DeLany 2000, Deig 2001, Jones 1981.

Gross positioning to relieve lumbar flexion stresses and strains takes the (usually supine) patient painlessly into flexion (by raising the flexed lower limbs to induce lumbar flexion), with the final position of ease being held for at least 90 seconds.

The 'position of ease' is determined by means of palpation of the tender point, with the patient reporting on the change in 'score' as the positioning is 'fine tuned'. A score of 3 or less is the objective, having commenced from a score of 10 before the repositioning starts.

- Jones (1981) reports that L1 has two tender points: one at the tip of the anterior superior iliac spine and the other on the medial surface of the ilium, just medial to ASIS.
- The tender point for 2nd lumbar anterior strain is found lateral to the anterior inferior iliac spine.
- The tender point for L3 lies 1 inch (2.5 cm) below a line connecting L1 and L2 points.
- L4 tender point is found at the attachment of the inguinal ligament on the ilium.
- L5 points are on the body of the pubes, just to the side of the symphysis.
- In bilateral strains, both sides should be treated. L3 and L4 usually require greater side-bending in fine-tuning than the other lumbar points.

---

the dysfunctional patterns associated with these (see notes on strain/counterstrain in Ch. 8 and also Box 7.4).

Lateral rectus sheath

The thumbs, or fingertips, may then be insinuated beneath the lateral rectus border at its lower margins, and deep pressure applied towards the midline. The hand or thumb should then slowly move cephalad, in short stages, whilst maintaining this medial pressure. This lifts the connective tissue from its underlying attachments and helps to normalise localised contractures and fibrous infiltrations. Additionally, when working on the right the ascending colon, and on the left the decending colon, will be receiving the 'lift' appropriate for release of mesenteric drag symptoms (see Fig. 7.3B).

Umbilicus

A series of strokes should then be applied around the umbilicus. Using thumb or flexed fingertips, a number of movements of a stretching nature should be performed, in which the non-treating hand stabilises the tissue at the start of the stroke, which first runs from approximately 1 inch (2.5 cm) superior and lateral to the umbilicus on the right side, to the same level on the left side. The non-treating hand then stabilises the tissues at this end-point of the stroke and a further stretching and probing stroke is applied inferiorly to a point about 1 inch (2.5 cm) inferior and lateral to the umbilicus, on the left side. This area is then stabilised, and the stroke is applied to a similar point on the right.

The circle is completed by a further stroke upwards, to end at the point at which the series began. This series of movements should have a rhythmical pattern so that, as the treating hand reaches the end of its stroke, the non-treating hand comes to that point and replaces the contact as a stabilising pressure whilst the treating hand begins its next movement. A series of three or four such circuits of the umbilicus is performed. Note that the superior mesenteric attachment, which supports the small intestine, is located 1 inch (2.5 cm) superior and 1 inch (2.5 cm) laterally to the left of the umbilicus.

Additional strokes may be applied along the midline and the sheaths of the recti muscles from the costal margins downwards.

A soothing culmination to the foregoing (which should take approximately 10–15 minutes) may be applied by a circular clockwise series of movements in which the palm of one hand and the heel of the other alternately circle the whole abdominal area. Thus, with the practitioner standing to the right of the patient, the palm and fingers of the left hand stroke deeply but gently down the left abdominal structures and then across the lower abdomen towards the practitioner where, using the heel and palm, the right hand takes over the stroke and proceeds up the right side to the costal margin. At this point it changes direction to run across the upper abdomen, where the left hand takes over to repeat this pattern several times. Alternatively, the positional releases, as described by Wallace et al (1997) and Kuchera (1997) (see Figs 7.3 & 7.4), may be performed.

Linea alba

Additional strokes should be applied along the midline, on the linea alba itself, while searching for evidence of contractions, adhesions, fibrotic nodules, oedema and sensitivity. Caution is always required to avoid deep pressure on the linea alba, especially if the patient has weakened this muscular interface via pregnancy, surgery or trauma. It should also be recalled that the linea alba is a place of attachment of the external obliques as well as transversus abdominis (Braggins 2000).

Finally, specific release techniques may be applied during or after this general treatment (see Fig. 8.21A,B and accompanying notes in Ch. 8). Abdominal treatment can be repeated several times weekly, if indicated, but normally once a week is adequate until improvement in function is achieved.

In chronic conditions of abdominal or pelvic dysfunction, the NMT approach as described, together with specific release movements, and appropriate spinal and whole body treatment, is capable of having a profound effect on function in the area.

With an improvement in circulation and drainage, and a reduction in tensions, contractions and reflex activities, homeostatic mechanisms are automatically enhanced.

REFERENCES

Baldry P 1993 Acupuncture, trigger points and musculoskeletal pain. Churchill Livingstone, Edinburgh

Barral JP, Mercier P 1988 Visceral manipulation. Eastland Press, Seattle

Beal M 1985 Viscerosomatic reflexes: a review. Journal of the American Osteopathic Association 85(12):786–801

Braggins S 2000 Back care: a clinical approach. Churchill Livingstone, Edinburgh

Chaitow L 2002 Positional release techniques. 2nd ed. Churchill Livingstone, Edinburgh

Chaitow L, DeLany J 2000 Clinical applications of neuromuscular technique. Churchill Livingstone, Edinburgh

Deig D 2001 Positional release technique. Butterworth Heinemann, Boston

Fielder S, Pyott W 1955 The science and art of manipulative surgery. American Institute of Manipulative Surgery, Salt Lake City, Utah

Grieve G 1994 The masqueraders. In: Boyling JD, Palastanga N, eds. Grieve's modern manual therapy. 2nd edn. Churchill Livingstone, Edinburgh

Gutstein R 1944 The role of abdominal fibrositis in functional indigestion. Mississippi Valley Medical Journal 66–114

Hoyt H 1953 Segmental nerve lesions as a cause of trigonitis syndrome. Stanford Medical Bulletin 11:61–64

Jones L 1981 Strain and counterstrain. Academy of Applied Osteopathy, Colorado Springs

Kuchera M, Kuchera W 1994 Considerations in systemic dysfunction. Greyden Press, Columbus, Ohio

Kuchera W 1997 Lumbar and abdominal region. In: Ward R, ed. Foundations for osteopathic medicine. Williams & Wilkins, Baltimore

Mackenzie J 1909 Symptoms and their interpretation. London

Melnick J 1954 Treatment of trigger mechanisms in gastrointestinal disease. New York State Journal of Medicine 54:1324–1330

Owen C 1980 An endocrine interpretation of Chapman's reflexes. American Academy of Osteopathy, Newark, Ohio

Ranger I et al 1971 Abdominal wall pain due to nerve entrapment. Practitioner 206:791–792

Simons D, Travell J, Simons L 1999 Myofascial pain and dysfunction: the trigger point manual. Vol. 1: Upper half of body. 2nd edn. Williams & Wilkins, Baltimore

Theobald G 1949 Relief and prevention of referred pain. Journal of Obstetrics and Gynaecology of the British Commonwealth 56:447–460

Thomson H, Francis D 1977 Abdominal wall tenderness: a useful sign in the acute abdomen. The Lancet i: 1053

Travell J, Simons D 1983 Myofascial pain and dysfunction – trigger point manual. Williams & Wilkins, Baltimore

Wallace E, McPartland J, Jones J, Kuchera W, Buser B 1997 Lymphatic system. In: Ward R, ed. Foundations for osteopathic medicine. Williams & Wilkins, Baltimore

Ward R, ed. 1997 Foundations for osteopathic medicine. Williams & Wilkins, Baltimore

Weiss J 2001 Pelvic floor myofascial trigger points: manual therapy for interstitial cystitis and the urgency–frequency syndrome. Journal of Urology 166:2226–2231

Zhao-Pu W 1991 Acupressure therapy. Churchill Livingstone, Edinburgh

8

Associated techniques

SOFT TISSUE APPROACHES

In Chapter 6 a detailed description was given of NMT in spinal, cervical, pelvic and intercostal structures, and abdominal techniques were described in Chapter 7. In this chapter a number of additional soft tissue approaches that are frequently employed alongside NMT (listed in Box 8.1) will be outlined in alphabetical order, rather than any other sequence.

Elbow technique

Caution – Direct pressure should be avoided, or performed with great care:

Box 8.1   Additional soft tissue approaches

- Elbow technique
- Chill-and-stretch technique
- Deep tissue release
- Induration technique
- Integrated neuromuscular inhibition technique (INIT)
- Ischaemic compression
- Muscle energy techniques
- Percussion technique
- Piriformis technique
- Proprioceptive adjustment
- Psoas technique
- Pump techniques (liver, lymphatics, spleen)
- Skin techniques
- S-contact technique
- Soft tissue manipulation (including massage)
- Special (abdominal) release technique
- Strain/counterstrain
- Tensor fascia lata technique
- Trigger point treatment methods.

---

1. if tissues are inflamed or in remodelling phase after trauma following injury is incomplete
2. in cases of malignancy
3. close to blood vessels and nerves
4. close to attachment sites
5. if pain (local or referred) is excessive.

In treating certain muscle groups, notably the gluteals and the sacrospinalis group, it is sometimes difficult, or even impossible, to impart adequate force via the thumb, owing to the degree of resistance in the tissues involved. Elbow technique treatment should not be given at the same time as NMT but should be preparatory to it, on a number of occasions, so that NMT can subsequently be applied effectively.

In treating sacrospinalis, for example, the entire spine should be lubricated and the practitioner should stand on the patient's left side (patient supine, pillow under thorax) (Fig. 8.1).

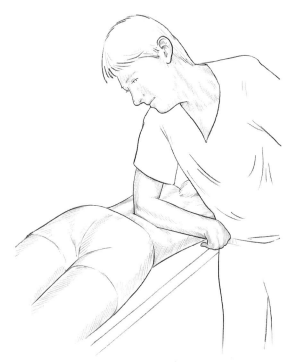

Figure 8.1 Elbow technique applied to paraspinal musculature.

The right elbow tip is placed just superior to the sacral base, with the forearm at right angles to the patient's body. By flexing the knees slightly and allowing weight to be transferred via the elbow, the practitioner can apply controlled pressure to the muscles. The elbow is allowed to glide slowly cephalad. If pain is reported, pressure is lessened. Several glides or strokes along the full length of the spine will greatly relax even marked contractions. Similar techniques can be applied to the gluteal area.

Treatment of piriformis muscle, and its central trigger points, is usefully achieved by means of elbow pressure, applied to the trigger point while the side-lying patient's leg is externally rotated, in order to achieve a lengthening of the muscle. (See details of this method later in this chapter and also Figs 8.11 and 10.13B,C).

Chill-and-stretch technique, trigger point technique

Chilling and stretching a muscle housing a trigger point rapidly assists in deactivation of the abnormal neurological behaviour of the site. Travell and Mennell have described these effects in detail (Mennell 1974, Simons et al 1999, Travell 1952, Travell & Simons 1992).

Travell & Simons (1992) and Simons et al (1999) have discouraged the use of vapocoolants to chill the area because of environmental considerations relating to ozone depletion, and have instead urged the use of stroking with ice in a similar manner to the spray stream to achieve the same effect. The objective is to chill the surface tissues while the underlying muscle housing the trigger is simultaneously stretched. They also point out that the spray is applied before or during the stretch and not after the muscle has already been elongated.

A container of vapocoolant spray with a calibrated nozzle which delivers a moderately fine jet stream, or a source of ice, is needed. The jet stream should have sufficient force to carry in the air for at least 3 feet. A mist-like spray is less desirable.

Ice can consist of a cylinder of ice formed by freezing water in a paper cup and then peeling this off the ice. A wooden handle will have been frozen into the ice to allow for its ease of application, as it is rolled from the trigger towards the referred area in a series of sweeps.

The author has found that a cold drink can that has been partially filled with water and then frozen is more suitable, because ice applied directly on to skin melts rapidly and, as Travell

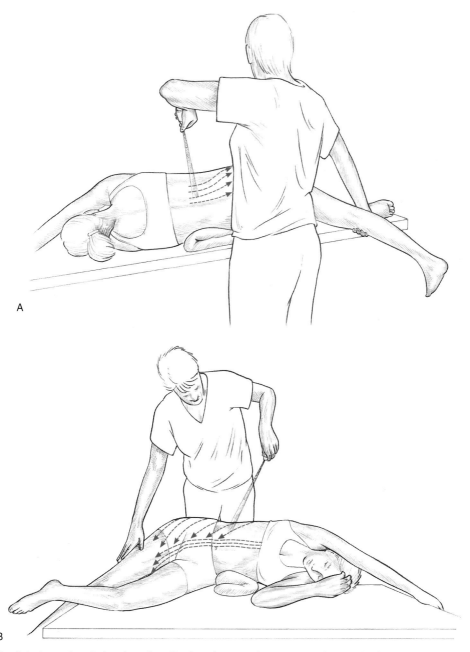

Figure 8.2A,B Anterior and posterior view of application of vapocoolant spray to trigger point (quadratus lumborum in this illustration). Muscles housing trigger points are placed at stretch while a coolant spray is utilised to chill the point and the area between it and the target reference area.

& Simons (1992) have pointed out, the skin must remain dry for this method to be successful because dampness slows the rate of cooling of the skin and may also delay rewarming. An ice-cold metal container, however, can be rolled over the skin and will retain its chilling potential for long enough to achieve the ends desired.

Whichever method is chosen, the patient should be comfortably supported to promote muscular relaxation. If a spray is used, the container is held about 2 feet away, in such a manner that the jet stream meets the body surface at an acute angle or at a tangent, not perpendicularly (Fig. 8.2). This lessens the shock of the impact. For the same reason, the stream is sometimes started in air or on the practitioner's hand and is gradually brought into contact with the skin overlying the trigger point.

The stream/ice massage/frozen canister is applied in one direction, not back and forth. Each sweep is started at the trigger point and is moved slowly and evenly outward over the reference zone. Probably it is advantageous to spray or ice-chill both trigger and reference areas, because secondary trigger points are likely to have developed within reference zones when pain is very strong. (The direction of movement is also in line with the muscle fibres towards their insertion.)

The optimum speed of movement of the sweep/roll over the skin seems to be about 4 inches (10 cm) per second. Each sweep is started slightly proximal to the trigger point and is moved slowly and evenly through the reference zone to cover it and extend slightly beyond it. These sweeps are repeated in a rhythm of a few seconds on and a few seconds off, until all the skin over trigger and reference areas has been covered once or twice. If aching or 'cold pain' develops, or if the application of the spray/ice/canister sets off a reference of pain, the interval between applications is lengthened. Care is taken not to frost or blanch the skin. During the application of cold or directly after it, the taut fibres should be stretched passively. The fibres should not be stretched in advance of the cold.

Steady, gentle stretching is usually essential if a satisfactory result is to be achieved.

As relaxation of the muscle occurs, continued stretch should be maintained for 20–30 seconds, and after each series of cold applications active motion is tested.

The patient is asked to move in the directions that were restricted before spraying, or that were painful to activate.

An attempt should be made to restore the full range of motion, but always within the limits of pain, as sudden overstretching can increase existing muscle spasm.

Travell & Simons (1992) have, however, pointed out that the skin should remain dry for this method to be successful as dampness retards the rate of cooling of the skin and may also delay rewarming. Wrapping the ice in thin plastic (bag or wrap) will prevent moisture from touching the skin, but reduces the efficacy somewhat compared with that of vapocoolants.

The treatment is continued in this manner until the trigger points (often several are present, or a 'nest' of them) and their respective pain reference zones have been treated.

The entire procedure may occupy 15–20 minutes and should not be rushed. The importance of re-establishing normal motion in conjunction with the use of the chilling is well founded. It may be that the brief interruption of pain impulses is insufficient and that input of normal impulses must also occur for the obliteration of trigger points to be successfully achieved. Simple exercises that utilise the principle of passive or active stretch should be outlined to the patient, to be carried out several times daily, after the application of gentle heat (hot packs, etc.) at home. Usual precautions should be mentioned, such as avoiding the use of heat if symptoms worsen or if there is evidence of inflammation.

Deep tissue release
(Fielder & Pyott 1955)

In using NMT it is often helpful to apply a local 'tissue release' technique to areas of marked contraction or spasticity. In areas overlying bone, the techniques suitable for use in the abdominal region (see Specific (abdominal) release techniques, later in this chapter) are not applicable.

The method recommended is as follows:

● The contact on the tissues involved is made by extending the digits of either hand and making firm contact with the area between the first and second metacarpophalangeal joints, taking out the slack of the tissues and engaging a resistance barrier.

● This contact is rotated clockwise or anti-clockwise in order to increase the tension in the underlying tissues, until the tissues with the greatest resistance are noted and combined barrier is engaged – downwards and in a torsional manner.

● The other hand is then placed over the contact hand so that the downward pressure and rotation are reinforced.

● In addition, a further direction of stretch should be introduced by the second hand – towards the direction laterally/medially or superiorly/inferiorly, whichever offers the greatest resistance.

● The tissues would therefore be receiving a direct downward pressure, a rotational stretch, and a further degree of stretch in another direction, all maintained by the two treating hands.

● The overlying hand should have been placed in such a way that the radial border of the metacarpal base of the thumb is directly over the contact point of the first hand's contact (i.e. over the second metacarpal joint area). See Fig. 8.3.

● The fingers of the overlying hand should be tightly in contact with the lateral border of the contact hand.

The final application of the release technique may be performed in one of two ways:

1. The overlying hand executes a short sharp squeeze by flexing the middle finger against the metacarpals of the contact hand. The resulting pressure in the intermetacarpal area provides the 'thrust' or release force. The line of force of this squeeze is towards the practitioner.

2. The second method of release, which is more suitable for deeper contractions of tissue, is applied via short sharp thrust by the overlying hand against the contact hand, with a simultaneous medial rotation of the contact hand. The

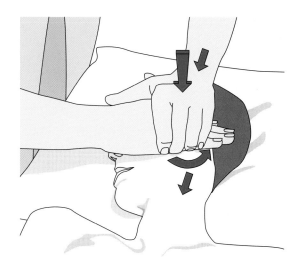

Figure 8.3   Deep tissue release technique applied, in this example, close to the temporomandibular joint area. The soft tissue slack will have been removed (i.e. barriers engaged) by a precise contact from the right hand (the area between the first and second metacarpophalangeal joints) in directions of greatest resistance (a) into the soft tissues, (b) into rotation (counterclockwise in this example) and (c) inferiorly, with the left hand, supported by the left hand contact, which then completes the release by means of either a sharp contraction of the contact or a short sharp thrust (see text for further detail). Redrawn from Fielder & Pyott (1955).

line of force in this technique is away from the practitioner.

This soft tissue approach, which emerged from American naprapathy (a form of soft tissue manipulation popular primarily in Sweden and the Chicago area of the United States) and an adhesion releasing method known as 'bloodless surgery' between the two World Wars, has been adapted for use in the UK by McTimoney chiropractic practitioners.

Induration technique
(Morrison 1969)

Note: This method is suitable even in cases of great fragility (osteoporosis) because pressure is not meant to exceed an ounce or two, at most.

As many patients are too frail or too ill to allow the full NMT treatment to be applied, a useful technique exists to aid in normalising reflex and local areas of the paraspinal musculature. Stoddard (1969) has pointed out that protective spasm in muscle can often indicate underlying pathology (osteoporosis, etc.) and, clearly, deep pressure techniques would be contraindicated in such conditions.

● With the patient sitting or lying, the practitioner, using a very light 'skin–skin' contact which evaluates 'drag' or hills/valleys (see Ch. 5), runs the fingertips longitudinally down the side of the spine (side of spine opposite that on which practitioner is standing) over the transverse processes.

● Any spot or area of hardened or indurated tissue that also palpates as tender to the patient is marked for attention.

● Treatment is applied by palpating the sensitive area with the tip of the thumb of one hand whilst applying light pressure towards the painful spot with the soft thenar or hyperthenar eminence of the other hand, which is resting on the spinous process of the vertebra alongside the indurated tissue (Fig. 8.4).

● Direct pressure (extremely light – ounces only) towards the pain should lessen the degree of tissue contraction and the sensitivity.

● If it does not do so, the angle of push on the spinous process towards the painful spot should

be varied slightly so that, somewhere within an arc embracing a half circle, an angle of push towards the pain will be found to abolish the pain totally and will lessen the objective feeling of tension.

● The 'position of ease' is held for around 20 seconds before moving on to the next sensitive area.

This technique, which has strong echoes of 'strain/counterstrain' (described later in this chapter) can be used with NMT or instead of deeper probing measures which, for practical reasons, may be contraindicated (for example if the patient's condition precluded it due to extreme sensitivity, inflammation or pathology).

Ischaemic compression

Caution – Direct pressure should be avoided, or performed with great care:

1. if tissues are inflamed or in remodelling phase after trauma
2. in cases of malignancy
3. close to blood vessels and nerves
4. close to attachment sites
5. if pain (local or referred) is excessive.

Direct inhibitory pressure has a long history of use in many forms of bodywork, including osteopathy, in order to achieve a release of hypertonically tense tissues, spasm, cramp, etc. Travell & Simons (1983, 1992) have suggested that trigger points receive ischaemic compression ('sustained digital pressure') for a period of between 20 seconds and 1 minute. The pressure is gradually increased as the trigger point's sensitivity (referred sensation as well as the local discomfort) reduces and the tension of the tissues housing the trigger ('taut band') eases. Stretching techniques should be applied following the compression; see integrated neuromuscular inhibition technique (INIT) below. The mechanisms involved, as seen from a Western perspective, would include 'neurological overload', the release of endogenous morphine-like products (endorphins, enkephalins) as well as 'flushing' of tissues with fresh oxygenated blood

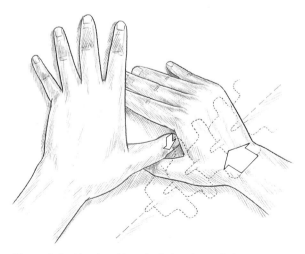

Figure 8.4 Hand positions for induration technique. Pressure used on the spinous process is measured in ounces (grams) at most.

following the compression. Oriental interpretations would include modulation of energy transmission.

See Chapter 3, Box 3.5, for more detail on compression effects.

Integrated neuromuscular inhibition technique (INIT)
(see Fig. 9.1 and Ch. 9) (Chaitow 1994)

INIT, when used to deactivate a trigger point, involves the application of a sequence that includes:

● inhibitory (ischaemic) compression until a change is reported or noted
● placing of the tissues into a position of ease, to encourage a muscle spindle release of excessive tone (see descriptions of 'positional release' below)
● introduction by the patient of an isometric contraction of the precise tissues housing the trigger point
● passive stretching of the local tissues
● active and passive stretching of the entire muscle (subsequent to another isometric contraction) (see notes on muscle energy technique (MET) below)
● activation of antagonists to muscle housing the trigger point may be used to complete the sequence.

This approach achieves a triple effect: inhibition/ischaemic compression, positional release, followed by an isometrically enhanced stretch. The sequence represents a significant advance in deactivating trigger points and the tissues that house them. The initial pressure application (and subsequent positional release and MET) may follow on from identification of the trigger point during NMT evaluation.

Muscle energy techniques (MET) – including isolytic stretch

Caution – Stretching of tissues should be avoided:

1. during the recovery and remodelling phase after injury (3 weeks)
2. if acutely painful before treatment
3. if pain is noted during stretching
4. if a joint is involved (instead of stretching soft tissues, 'slack' should be taken out until new barrier(s) have been engaged)
5. if tissues are inflamed.

Thanks to the influence on their work by Karel Lewit (1992), the more recent editions of Travell & Simons (1992) and Simons, Travell & Simons (1999) classic books on myofascial trigger points advocate the use of variations on the theme of MET.

The terms isometric and isotonic contraction, used in MET, require clear definition and emphasis.

Isometric contraction (Figs 8.5 & 8.6)

An isometric contraction is one in which a muscle, or group of muscles, or a joint or region of the body is called upon to contract, or move in a particular direction, and in which that effort is matched by the practitioner's effort, so that no movement is allowed to take place. Following a sustained (7–10 seconds) isometric contraction, two effects are noted:

1. The muscle that was contracted isometrically will display a period of approx-

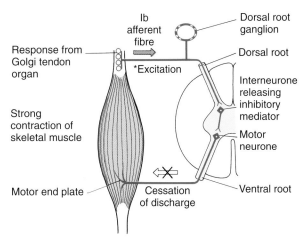

Figure 8.5A Schematic representation of the neurological effects of the loading of the Golgi tendon organs of a skeletal muscle by means of an isometric contraction, which produces a post-isometric relaxation effect in that muscle.

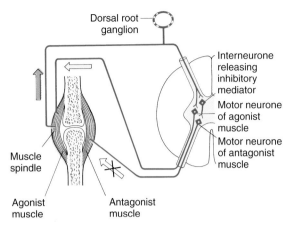

Figure 8.5B Schematic representation of the reciprocal effect of an isometric contraction of a skeletal muscle, resulting in an inhibitory influence on its antagonist.

imately 20 seconds of post-isometric relaxation, during which time it will be stretched more easily, or its deeper tissues accessed by palpating contacts (Fig. 8.5A).

2. The antagonist to the muscle that has been contracted isometrically for 7–10 seconds will be inhibited reciprocally (Fig. 8.5B), with similar reduction in tone and opportunity for stretching or deeper access.

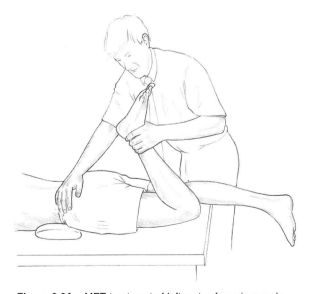

Figure 8.6A MET treatment of left rectus femoris muscle. Note the practitioner's right hand stabilises the sacrum and pelvis to prevent undue spinal stress during the stretching phase of the treatment.

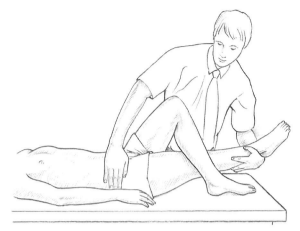

Figure 8.6B MET treatment of tensor fascia lata. If a standard MET method is being used, the stretch will follow the isometric contraction in which the patient will attempt to move the right leg to the right, against sustained resistance. It is important for the practitioner to maintain stability of the pelvis during the procedure (see pp 181/2).

Lewit (1992) advocates the therapeutic benefits of those aspects of MET (physiological use of patient-generated isometric and isotonic contractions) that are related to the achievement of post-isometric relaxation and/or reciprocal inhibition. He says:

> By involving muscular physiology we have increasingly engaged the patient's own activity; originally passive manipulative techniques became semi-active, until finally the patient began to learn self-treatment, independent of the therapist. Since these techniques are very effective in producing muscular relaxation, they can also be used to treat muscular spasm, trigger points and even referred pain.

Isotonic contraction

An isotonic contraction is one in which movement does take place, in that the counterforce offered by the practitioner is either less than that of the patient (isotonic concentric) or is greater (isotonic eccentric):

1. With an *isotonic concentric contraction* there would be an approximation of the origin and insertion of the muscle(s) involved, as the effort exerted by the patient more than matches that of the practitioner. This has a tonic effect on the

muscle(s) and is useful in toning weakened musculature.

2. With a *rapid isotonic eccentric contraction*, the origin and insertion of the muscles involved are taken further apart while the muscle is contracting, due to the greater effort of the practitioner's counterforce overcoming the muscular effort. When such a manoeuvre is performed rapidly, it is known as an *isolytic contraction*. Isolytic stretches are useful in cases where a marked degree of fibrotic change is present in the soft tissues. The effect is to create microtrauma during the rapid stretch, subsequently allowing an improvement in elasticity and circulation.

To achieve an isolytic contraction (eccentric isotonic), the patient should be instructed to use no more than 20% of possible strength on the first contraction, which is resisted and overcome by the practitioner, in a contraction lasting 2–3 seconds. This is then repeated, but with an increased degree of effort on the part of the patient (assuming the first effort was relatively painless). This continuing increase in the amount of force employed in the contracting musculature may be continued until, hopefully, a fairly strong but painless contraction effort is possible, again to be resisted and overcome by the practitioner. In some muscles, of course, this may require a heroic degree of effort on the part of the practitioner, and alternative methods would need to be found. NMT would seem to offer one such alternative. The isolytic manoeuvre should have as its ultimate aim a fully relaxed muscle, able to reach its normal resting length. This will seldom be possible in one treatment session.

3. A *slow isotonic eccentric contraction* offers various important clinical benefits (Lewit 1999, Liebenson 2001, Norris 1999):

● To tone postural (type I) muscles that may have lost their endurance potential, a slow isotonic eccentric contraction should be performed, involving increasing degrees of effort. For example, slowly overcome flexion of the wrist forcing it into extension (i.e. the arm flexors, which are postural type I muscles, are stretched while contracting).

● To relax hypertonic postural (type I) muscles, a slow isotonic eccentric stretch should be performed of their inhibited antagonists (using 40–80% strength). For example, slowly overcome the extended wrist, forcing it into flexion (i.e. the arm extensors, which are phasic type II muscles, are contracting but their effort is overcome). See Fig. 8.7.

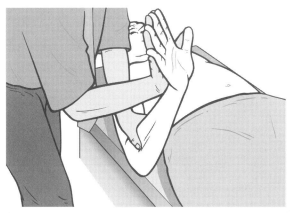
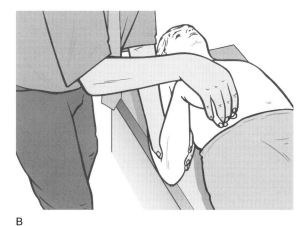

A   B

Figure 8.7 Slow eccentric isotonic stretch of inhibited extensor muscles in order to tone them and release tense flexor muscles. From Chaitow (2001), with permission.

Percussion technique or spondylotherapy

For soft tissue treatment

Trigger points can be treated effectively using a series of percussive strokes according to Travell & Simons (1992):

1. The muscle is lengthened to the point of onset of passive resistance.
2. The clinician or patient uses a hard rubber mallet or reflex hammer to hit the trigger point at exactly the same place approximately 10 times.
3. This should be done at a slow rate of no more than one impact per second, but at least one impact every 5 seconds; slower rates are likely to be more effective.

Travell & Simons suggest that this enhances, or substitutes for, intermittent cold with stretch ('spray and stretch') methods, as described above.

The muscles that they list as benefiting most from percussion techniques include quadratus, brachioradialis, long finger extensors and peroneus longus and brevis.

Caution – It is specifically suggested that anterior and posterior compartment leg muscle should not be treated by percussion, owing to the risk of compartment syndrome, should bleeding occur in the muscle.

TCM percussion

Contraindications:

- acute disease
- severe heart disease
- tuberculosis
- malignant tumours
- haemorrhagic disease
- skin disease in area to be treated
- poor constitutional states such as malnutrition or asthenia.

In recent years, Chinese methods involving percussion have added dramatically to our knowledge of the potential of these methods

(Zhao-Pu 1991). In traditional Chinese medicine (TCM), percussion methods are incorporated into a broad heading of 'acupressure'. Zhao-Pu states:

Acupressure is based on the same theory as acupuncture and uses the same points and meridians . . . the therapeutic effect of acupressure technique lies in the way in which it regulates and normalises blocked functions.

Included in these functions (as well as hypothesised energy transmission) are, 'stimulating circulation of blood . . . and improving conductivity of nerves.'

In TCM, percussion techniques involve one of three variations (Fig. 8.8):

1. One-finger percussion, using the middle finger braced by the thumb and index finger.
2. Three-finger percussion, using the thumb, index and middle fingers.

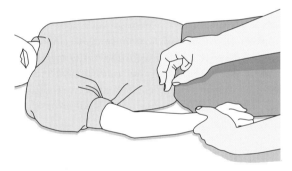

Figure 8.8A One-finger percussion uses middle finger braced by thumb and index finger. Redrawn from Zhao-Pu (1991), with permission.

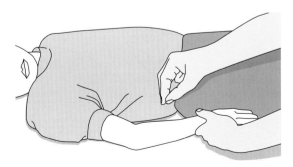

Figure 8.8B Three-finger percussion uses thumb, index and middle finger. Redrawn from Zhao-Pu (1991), with permission.

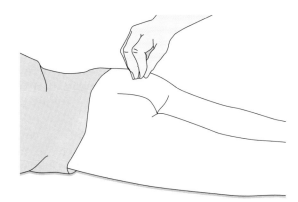

Figure 8.8C Five-finger percussion uses thumb and all fingers. Redrawn from Zhao-Pu (1991), with permission.

3. Five-finger percussion, using the thumb and all fingers.

The degree of force applied during percussion is also of three types:

1. Light, which involves a movement of the hand from the wrist joint
2. Medium, which involves a movement from the elbow joint with wrist fairly rigid
3. Strong, which involves a movement of the the upper arm, from the shoulder, with a rigid wrist.

Treatment is offered daily, on alternate days or once every 3 days, and a course would involve 20 sessions. Patients often receive three courses or more.

Professor Wang Zhao-Pu (whose work using this approach was based on his extensive experience as an orthopaedic surgeon) describes remarkable clinical results involving patients with paralysis and cerebral birth injuries. He states (Zhao-Pu 1991):

Research was carried out on the cerebral haemodynamics of patients with cerebral birth injury before and after acupressure (percussion and pressure techniques) therapy. Scanning techniques were used in monitoring the short half-life radioactive materials through the cerebral circulation; in almost one-third of the patients the regional cerebral blood flow was increased after acupressure therapy ranging from 28 to 60 sessions.

In an introduction to Zhao-Pu's book, Graeme Schofield states:

After cerebral birth injury, significant though the damage may be, there are large areas of the brain and many millions of nerve cells which are still intact. These areas and the cells they contain are the targets of education for future living.

This approach is, therefore, not one that produces instant results, but that influences and gradually harnesses the potential for recovery and improvement that is latent in the tissues of the patient. For more information on oriental bodywork approaches, a complete manual of Chinese therapeutic massage (with many aspects that echo NMT methodology) edited by Sun Chengnan is highly recommended (Chengnan 1990).

Western percussion

Contraindications:

- osteoporosis
- malignancy
- inflammation in the area to be treated
- recent trauma in the area to be treated
- pain during application of percussive treatment.

In order to stimulate organs via the spinal pathways, direct percussion techniques have long been employed by osteopathic and chiropractic practitioners.

Over the past century in the USA, a number of mechanical methods of percussion has evolved (Abrams 1922), as have effective manual systems in which the middle finger is placed on the appropriate spinous process(es) while the other hand concusses the finger with a series of rapidly rebounding blows. This approach is known as spondylotherapy (Johnson 1939) (see Fig. 8.9). One or two percussive repetitions are applied per second. Spondylotherapy percussion is usually applied to a series of three or four (or more) adjacent vertebrae.

An example of this is the treatment, as above, of the 5th thoracic spinous process, proceeding downwards to the 9th, in the case of liver dysfunction. Treatment would be applied only if the area were painful to palpating pressure. Similarly, concussion over the 10th, 11th and

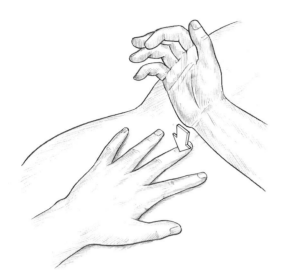

Figure 8.9 Percussion technique (spondylotherapy) for reflexive effects or treatment of trigger points (slow percussion).

12th thoracic spinous processes would stimulate kidney function.

In order to stimulate the organ or tissues using the spinal reflexes, percussion would involve only a short amount of time: 15–30-second applications repeated three or four times, over approximately 4–5 minutes. A mild 'flare up' of symptoms and increased sensitivity in the area treated would normally indicate that the desired degree of stimulation had been achieved. In order to inhibit function or to produce dilatation of local blood vessels, Johnson (1939) suggests that percussive repetitions be repeated for prolonged periods to fatigue the reflex.

Manual spondylotherapy complements NMT by virtue of its reflex influences and its ease of application. Needless to say, a sound knowledge of spinal mechanics and neurological connections is a prerequisite to its usage.

Piriformis muscle technique
(Retzlaff et al 1974)

Contraindications:

- severe pain on application of pressure
- pain on rotation of hip joint as described
- sciatic inflammation.

The piriformis muscle syndrome results from contraction of the muscle either due to trauma or repetitive mechanical or postural stress, or due to the presence in the muscle of active trigger points. The effects of piriformis shortening can be circulatory, neurological, reflex or functional, inducing pain and paraesthesia of the affected limb as well as alterations to pelvic and lumbar function, as the muscle anchors the sacrum to the femur. Diagnosis usually hinges on the absence of spinal causative factors for the symptoms.

Piriformis muscle syndrome is frequently characterised by such bizarre symptoms that they may seem to be unrelated. One characteristic complaint is a persistent, severe, radiating low-back pain extending from the sacrum to the hip joint, over the gluteal region and the posterior portion of the upper leg and down to the popliteal space. In the most severe cases the patient will be unable to lie or stand comfortably, and changes in position will not relieve the pain. Intense pain will occur when the patient sits or squats.

A common sign of the piriformis syndrome is a persistent external rotation of the upper leg. This indication, which is known as the positive piriformis sign, is easily detected when the patient is examined in the supine position.

The buttock on the same side as the piriformis lesion is usually sensitive to touch or palpation. Severe pain may occur when pressure is applied to the area over the piriformis muscle and its tendinous insertion on the head of the greater trochanter.

Another diagnostic sign may be the shortening of the leg on the affected side due to contraction of the piriformis muscle. In cases where the leg on the opposite side appears shortened, it is probable that some other dysfunction exists, and that the condition is not directly related to the piriformis syndrome.

The patient may also mention pain that follows the distribution pattern of the sciatic nerve to the level of the popliteal space and sometimes to the more distal branches of this nerve. When the common perineal nerve is involved, there may be a paraesthesia of the posterior surface of the upper leg and some portions of the lower leg.

One of the most perplexing problems arising from the piriformis syndrome is the involvement of the pudendal nerve and blood vessels. This nerve, with its branches, provides the major sensory innervation of the perineal skin and the somatic motor innervation of much of the external genitalia and related perineal musculature in both women and men. The pudendal blood vessels supply essentially the same areas. The pudendal nerve, after passing through the greater sciatic foramen, re-enters the pelvis by way of the lesser sciatic foramen. In a significant proportion of people, the perineal and tibial components of the sciatic nerve actually pass through the piriformis muscle, giving rise in these individuals to a greater likelihood of severe symptoms if the muscle shortens or is stressed (Polstein 1991). Compression of the pudendal nerve and blood vessels can result in serious problems involving the functioning of the genitalia in both sexes. Since external rotation of the upper legs is required for women during coitus, if there were interference with the blood supply and innervation of the genitalia, it is understandable that a female patient might complain of pain during sexual intercourse. This could also be a basis for impotency in men. Ischaemic compression applied by thumb or elbow, together with stretching of the muscle to its normal resting length (with or without MET), is usually sufficient to remedy the problem.

Precise localisation of piriformis trigger points/landmarks

The patient is side-lying, tested side uppermost. The practitioner stands at the level of the pelvis in front of, and facing, the patient and, in order to contact the femoral attachment of piriformis, draws imaginary lines between:

- ASIS and the ischial tuberosity, and
- PSIS and the most prominent point of trochanter.

Where these reference lines cross, just posterior to the trochanter, is the insertion of the

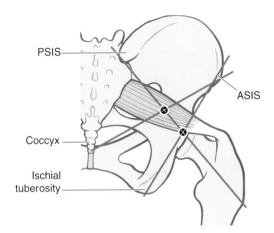

Figure 8.10 Using bony landmarks as coordinates, the commonest tender points are located in piriformis, in the belly and at the attachment or the muscle. From Chaitow (2001), with permission.

muscle, and pressure here will produce marked discomfort if the structure is short or irritated.

If the most common piriformis trigger point site, in the belly of the muscle, is sought, then the line from the ASIS should be taken to the tip of the coccyx rather than to the ischial tuberosity.

Pressure where this line crosses the other will access the midpoint of the belly of piriformis, where triggers are common. Light compression here that produces a painful response is indicative of a stressed muscle and possibly an active myofascial trigger point (Fig. 8.10).

Piriformis treatment

Piriformis method 1

1. The patient is side-lying, close to the edge of the table, affected side uppermost, both legs flexed at hip and knee.

2. The practitioner stands facing the patient at hip level.

3. The practitioner places his or her cephalad elbow tip gently over the point behind trochanter, where piriformis inserts, or on to the central area of the muscle belly, where an active trigger point is common.

4. The patient should be close enough to the edge of the table for the practitioner to stabilise the pelvis against his or her trunk (Fig. 8.11).

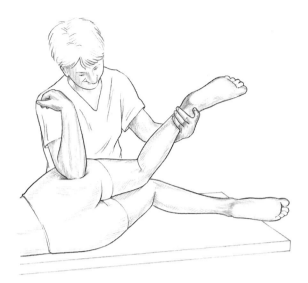

Figure 8.11 Combined ischaemic compression (elbow or thumb) and MET applied to piriformis muscle.

5. At the same time, the practitioner's caudad hand grasps the ankle and uses this to bring the upper leg/hip into internal rotation, taking out all the slack in piriformis.

6. A degree of inhibitory pressure (sufficient to cause discomfort but not pain) is applied via the elbow for 5–7 seconds while the muscle is kept at a reasonable but not excessive degree of stretch.

7. The practitioner maintains contact on the point, but eases pressure, and asks the patient to introduce an isometric contraction (25% of strength, for 5–7 seconds) to piriformis by bringing the lower leg towards the table against resistance, attempting to rotate the hip externally.

8. After the contraction ceases, and the patient relaxes, the lower limb is taken to its new resistance barrier, and elbow pressure is reapplied.

9. This process is repeated until no further gain is achieved.

This method is a variation on the method advocated by Te Poorten (1969), which calls for longer and heavier compression, and no intermediate isometric contractions.

Piriformis method 2

1. In the first stage of this alternative method, the patient lies on the non-affected side with knees flexed and hip joints flexed to 90°.

2. The practitioner places his or her elbow on the piriformis musculotendinous junction and a steady pressure of 20–30 lbs (9–13 kg) is applied.
3. With the other hand, the practitioner abducts the foot so that it will force an internal rotation of the upper leg.
4. The leg is held in this rotated position, at its elastic barrier, for periods of up to 2 minutes.
5. This procedure is repeated two or three times.
6. The patient is then placed in the supine position and the affected leg is tested for freedom of both external and internal rotation.

Proprioceptive adjustment (applied kinesiology)
(Figs 8.12 & 8.13) (Walther 1988)

Kinesiological muscle tone correction utilises two key receptors in muscles to achieve its effects. These are the muscle's spindles, which are responsible for reporting on muscle length and changes in length, and the Golgi tendon organs, which report on the load on, or tension of, the muscle (Fig. 8.13).

A muscle in spasm may be helped to relax by the application of direct pressure (using 1–7 kg (2–15 lbs) of pressure:

STRENGTHEN

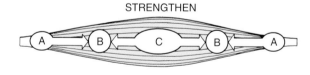

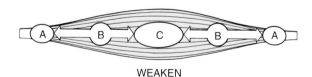

WEAKEN

A = golgi tendon organs

B = belly of muscle

C = muscle spindle

Figure 8.12 Proprioceptive manipulation of muscles (see text).

- away from the belly of the muscle, in the area of the Golgi tendon organs; and/or
- application of the same amount of pressure towards the belly of the muscle, in the area of the muscle spindle cells (see Fig. 8.12).

The precisely opposite effects (i.e. toning or strengthening the muscle) are said to be achieved by applying pressure:

- away from the belly of the muscle, in the muscle spindle region; and
- towards the belly of the muscle in the Golgi tendon organ region.

Note that Janda (1990, 1992), in particular, takes the view that weakness in a muscle can best be addressed by dealing with (stretching, etc.) hypertonicity in its antagonist(s). Similarly, strength can be restored to a muscle by slowly stretching it during an isotonic eccentric contraction (which will simultaneously reduce tone in hypertonic antagonist). (See section on Muscle energy techniques, above.)

Psoas techniques

In postural distortion such as scoliosis, or marked lumbar lordosis, as well as in many

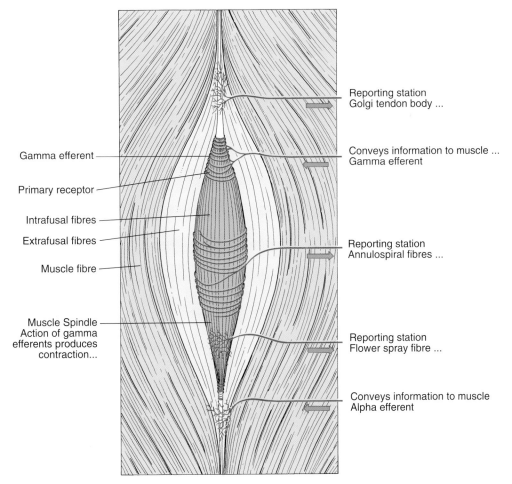

Figure 8.13   Illustration of muscle spindles, showing Golgi tendon organ and neural pathways to and from these reporting stations.

acute low back and sciatic cases, the iliopsoas muscle is found to be involved (Lewit 1996, 1999).

Contraindications to methods listed below:

- aortic disease (e.g. aneurism, calcification)
- inflammatory bowel or pelvic disease
- pain on application of palpatory pressure, as described below.

Test for psoas shortness

A simple test involves the patient lying at the end of the bed with the unaffected (non-tested) side leg in full flexion at hip and knee, and the tested leg hanging freely. If the thigh is parallel with the floor/table, and has sufficient flexibility to allow for an easy depression into slight extension, the iliopsoas is considered normal; however, if it is elevated, or is parallel with the floor but has no 'give' when pushed lightly into extension, shortness is presumed.

Psoas technique – direct inhibitory pressure

Method (a)

1. The patient lies supine with knees flexed, hands at side.
2. The practitioner stands on the side opposite the contracted psoas.
3. One hand presses down firmly through the linea alba, 3–4 inches (7–10 cm) below the umbilicus, until the gently probing fingers contact the body of the 4th to 5th lumbars.
4. The practitioner then eases fingers over the curved anterior surface of the lumbar body, towards the contralateral side, until the attachment of psoas is located.
5. Firm but gentle pressure is maintained for about 1 minute (Fig. 8.14A, B).

Method (b)

1. Same as method (a), practitioner is standing on opposite side to contraction.
2. Same contact with fingers through linea alba but with the other hand bringing the flexed leg towards the opposite shoulder and rotating the pelvis against probing fingers.

Method (c)

1. Same as method (a), except practitioner places flexed leg on the table to support the patient's leg on contracted psoas side.
2. In this manner, both hands are free to support each other as they penetrate heavier abdomens (Fig. 8.14C).

Method (d)

1. Same as method (a), except practitioner's flexed leg supports both of the patient's legs.
2. This is especially useful when there is a contraction of both psoas muscles (Fig. 8.14D).

Instead of accessing psoas directly through the linea alba, an oblique contact to the belly of the muscle can be made by applying fingertip pressure towards the spine from the lateral border of rectus abdominis (not illustrated).

In addition, MET may be used by having the patient briefly contract the muscle against resistance ('bring your knee toward your face'), after which easier access, and a more relaxed muscle, should be noted. Additional tactics include having the patient slowly lengthen (extend) and flex the hip, while direct pressure is maintained on the attachment, or the belly, or psoas.

Note: To apply the methods, as described, the practitioner stands contralaterally when using the linea alba access, and ipsilaterally when applying the oblique access contact.

A number of additional MET and strain/counterstrain approaches exist for safely treating psoas, and appropriate texts should be consulted for details of these (Chaitow 2001, 2002).

Pump techniques – lymphatics, liver or spleen
(Arbuckle 1977, Fielding 1983)

Indications for the use of lymphatic pump techniques include all conditions that involve congestion, lymphatic stasis and infection (apart from those listed under 'Contraindications'). Wallace et al (1997) report:

Lymphatic pump techniques are designed to augment the pressure gradients that develop between the

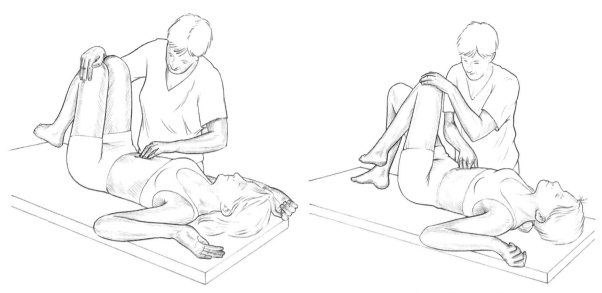

Figure 8.14A Direct finger pressure applied to left side of psoas attachment to spinal structures.

Figure 8.14B Use of altered knee positions to enhance access to left side of psoas attachments.

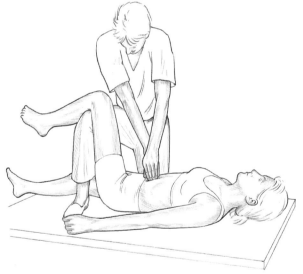

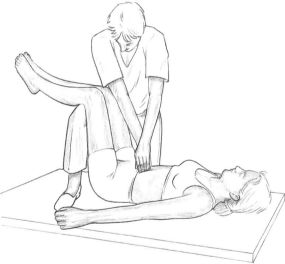

Figure 8.14C Two-handed contact to reinforce psoas contact, with use of practitioner's leg to support patient's contralateral leg in order to modify overlying muscle and psoas tension (left).

Figure 8.14 Psoas techniques.

Figure 8.14D Both patient's legs supported by practitioner's leg as a means of modifying psoas tension in cases of bilateral psoas dysfunction.

thoracic and abdominal regions during normal respirations.

The benefits of enhanced lymphatic movement – encouraged by the various techniques described in this section – include (Wallace et al 1997):

- increased resorption of fluids
- increased circulation and respiration

- decreased proteins in the interstitium
- facilitation from a more beneficial pH balance.

Caution – It is important to make sure that the patient has no food, chewing gum or loose dentures in the mouth when these procedures are being applied.

Contraindications to pump techniques:

- malignant or other serious diseases of the lungs, liver, spleen or associated organs
- recent abdominal or thoracic surgery
- hepatitis
- infectious mononucleosis
- osteoporosis
- fracture, dislocation or other painful dysfunction involving the joints of the thoracic cage or spine
- avoid thoracic pump techniques where the patient has a reduced cough reflex.

Pectoralis release

Release of pectoralis minor produces an increased range of movement for the upper ribs, and a consequent increase in thoracic volume (Wallace et al 1997). This allows subsequent pump techniques (see below) to be applied more effectively. Kuchera & Kuchera (1994) note that 'a one centimeter increase in the diameter of the chest increases air intake by 200 to 400 cc'. The effect on lymphatic drainage is profound, because the pumping action involved in the breathing process impacts directly on lymph motion. Kuchera & Kuchera (1994) also note:

This is an efficacious technique that can be used with relative ease with patients with brittle bones, with patients in the intensive care unit, where multiple tubes and monitoring devices may be in place, and with post-surgical patients.

In other words, it is a safe procedure!

Method for pectoralis minor release

- The patient is supine with the arms comfortably at the side.
- The practitioner, while standing at the head of the table, places the palms of the hands (having ensured nails are well clipped) into the

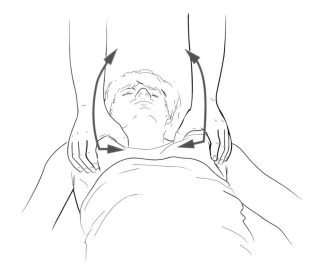

Figure 8.15 Direct myofascial stretch for pectoralis minor.

axilla, palms touching the medial humerus, thumb side of index fingers touching the axilla.

- In this way the dorsum of the fingers are located under the lateral border of each pectoralis minor.
- The practitioner then slowly externally rotates the arms and, using gentle pressure, insinuates fingertips under the lateral border of the muscle.
- The hands, the palms of which are now facing medially, are then drawn lightly toward each other (medially) until all the slack in pectoralis minor has been removed (Fig. 8.15).
- The practitioner's hands then slowly, deliberately and painlessly lift the tissues towards the ceiling, to their elastic barrier, easing the muscle away from its attachments, until all slack has been removed (i.e. no actual stretching is taking place at this stage, merely a removal of all slack).
- The practitioner should then transfer body weight backwards to introduce a lean, which removes the slack further, by tractioning the muscles in a superior direction (toward the head).
- The muscle fibres will now have been eased medially, anteriorly and superiorly, and should be held at these combined barriers as they

slowly release over the next few minutes, as the patient breathes deeply and slowly.

● If correctly applied, this procedure should not be painful. Wallace et al (1997) note: 'The combination of traction and respiratory motion releases the upper thoracic muscle tension.'

Lymphatic pump method (a)

1. Patient is prone, pillow under chest, arms over the side, with the practitioner standing at the head of the table, facing caudad.
2. The practitioner's thumbs are pressed, bilaterally, on to the intertransverse spaces, starting at the base of the neck (Fig. 8.16A).
3. Pressure is exerted towards the floor as the patient swings the arms forwards.
4. This swing is repeated each time the thumbs move down one intervertebral space.
5. This will have a stimulating effect on the lymphatic drainage of the body as a whole.
6. The effect is enhanced if the patient inhales deeply during the procedure and coincides the strong swing of the arms with the cycle of the breath.

Lymphatic pump method (b)
(Sleszynski & Kelso 1993, Wallace et al 1997)

1. The patient lies supine, knees and hips flexed.
2. The practitioner is at the head of the table with hands spread across the patient's chest, below the clavicles, with thumbs resting next to each other on the sternum, fingers spread laterally. The arms should be more or less straight for ease of transmission of force from the shoulder to the hands.
3. Pressure is introduced by the practitioner, in a downwards and caudad direction, which is just sufficient to overcome resistance, by means of a repetitive, minimal, flexion and extension of the elbows.
4. The patient continues to breathe normally and does not resist the repetitive pressure applied by the practitioner, which should be between a rate of 100 and 120 per minute.
5. The patient breathes through the mouth, and the pumping action takes over the respiratory

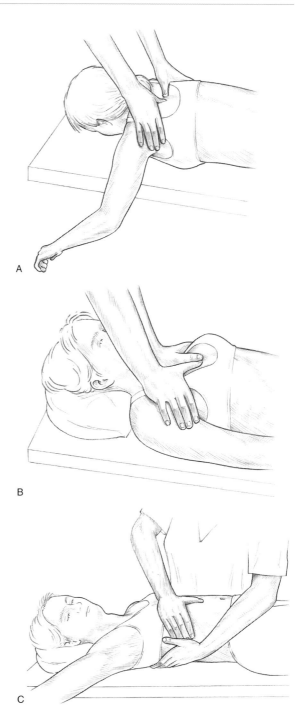

A

B

C

Figure 8.16 Lymphatic pump techniques. (A) Patient prone. (B) Patient supine. (C) Liver pump technique.

function (Fig. 8.16B). This should continue for at least 3 minutes, and for up to 5 minutes.

In babies, the method can be used with one hand over the sternum, the other under the spine, with the baby cradled or seated on the practitioner's lap. The effect of this is to improve lymphatic drainage dramatically. This method is useful in all cases of oedema and infection. It also has a beneficial effect on immune function (Hoag 1969).

Treatment using Chapman's reflexes (see Ch. 4) provides additional localised drainage, which supports the general drainage and stimulation of lymphatic function. These methods are particularly useful in children. None of the procedures described should be painful.

Lymphatic pump method (c)

1. The patient, practitioner and the hand positions are as in method (b) above.
2. The patient inhales and exhales fully through an open mouth.
3. As the patient exhales, the practitioner, elbows straight, encourages exhalation by applying pressure to the upper thorax, and maintains the degree of compression achieved at the full exhalation.
4. This process is repeated three or four times, with the degree of sustained compression increasing slightly after each exhalation (i.e. the patient commences each subsequent breath with the upper chest held in compression).
5. Approximately a third to a half of the way through the fourth or fifth inhalation, as pressure builds up against the restraining hands, these should be removed extremely rapidly, releasing pressure from the chest. A vacuum will have been created and a sound of in-rushing air should be heard. A byproduct of this should be a major shift in lymphatic movement.

Liver/spleen pump method

1. A simple measure, via which function of either the liver or the spleen may be enhanced, involves the practitioner standing on the side opposite the organ that is being stimulated (left side of patient, reaching across for the liver, and vice versa for the spleen).
2. The patient is supine, knees and hips flexed, and the practitioner's caudad hand is placed under the lower ribs, and the other is placed anteriorly, just medial to the costal cartilages of the lower five ribs (Fig. 8.16C).
3. Bimanual compression should initially be carried out in a direct anterior–posterior direction, in a rhythmic manner in which the hands squeeze the tissues together approximately 20 times per minute, for 1–2 minutes.
4. After this, the direction of the pumping action should be in a more anterolateral direction, for a further minute.
5. The effect on the spleen is such as to increase the leucocyte count by an average of 2200 cells per cubic millimetre (Castlio 1955, Wallace et al 1997).

SKIN TECHNIQUES

Skin rolling

Skin rolling (see Figs 8.17 and 5.5) is a useful all-purpose approach that involves the use of either or both hands. The fingers draw tissue towards the practitioner whilst the ball(s) of the thumb(s) roll over the gathered mound of tissue. In this way the tissue is effectively lifted, stretched and squeezed. The most useful areas of application

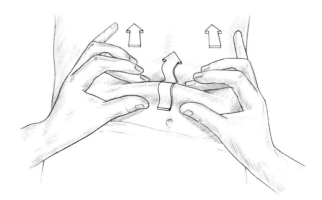

Figure 8.17 Skin rolling method.

occur where the tissues lie tight to the underlying structures, such as directly over the shoulder joint and on the lateral aspect of the thigh. The squeezing pressure imparted by the roll of the thumb can be extremely uncomfortable, and care should be exercised during its application. The angle of stretch, pull and roll may be varied and repeated several times to impart maximum stimulus to the reflex effects and to stimulate circulation and drainage. The degree of stretch and/or pinch employed during rolling of the tissues is a variable factor that the practitioner may decide upon, depending upon the amount of stimulus called for. Either skin alone, or skin and underlying tissue, may be lifted, stretched and stimulated (pinched) in this way.

Stanley Lief and Boris Chaitow employed this simple, yet effective, manoeuvre as part of their general treatment. The latter described its usefulness as follows (B. Chaitow, personal communication, 1983):

One of my favourite techniques to enhance nerve and blood circulation is 'skin rolling'. Between the skin and the muscular and bony structures it covers, is a veritable network of blood and nerve structures and functions which can, and often do, fail to achieve their full, effective circulation for high efficiency and health because the skin is often so adhered to its lower structures (fascia) that circulation and function is appreciably reduced. This of course adversely affects the efficiency and health of the patient. There is probably no formula that will enhance this aspect of function more effectively than 'skin rolling'. A specific example of its effective benefit is to skin-roll a major joint such as a shoulder in conditions of articular rheumatism, arthritis, neuritis, frozen shoulder etc.

Traditional Chinese medicine calls for this procedure to be undertaken from the base of the spine upwards, for a tonifying effect, and from the neck downwards, for a sedating effect.

Treating hyperalgesic skin zones – stretching
(Lewit 1992)

As noted in earlier chapters, the skin overlying regions or points of reflex activity will frequently be found to have markedly reduced elasticity and to adhere to underlying structures (see Fig. 5.6 and the text that discusses assessment of these areas in Ch. 5).

1. To treat hyperalgesia, the fingertips (for a small area) or the ulnar aspects of the crossed hands (for a larger area) are placed together on the skin surface overlying the affected area, and the tissues are stretched apart, to their easy resistance barrier, as the fingers, or hands, separate.
2. To establish the presence or lack of physiological elasticity, the skin is stretched in various directions.
3. If restriction is noted, the tissues are held in a painlessly stretched position until a degree of release is noted. This commonly takes 10–20 seconds.
4. The same area may be stretched in this manner in various appropriate directions, each time being held at its barrier of resistance until a release occurs (see Fig. 5.7A,B).
5. The release of the tissues is itself the therapeutic effort, providing reflex stimulus to underlying structures.
6. The subsequent maintenance of the free elastic state of the tissues is evidence of an improvement in the causative factors. Naturally, if underlying factors maintain the reflex activity, whether this be musculoskeletal or visceral dysfunction, the improvement will be short lived.

Hyperalgesic skin zones (HSZs) are useful diagnostically and prognostically. Lewit (1992) states:

If pain is due to the HSZ, this method is quite as effective as needling, electrostimulation and other similar methods. Moreover, it is entirely painless, and can be applied by the patient himself.

Such zones are frequently noted with musculoskeletal conditions and in chronic pain syndromes. In cases of recurrent headache, HSZs are found medially below the mastoid process, at the temples and eyebrows, and on the forehead above the eyebrows, and on both sides of the nose. This correlates with many of Bennett's neurovascular reflexes, as discussed in previous chapters.

Treating hyperalgesic skin zones – positional release

1. The practitioner places a contact (finger pad(s) or whole hand) on to the skin, which appears less pliable, more adherent (to underlying fascia; see Ch. 5) or palpates as 'different' to, or more sensitive than, surrounding tissues, suggesting that it is a HSZ.

2. The contact hand or finger pad(s) should slide the skin superiorly and inferiorly, medially and laterally, and should turn in a clockwise and then an anticlockwise direction, and with each of these movements should seek the direction of most comfort and least tension/bind.

3. The motion of the contact fingers or whole hand on the tissues is asking: 'In which direction do the tissues move most easily?' (Fig. 8.18).

4. When the various positions of ease, evaluated in this way, are 'stacked' together, this produces the combined 'preference pattern' – the skin and fascia will have been taken in their respective directions of motion away from whatever restriction barriers they currently exhibit.

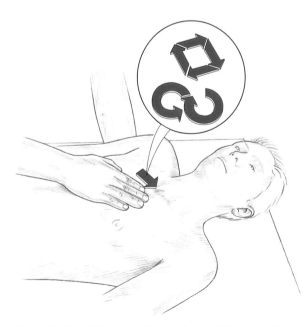

Figure 8.18 Achieving positional release of tissues – skin and fascia – by holding them in their preferred 'ease' directions. From Chaitow (2002), with permission.

5. Normal, unstressed, tissues exhibit an equal excursion in all directions of rotation, although this is seldom found in adults, even if surgical trauma has not been a factor (Zink & Lawson 1979).

6. The final position of ease should be held until tension releases spontaneously, usually a period of 30–90 seconds. This will commonly release recently acquired stress patterns in the fascia, possibly revealing older patterns, which can then be treated.

Lengthening soft tissues: 'C' and 'S' bends, and myofascial release

Lederman (1997) has described the relatively few ways in which tissues can be modified by forms of direct therapeutic pressure. These involve:

● Tension loading – including traction, stretching and other lengthening approaches are involved, resulting in changes in connective tissue status (see 'C' bends below).
● Compression loading, on the other hand, shortens and widens tissues. See Chapter 3, Box 3.5, for a summary of these effects, which include fluid changes as well (possibly) as changes in length.
● Rotation loading elongates some fibres while compressing others (see 'S' bend description below).
● Bending loading combines compression loading (on the concave side) and tension loading on the convex side (see 'C' bend description below).
● Shearing loading involves shift or translation movements and is used primarily in joint mobilisation, while elongating and compressing associated soft tissues.
● Combined loading incorporates a variety of the models listed above (see Fig. 8.21).

Other variables to be considered when evaluating therapeutic 'pressure' include:

● The degree of pressure (see Box 3.6).
● How great an area of contact is involved and/or how large an area is receiving one or other form of loading.

- How great an amplitude is involved – in other words, how far are the tissues being taken, stretched? (The degree of force largely determines the amplitude.)
- How rapid is the application of force – does it involve high velocity or low velocity?
- For how long are the tissues loaded?
- Is the application of force static or rhythmic, and, if rhythmic, is it rapid or slow, perhaps coinciding with the breathing cycle?
- How steady is the force application, static or moving (gliding)?
- Is the patient participating in the process, actively moving, or resisting the force application?

Examples of the application of force include the 'C' and 'S' bend techniques.

 'C' bend technique

In order to lengthen local areas of muscle and/or connective tissue, the tissues may be bent (into a 'C' shape) to a first barrier of resistance, so that the thumbs engage the barrier, waiting for this to release and retreat, over a period of 5–30 seconds. Lewit (1996) points out:

Shortness of the connective tissue is most characteristic for short (taut) muscles, usually overactive muscles. Producing a tissue fold and stretching it is the most effective way to obtain lengthening because the stretch reflex can be avoided.

See Fig. 8.23A for an example of a 'C' bend, fold, applied to the distal aspects of the iliotibial band. In that example, as described and illustrated later in this chapter (under the heading Tensor fascia lata techniques), the method involves a series of rapid, high-velocity, low-amplitude 'snapping' bends of the tissues. For structures that are less rigid than the iliotibial band, the 'C' bend is performed slowly, allowing a lengthening to occur (Lewit 1996).

'S' bend technique

To achieve a relaxation of a specific area of muscle tension using an 'S' bend, the hands should be positioned in such a way as to allow thumb or hand pressure to be applied across the

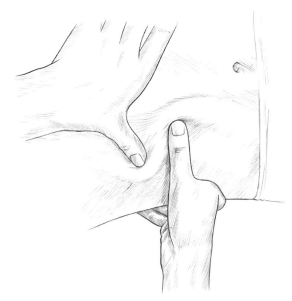

Figure 8.19 'S' bend pressure applied to tense or fibrotic musculature.

fibres of a contracted or indurated muscle, so that the contacts are travelling in opposite directions to each other (Lewit 1992). As pressure is applied simultaneously with each thumb or hand (see Figs 8.19 and 8.23B), the tissues between the two contacts will progressively have the slack removed, and be placed in a slightly lengthened situation, in which they can be held until release occurs (or 'springing' is introduced).

This technique can be applied along the course of particularly spastic, and hard unyielding, tissues, in addition to the basic NMT thumb technique (see Chs 6 & 7). Additionally the 'S' bend may be used with a flicking action of the thumb to complete the stroke, once effective tension has been created in the tissues by the opposing thumbs. This 'springing' has the effect of stimulating local circulation most effectively and, if the tissues are not too sensitive, may be effective in breaking down infiltrated or indurated tissues.

The 'S' contact is so named because the tissues being treated form that shape as the strokes are performed. If used in its 'slow' mode, the tissues are held in this opposition lengthening state for upwards of 30 seconds, before slightly different fibres are selected for the same procedure. Alternatively a rapid, heel of hand, thrust, across the tissues (see Fig. 8.23B), may be used on particularly rigid structures such as the iliotibial band. This approach is described later in the chapter.

Stretching fascia – myofascial release

The skin stretching methods described above under the heading 'Treating hyperalgesic skin zones – stretching' are, in effect, examples of miniature myofascial release. Whenever skin, or other soft tissues, fails to present symmetrical freedom of movement, either in terms of lengthening potential, range of motion or ability to glide on underlying tissues, a degree of dysfunction can be assumed (Lewit 1996). Lewit describes releasing these tightened, often fascial, tissues as 'shifting', rather than stretching. Tissues are taken to their painless elastic barrier, by application of a separation force between the hands or fingers, and held until a lengthening occurs. For examples, see Fig. 8.20A,B.

SOFT TISSUE MANIPULATION – INCLUDING MASSAGE

The term 'soft tissue manipulation' (STM) can be used to incorporate all manual methods (including massage) that address tissues other than bone. STM therefore incorporates the main topics of this book. Neuromuscular technique, muscle energy techniques and positional release methods (e.g. strain/counterstrain) can (with other modalities such as chilling agents) all be used as effective measures to detect, and help normalise, dysfunctional soft tissues, including areas housing noxious trigger points, which can themselves be associated with, and at times be responsible for, the promotion or maintenance of muscular weakness, muscular contraction, pain, vasodilatation, vasoconstriction, tissue degeneration, gastrointestinal, respiratory and a myriad other disorders, including emotional and 'psychological' disorders (Baldry 1993, Lewit 1999, Simons et al 1999).

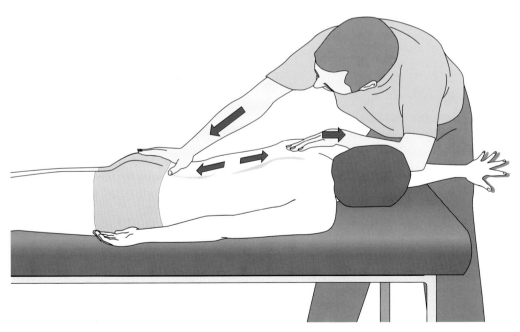

Figure 8.20A   Myofascial release of the thoracic fascia. Redrawn from Lewit (1996).

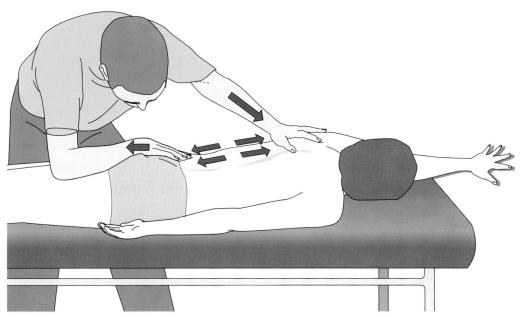

Figure 8.20B   Releasing the axillary lateral thoracic fascia and pectoralis fibres (abdominal attachments). Redrawn from Lewit (1996).

The logical approach to correction of dysfunction involving shortened tight musculature, is to identify the reasons for their dysfunction, and possibly to lengthen and stretch these tissues. NMT and muscle energy techniques are useful in achieving this, as are positional release methods, especially in more acute settings. Such an approach may involve any combination of the many variations of these techniques, and could include deep NMT followed by MET methods, which employ post-isometric relaxation, as well as reciprocal inhibition, and also isotonic (isolytic) methods that contribute towards breaking down fibrotic contractions.

Is there a 'correct' sequence of therapy?

Treatment of dysfunction associated with muscles that have become weak could involve initial attention to their antagonists, which may be inhibiting them, as well as to isotonic concentric MET methods applied to weakened muscles, plus exercises specific to the area. Possible joint influences on dysfunctional soft tissues should be addressed, either through mobilisation or, in instances where true joint blockage exists, by active (high-velocity thrust) manipulation. It is a contention of many practitioners who work with somatic dysfunction that in most instances soft tissue normalisation leads to joint normalisation; however, the reverse is not a rarity, and at times the joint restriction is primary (Lewit 1996, 1999, Chaitow 2001).

General postural re-education and body-toning exercises could follow. Before such exercise is initiated, it is important to discover and treat local dysfunction within shortened or weakened muscles – such as trigger points – and NMT will usefully help towards achieving this. It is often useful to allow the results of normalisation of shortened muscles to unfold without confusing the issue by focusing on the weakened antagonists too soon, as a natural toning effect will occur when inhibitory influences are removed.

If, after several weeks of treatment (and possibly home stretching) of the shortened, contracted, postural muscles and their trigger points, there is not an observable and measurable improvement in the weak antagonists, then MET and exercise could usefully be introduced to these as well. The use of gentle functional techniques, such as those of Lawrence Jones (e.g. strain/counterstrain), are suitable for combining with NMT and MET methods. By using MET to help to lengthen shortened structures, and NMT to aid in this, as well as in identifying localised areas of soft tissue dysfunction (myofascial trigger points or other forms of soft tissue dysfunction), the practitioner has a wide range of diagnostic and therapeutic methods, literally at his or her fingertips. Correct sequencing will be individual, but requires a correct (or at least reasonable) understanding of the causes of the dysfunction, and that treatment takes account of local and bodywide biomechanical influences, as well as psychosocial and lifestyle features (nutrition, exercise, sleep and breathing patterns, etc.).

Massage

Using standard massage protocols, Field (2000) has demonstrated, in hundreds of research projects, that significant benefits occur in the following conditions and patient populations: enhanced growth in preterm infants, cocaine and human immunodeficiency virus (HIV)-exposed infants, pain reduction, during labour, pre-debridement for burn patients, juvenile rheumatoid arthritis, fibromyalgia, premenstrual syndrome, migraine, children with autism, adolescents with attention deficit hyperactivity disorder (enhanced attentiveness), anxiety (e.g. exam settings), depression, post-traumatic stress, adolescent psychiatric patients, adolescent mothers, bulaemia and anorexia, chronic fatigue syndrome, autoimmune and immune disorders, diabetes mellitus (reduced glucose levels), asthma, cystic fibrosis, atopic dermatitis, HIV-positive adults, oncology patients.

Field's explanations for the benefits of massage are summarised later in this section.

We should also not lose sight of the tried and tested effects of massage on the soft tissues. The degree of that effect will vary with the type of soft tissue manipulation employed, and the nature of the patient and the problem. Soft tissue techniques, apart from those specifically associated with NMT, may include the following.

Petrissage

This involves wringing and stretching movements that attempt to 'milk' the tissues of waste products, and assist in circulatory interchange. The manipulations press and roll the muscles under the hands. Petrissage may be performed with one hand, where the area requiring treatment is small, or, more usually, with two hands. In extremely small areas (e.g. base of the thumb), it can be performed by two fingers, or finger and thumb. It is applicable to skin, fascia, muscle, etc. In a relaxing mode, the rhythm should be around 10–15 cycles per minute, and to induce stimulation this can rise to around 35 cycles per minute. It is usually a cross-fibre activity.

Unhurried, deep pressure is the usual mode of application in large muscle masses that require stretching and relaxing. The thenar eminence and the hyperthenar eminence are the main strong contacts, but fingers, or the whole of the hand, may be involved. An example of this movement, as applied to the low back, would be as follows.

Method. Both hands are placed on one side of the prone patient, one at the level of the upper gluteals, the other several inches higher; each hand will describe circles, counterclockwise, but they will do so in such a manner that, as one hand moves laterally from the spine, the other hand will begin to move towards the spine from a point a little higher on the back. The contact can be the flat hand, or the thenar or hyperthenar eminence.

One-handed petrissage may involve treatment of an arm, for example. In this, the hand lifts and squeezes the tissues, making a small circular motion. Many other variations exist in this technique, which is aimed mainly at achieving general relaxation of the muscles, and improved circulation and drainage.

Kneading

This is used to improve fluid exchange and to achieve relaxation of tissues. The hands shape themselves to the contours of the area being treated. The tissues between the hands, as they approximate each other, are lifted and pressed downwards and together. This squeezes and kneads the tissues. Each position receives three or four cycles of this sort before the lower hand takes the place of the upper hand, and it glides upwards to its next position. Little lubricant is required, as the hands should cling to the part being manipulated, lifting it, and pressing and sliding only when changing position. A degree of deep stroking is used to move fluid contents.

Inhibition

This involves application of pressure directly to the belly or origins or insertions of contracted muscles, or to local soft tissue dysfunction, for a minute or more, or in a 'make and break' manner, to reduce hypertonic contraction or for reflex effects.

Effleurage

Effleurage (stroking) is used to induce relaxation and reduce fluid congestion – applied superficially or at depth. This is a relaxing drainage technique, which should be used, as appropriate, to initiate or terminate other manipulative methods. Pressure is usually even throughout the strokes, which are applied with the whole hand in contact. Any combination of areas may be thus treated. Superficial tissues are usually treated rhythmically by this method. As drainage is one of its main aims, peripheral areas are often treated, in order to drain venous or lymphatic fluid towards the centre. Lubricants are usually used.

A useful low back variation is the use of stroking horizontally across the tissues. The practitioner stands facing the side of the patient, at waist level. The caudad hand rests on the upper gluteals, and the cephalad hand on the area just above the iliac crest. One hand strokes from the side closest to the practitioner away to the other side, as the other hand applies a pulling stroke, from the far side towards the practitioner. The two hands pass and then, without changing position, reverse direction and pass each other again. The degree of pressure used is optional, and the technique can be continued in one position for several strokes, before moving the hands upwards on the back. This is but one of many variations on the theme of stroking – a technique that is relaxing to the patient and useful in achieving fluid alteration.

Vibration and friction

Vibration and friction are used near origins and insertions, and near bony attachments, for relaxing effects on the muscle as a whole. This is used to reach below superficial tissues. It is performed by small circular or vibratory movements, with the tips of fingers or thumb. The heel of the hand may also be used. The aim is to move the tissues under the skin, and not the skin itself. It is applied, for example, to joint spaces, around bony prominences and near well-healed scar tissue to reduce adhesions. Pressure is applied gradually, until the tolerance of the patient is reached. The minute circular or vibratory movement is introduced, and this is maintained for some seconds before gradual release and movement to another position.

Stroking techniques are used subsequently, to drain tissues and relax the patient.

Stretching

Stretching can be used along or across the belly of muscles using heel of hand, thumb or fingers applied slowly and rhythmically. Cross-fibre friction is one such approach which involves pressure across the muscle fibres, and in this form the stroke moves across the skin, in a series of short deep strokes. One thumb following the other, in a series of such strokes, laterally from the spinous processes, aids in reduction of local contraction and fibrous changes. Short strokes along the fibres of muscle may also be used, in which the skin contact is maintained, and the tissues under the skin are moved. This requires deep short strokes, and is useful in areas of fibrous change. Thumbs are the main contact in this variation.

Another choice in the treatment of fibrotic change is the use of deep friction, which may be applied to muscle, ligament or joint capsule, across the long axis of the fibres, using the thumb or any variation of the finger contacts. The index finger, supported by the middle finger, or the middle finger with its two adjacent fingers supporting it, makes for a strong treatment unit. Precise localisation of target tissues is possible with this sort of contact.

The methods listed above do not represent a comprehensive description of massage-based soft tissue techniques, but are meant to indicate some of the basic movements available from this source. Some, or all, of these are bound to be involved in any attempt to deal with soft tissue problems.

Other methods that we would associate with the above techniques of traditional massage might include the various applications of NMT, as described in this text, as well as connective tissue massage techniques, which are used primarily for reflex effects.

Massage effects explained

How are the various effects of massage and soft tissue manipulation explained? Field (2000), discussing her many research findings, states:

In all these studies depression, anxiety, and stress hormones significantly decreased following massage therapy. Because depression, anxiety and stress hormones (particularly cortisol) are notably elevated in autoimmune and immune disorders, we hypothesized that massage therapy might also reduce these problems.

Field further suggests that the evidence from her studies points to enhanced homeostatic function, in both infants and adults, following massage therapy, as evidenced by improved sleep patterns (and therefore higher levels of somatostatin), as well as increased serotonin levels. These thoughts are supported by the work of other researchers (Acolet 1993,

Ferel-Tory 1993, Ironson et al 1993, Weinrich & Weinrich 1990).

Apart from the undoubted anxiety- and stress-reducing influences, a combination of physical effects also occurs (Sandler 1983):

1. Pressure, as applied in deep kneading or stroking along the length of a muscle, tends to displace its fluid content.
2. Venous, lymphatic and tissue drainage is thereby encouraged.
3. The replacement of this with fresh oxygenated blood aids in normalisation via increased capillary filtration and venous capillary pressure.
4. This reduces oedema and the effects of pain-inducing substances that may be present (Hovind & Nielson 1974, Xujian 1990).
5. Massage also produces a decrease in the sensitivity of the γ-efferent control of the muscle spindles, and thereby reduces any shortening tendency of the muscles (Puustjarvi et al 1990).
6. Pressure techniques, such as are used in NMT, and the methods employed in MET have a direct effect on the Golgi tendon organs, which detect the load applied to the tendon or muscle.
7. These have an inhibitory capability, which can cause the entire muscle to relax.
8. The Golgi tendon organs are set in series in the muscle, and are affected by both active and passive contraction of the tissues. The effect of any system that applies longitudinal pressure or stretch to the muscle will be to evoke this reflex relaxation. The degree of stretch has, however, to be great, as there is little response from a small degree of stretch.
9. The effects of MET, articulation techniques and various functional balance techniques depend to a large extent on these tendon reflexes (Sandler 1983).

Soft tissues at centre stage

We are in the midst of a change in the concepts of manual therapy that has far-reaching implications. One of the major changes is the restoration of the soft tissue component to centre stage, rather than the peripheral role to which it has been assigned in the past as ever more general health problems are found to involve musculoskeletal dysfunction, for example chronic fatigue conditions (Chaitow 1990).

Lewit (1985) discusses aspects of what he describes as the 'no man's land' that lies between neurology, orthopaedics and rheumatology, which, he says, is the home of the vast majority of patients with pain derived from the locomotor system, and in whom no definite pathomorphological changes are found. He makes the suggestion that these be termed cases of 'functional pathology of the locomotor system'. These include most of the patients attending osteopathic, chiropractic and physiotherapy practitioners.

The most frequent symptom of individuals involved in this area of dysfunction is pain, which may be reflected clinically by reflex changes such as muscle spasm, myofascial trigger points, hyperalgesic skin zones, periosteal pain points, or a wide variety of other sensitive areas that have no obvious pathological origin. As the musculoskeletal system is the largest energy user in the body, it is no surprise that fatigue is a feature of chronic changes in the musculature. It is a major part of the role of NMT to help in identifying such areas, and also in offering some help in differential diagnosis. NMT and other soft tissue methods are then capable of normalising many of the causative aspects of these myriad sources of pain and disability.

 ## Specific (abdominal) release techniques

Boris Chaitow, who worked closely with Stanley Lief, wrote (B. Chaitow, personal communication, 1983):

Stanley Lief taught that manipulation (bony or soft tissue) should not only be confined to the spine itself

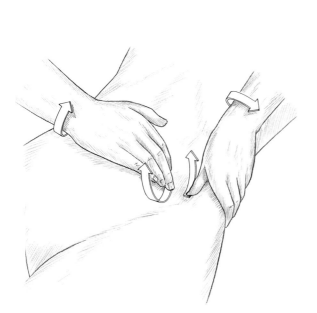

Figure 8.21A Both hands release tissue that has been taken to its elastic barrier in various directions: compressed, stretched apart, counter-rotated and finally 'sprung'.

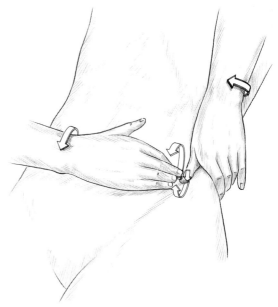

Figure 8.21B The right hand springs the restricted tissues after all slack has been removed and some stretch applied, while the left hand acts mainly to produce a stabilising contact against which a precisely controlled force is applied.

Figure 8.21 Specific release technique as used in treatment of adhesions and tensor fascia lata restrictions.

but also locally to every possible area related to the particular symptom or stress. On the whole the neuromuscular technique he devised is applied with the thumb, as this universally useful digit lends itself to the pattern of pressure and technique required, and is at the same time highly sensitive in diagnostic palpation.

One of the areas of the body which Stanley Lief found uniquely amenable for his soft tissue technique was the abdomen. It can be safely asserted that there is no one in middle age and older who has not, unfortunately, developed some of the tensions, contractions, adhesions, nerve and muscle spasms in various parts of the gastro-intestinal tract and abdominal cavity, so common today. All these would normally be outside the scope of the conventional manual therapist. But, with the neuromuscular technique, a practitioner can achieve almost dramatic benefits in local stresses, and in health in general. He devised for the abdomen the special technique he called 'bloodless surgery' – a method of breaking up deep-seated adhesions and contractions. It also enables the practitioner to improve function and circulation related to female problems such as dysmenorrhoea, menorrhagia and amenorrhoea, fibroids etc.

Lief used methods derived from an American system of manipulative or 'bloodless' surgery to amplify his abdominal techniques. His, and Boris Chaitow's, technique is presented here. These 'release' techniques can be applied to soft areas of the body (e.g. the throat) as well as to the abdomen. The original concept of 'bloodless surgery' was that adhesions were being 'peeled' away from their anchorage by the technique, and in some cases this might have been so. However, its current application is to any area of tight, fibrosed, spastic, contracted or adhering soft tissue in the abdominal region, or elsewhere – for example, on the lateral thigh in tense and contracted fascial tissues (Fig. 8.21A,B).

The most dramatic improvements in function were noted by Lief and Chaitow after its use in such conditions as spastic or atonic constipation, visceroptosis, dysmenorrhoea and menorrhagia, as well as ill-defined abdominal congestion and pain. The author confines its use to deeply indurated muscle and fascial structures such as are found in tensor fascia lata (see below).

Precisely what takes place after abdominal release technique is open to conjecture. An improvement in tone and circulation, and usually of general function, is the most obvious result. It is a matter of debate whether this is because of a release of a long-held contracted state in the soft tissues, or because of an actual breaking of adhesions, or because of some other mechanism.

A general abdominal neuromuscular treatment (see Ch. 7) precedes the first specific release technique (technique A below). This serves both to relax and to tone the abdomen in a general manner, while enabling the practitioner to localise areas that feel indurated or contracted objectively, as well as noting all areas of subjective sensitivity as reported by the patient. It is these (a) tight, contracted and (b) sensitive areas that receive the release technique.

Localising dysfunction

The ability of the practitioner to localise accurately such areas is obviously critical and needs to be a matter for constant practice until the hands and fingers feel such abnormalities as a matter of course. To this end, it is suggested that the middle finger of the right hand (in a right-handed practitioner) be trained to seek and mark those areas that will require specific release techniques. This requires practising the use of the hand in a position where the fingers are flexed, so that the middle finger is slightly more prominent than its neighbours. This aids its task of palpating specifically the tissues being probed. The non-searching fingers support the hand, and are involved in assessing tissue tension, as well as distracting surrounding soft tissues, as an aid to the palpating finger.

The patient should be supine with knees flexed and feet as close to the buttocks as possible, for maximum abdominal relaxation, and with the head on a small pillow.

The practitioner should stand facing the patient, on the side opposite that being treated, i.e. to treat the left inguinal area the practitioner stands, knees flexed, leaning across from the patient's right side. This allows the tissues being manipulated to be drawn towards the practitioner in a controlled manner, whereas such a procedure performed with the hands being pushed away from the practitioner, as would be the case if working from the side being treated, would cause a degree of pushing of the tissues, resulting in a lack of fine control, and possibly causing discomfort.

Technique A

1. Having located an area of contracted (often sensitive) tissue, the middle finger locates the point of maximum resistance and the tissues are drawn towards the practitioner, to the limit of pain-free movement.

2. The middle finger (right hand) and its neighbours should be flexed, fairly rigid, and be imparting force in two directions at this stage, i.e. downwards (towards the floor) and towards the practitioner. (In 'bloodless surgery' techniques, the right hand is always on the 'adhesion' and the other contact on the organ to which the lesion is attached.)

3. With the fingers maintaining the above position, the thumb of the left hand is placed almost immediately – no more than $1/4$ inch (6 mm) away – adjacent to the middle finger of the right hand, in such a way that a downward pressure (towards the floor) will provide a fulcrum point against which force can be applied via the right hand, in order to stretch or reduce the degree of contraction in the tissue (or indeed to break or 'peel' adhesions).

4. The thumb should also be flexed, and the contact can be via its tip or its lateral border, or a combination of both.

5. The idea of a fulcrum is important because the two points of contact are both on soft tissue structures, and the effect of the manipulation is achieved, not by pulling or twisting these apart, but by a combination of movements that impart force in several directions at the same time.

6. This is accomplished by a rapid clockwise movement of the right hand (middle finger contact) against the stabilising anchorage of the left thumb (see Fig. 8.21A).

7. Synchronous movement of the thumb, during this release, is not essential or necessary. However, Boris Chaitow does impart a degree of additional torsional force by releasing the thumb contact in an anticlockwise direction at the moment of manipulation.

8. With both hands in contact, as described, and the contact digits flexed and rigid, the practitioner should be so positioned that he or she is leaning over the affected area, knees flexed with the legs separated for stability, and elbows flexed and separated to a point of 180° separation. The force that will be present at the point of contact is a downward one, to which is added a slight separation of the hands, which increases the tension on the affected tissues. The manipulative force is imparted by a quick flicking of the right contact in a clockwise direction, whilst maintaining the left thumb contact (or taking it in an anticlockwise direction).

9. The effect of the right hand movement would be to snap the right elbow towards the practitioner's side. If a double release is performed, then both elbows will come rapidly to the sides.

10. The amount of force imparted should be controlled so that no pain is felt by the patient.

The essence of this technique is the speed with which it is applied. This very high velocity release involves tissues that have been 'wound up', by being taken in at least two directions of distraction – compression, separation and a degree of torsion – and its success depends upon this as much as the correct positioning of the hands, and the exact location of the area of tissue dysfunction.

The same procedure can be repeated several times on the same area, and the release of a number of such areas of contracted or indurated tissue at any one treatment is usual. The same thumb contact is often maintained whilst variations in the direction of tissue tension are dealt with by slightly altering the angle of the right hand contact and manipulative effort.

If, after manipulation, no objective improvement is noted on palpation, the angle of the contacts should be varied. Nothing will be gained, however, by attempting to use excessive force in order to achieve results. As the degree of soft tissue trauma to the patient is minimal, the after-effects should not include bruising or much discomfort. Any such after-effect would indicate undue pressure or force.

Boris Chaitow (personal communication, 1983) describes the above method as follows:

For the technique of NMT on the abdomen referred to already as 'bloodless surgery', palpate with the tips of the fingers of the right hand, and having located the area of abnormal feel, place those four fingers as a group at the distal border of the lesioned area, and place the thumb of the left hand alongside the nails of the right fingers. Give a sharp flick with both hands simultaneously, the left hand thumb being twisted anticlockwise, and the fingers of the right hand clockwise (difficult if not impossible to describe on paper). This achieves an appreciable breaking-up, without trauma or hurt to the patient, of tensions, adhesions, congestions etc., both on the wall of the abdomen and structures within the cavity. Obviously these flicks with the hands have to be repeated a number of times to feel a discernible difference in the lesioned tissue. Stanley Lief achieved dramatic changes in tissue structure and functional improvements in many types of abdominal stresses including digestive problems, gall bladder blockage, gall stones, constipation, spastic colon, colic, colitis, uterine fibroids, dysmenorrhoea, menorrhagia, small non-malignant abdominal tumours, postoperative adhesions etc.

Technique B A second method for the release of tense, contracted, indurated connective and muscular tissue is sometimes employed. This requires the same positioning of the patient and the practitioner, as in method A.

It is worth recalling that thickening will occur in fascia in accordance with the degree of stress imposed upon it. As enormous gravitational stress occurs in the abdominal region, as a result of postural embarrassment, it is frequently the case that tight 'stress bands' will be felt inferior, superior or lateral to internal organs (e.g. intestinal structures) that have sagged and become displaced. Such contracted tissue is often the source of reflex trigger activity, and is often, in itself, the cause of mechanical interference with normal venous and lymphatic drainage, as well as being a possible source of pain.

Any procedure that helps to normalise such tension should be accompanied by a programme of postural re-education and exercise, if it is to have any lasting beneficial effects.

1. The practitioner's right hand, fingers flexed and middle finger slightly in the lead, probes through the surface abdominal musculature and attempts to 'lift' the structures.

2. In this way, areas of abnormal resistance will be traced quite easily by the tip of the middle finger of the right hand. The most inferior point of attachment of such a band is located and held firmly by this flexed digit.

3. The tip and lateral border of the thumb of the left hand is then placed adjacent to this contact, so that the right hand contact is on the tension band and the left contact is on the structure to which it attaches.

4. The manipulative force is achieved by a rapid anticlockwise movement of the right contact, whilst firm, stabilising pressure is maintained by the left thumb (Fig. 8.21B).

5. The closer the two contacts are to each other at the moment of release, the less force is required and the less danger of injury to the tissues there will be.

6. It is suggested that, by visualising an attempt to tear an envelope held between thumbs and forefingers, this concept will be better understood. The closer the holding digits are to each other, the easier such an operation would be. As the manipulative effort is attempting to, at least, stretch and, at most, separate the fibres involved, it is necessary to impart a high-velocity, low-amplitude torsional force and not a vague stretching effort imparted over a large area of unyielding tissue.

7. The actual manipulative force is imparted by the tip of the middle finger of the right hand, but is, of course, the result of the movement of the whole hand. The wrist snaps medially and the elbow outwards at the moment of release.

8. This speedy 'flicking' action is one that should be practised over and over again so that its execution is a matter of routine. A release of contracted tissue will be followed by an immedi-

ate freedom of mobility of tissues and of organs formerly 'bound' and immobile.

Such 'release' procedures (technique A or B) should be performed throughout the abdominal area and preceded by the general neuromuscular treatment (Chs 6 & 7), and be followed by a general procedure to 'lift' the abdominal contents back to a physiologically correct position.

Instructions should be given of abdominal and postural exercises to be performed by the patient, as should improved postural and breathing rehabilitation techniques.

A series of six to ten such 'specific release' treatments, over a period of a month or so, is suggested in chronic conditions involving visceroptosis and abdominal congestion. The application of these techniques to the hypogastric and inguinal regions may be of benefit to patients suffering from menstrual irregularities. Local function can often be improved as a result of the structural and circulatory improvements following specific release techniques.

Strain/counterstrain and positional release techniques (Fig. 8.22)

In spinal and appendicular strains, injuries or lesions there is often an evident distortion from the normal anatomical posture or position. This eccentric state is often relieved by placing the joint or patient in an exaggerated degree of the deformity or distortion found at examination. If this is held for 90–120 seconds, a spontaneous release will often occur. Jones (1963, 1977) states that this technique depends on the ability to produce relaxation of reflex muscle tension that limits and binds the joint(s).

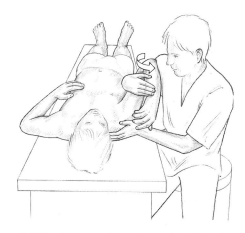

Figure 8.22B   A degree of ease is produced from that point by the initial positioning of the arm.

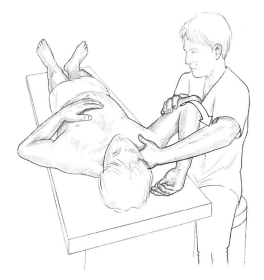

Figure 8.22C   A final position of ease is found by fine tuning to relieve pain in the tender point, and the position is held for 20–90 seconds.

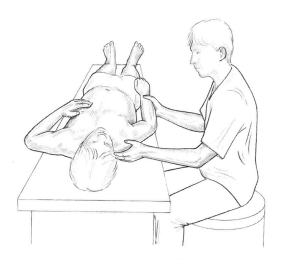

Figure 8.22A   A tender point is identified by the operator's left hand.

Figure 8.22   Application of positional release (strain/counterstrain) to the supraspinatus muscle.

The art lies in finding the specific direction in which a painful joint can be moved that will release muscular tension as well as relieve pain (the position of 'ease' or 'comfort'). When passively placed in such a position, inhibition of painful stimuli results, and the range of motion of the area will usually be significantly enhanced subsequently. There are two mechanisms thought to be involved in the resolution of hypertonicity when strain/counterstrain is used: a neurological resetting involving the muscle spindles and a circulatory 'flushing' of previously ischaemic tissues (Chaitow 2002, D'Ambrogio & Roth 1997, Deig 2001, Rathbun & MacNab 1970).

Jones' tender points

Jones has compiled lists of specific tender point areas relating to every imaginable strain of most joints, and many muscles, of the body. These are his 'proven' (by clinical experience) points, and he provides strict guidelines for achieving 'ease' in the tender point that is being palpated (locating the position of ease usually involves a 'folding' or crowding of the tissues in which the tender point lies). A number of variations exist as to the use of the concepts that Jones developed, and these are fully explained in *Positional Release Techniques* (Chaitow 2002). Additional texts by Deig (2001) and D'Ambrogio & Roth (1997) are also recommended (see Figs 4.5A,B,C).

An example is offered of the use of positional release in Fig. 8.22A,B,C.

Tensor fascia lata (iliotibial band) techniques

The iliotibial band, when contracted or pathologically tight, is often misdiagnosed as a sacroiliac problem. The symptoms associated with its dysfunction may include pain, localised in the region of the medial or posterior superior iliac spine. There may be radiating pain to the anterior, lateral or posterior aspects of the thigh, and also in the iliac fossa, which may suggest visceral disease. The symptoms frequently arise in the sacroiliac joint, but its dysfunction is the result, in many cases, of tightness in the iliotibial band, the tissues of which may have numerous trigger points present.

Test. A test for a tight iliotibial band involves having the patient lie on the unaffected side, with hip and knee flexed to 90°. The patient is asked to hold that leg to the table. The other leg is supported by the practitioner, who is standing behind the patient. The straight leg is extended, to the point where the iliotibial band lies over the greater trochanter. The practitioner's cephalad hand will be supporting the leg at the knee, while the caudad hand supports the ankle. The knee is then flexed to 90° and the hand supporting the leg at the knee is removed, allowing the knee to fall towards the table. If the iliotibial band has shortened, this will not occur and the leg will remain suspended. The band will palpate as tender under such conditions, as a rule.

 Treatment method 1

Treatment may employ a direct approach, as advocated by Mennell (1969) or by use of MET methods, as described below.

(a) 'Twig snap' method. First the patient is placed side-lying, with both legs flexed comfortably. The first contact is with that part of the band distal to the greater trochanter. The anterior fibres are stretched first, in a manner similar to that which would be used were the hands attempting to snap a stick (Fig. 8.23A). The fingers are laid over the anterior fibres of the band, distal to the trochanter, just above the knee. The thumbs rest, as a fulcrum, and are placed against the posterior aspect of the anterior fibres, and the snapping action is achieved by a rapid ulnar deviation of the hands (away from each other). The main force is transmitted through the thumbs, which should stretch the fibres without pressing them against the osseous structures (this would bruise the tissues). A rapidly applied series of movements such as this, starting at the knee and working up and down the band, is carried out.

(b) 'Piston thrust' method. The posterior fibres are then treated. The heel of each hand is pushed

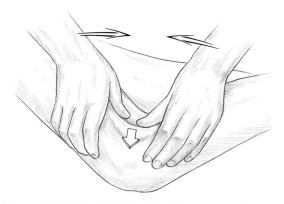

Figure 8.23A Anterior iliotibial band treatment, using a 'twig snapping' approach to address extreme shortness and fibrosity of these tissues. This is applied sequentially up and down the band using a degree of force that is easily tolerated.

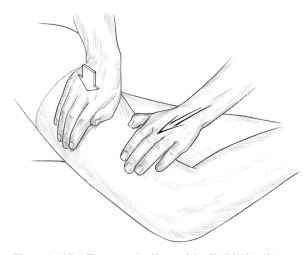

Figure 8.23B The posterior fibres of the iliotibial band are treated using the heel of one hand alternately to thrust against the band while it is stabilised by the other hand. An alternating sequence of this sort, applied up and down the band, produces marked release of hypertonic and shortened fibres.

in a piston-like manner against the fibres, alternately. As the heel (thenar or hyperthenar eminence) of one hand thrusts against the fibres, the other stabilises them by grasping the anterior aspect (Fig. 8.23B). A series of thrusts is made from above the knee to the trochanter and back again. The thrust must be against the fibres and

not against osseous structures, or bruising will ensue.

(c) 'C' bends over the trochanter. The region overlying the trochanter is treated by rolling it backwards and forwards over the bony prominence. The thumbs are the motive force, being pressed downwards and backward or forward, to achieve this. The roll is attempting to take the band posteriorly, and then anteriorly, over the trochanter. As the trochanter rolls backwards, the heel of the foot on the treated leg should rise from the table (but only if the band is tight).

(d) NMT. The area above the trochanter is treated by deep, kneading massage or NMT. This is often easily achieved when the patient is prone, and the tissues are contacted by the fingers of the treating hand, with the practitioner standing on the side opposite the area being treated. The fingers may be insinuated into the tissues, and a degree of lifting, drag, as well as pressure medial-wards, is achieved by the practitioner leaning backwards and drawing the treating hand towards him or her (see Figs 6.8A,B) This may be done as part of NMT treatment. These structures require maintenance stretching, via exercise, if improvement is to be held.

Treatment method 2

This involves either isometric or isolytic contraction (see Fig. 8.6B).

Isometric contraction. In the first instance the patient is supine, with the unaffected leg flexed and the affected leg extended. The practitioner takes the extended leg into maximum adduction, placing a maximum degree of stretch on to the lateral fibres (the abductors and fascia). To achieve this, the leg will be adducted and brought under the other, flexed, leg. Standing on the side of the unaffected leg, against which the practitioner applies stabilising pressure, the practitioner adducts the treated leg, taking out the slack, and asks the patient to make an attempt to abduct the affected leg using 25% of available strength. This is resisted for 10 seconds as the patient inhales. Release coincides with exhalation, at which time a little more slack is taken out and the affected leg is adducted slightly beyond its resistance barrier. The procedure is repeated two or three more times.

Isolytic contraction. The position is the same as that given above. Should the above method be only partly effective, then, as the patient attempts to abduct the affected leg (commencing with only a portion – say 25% – of available strength, but with increasing degree of effort, if the procedure is repeated several times) the practitioner overcomes this, and forces it further into adduction. This process may be uncomfortable, and the patient should be forewarned. This will produce microtrauma and reduce fibrous contractions. Progressively more effort on the part of the patient should be introduced on subsequent isotonic eccentric contractions.

Trigger point techniques

(see also discussion on ischaemic compression earlier in this chapter, Box 3.5, and INIT in Ch. 9)

There are a number of different pressure techniques used for dealing with trigger points. Where underlying (i.e. bony) tissues allow direct pressure on to such points, so that the trigger is squeezed between thumb and the underlying tissue, the variables will be the duration of such pressure, and degree of continuous or variable pressure employed. Where no such suitable underlying tissues exist, or where it would be dangerous to exert direct pressure through the muscle to the underlying structures (e.g. trigger points lying in sternocleidomastoid), then squeezing (compression) or pinching techniques can be employed. These will also vary in terms of the duration and nature (e.g. variable pressure) of the force imparted.

A combination of chilling and stretching of the tissues housing trigger points is known as 'spray and stretch' or chill-and-stretch technique treatment; this was discussed above.

Nimmo (1969) suggested a 5–7-second direct inhibitory pressure with a recheck of the tissues subsequently to assess reduced reflex activity.

The approach used until fairly recently by the author, was to apply a 5-second inhibitory pressure sufficient to reproduce the referred symptoms, followed by a short (2–3 seconds) rest phase, followed by a repeat of the initial pressure. This 'make and break' approach was continued until there was a reduction in the referred pain pattern intensity, or a significant alteration in the tone of the tissues, or until a minute or so had passed (with cessation if the symptoms were intensifying rather than diminishing).

This was usually followed by an isometrically induced release of tone followed by stretching of the tissues housing the trigger point.

A more recent evolution involves use of an integrated neuromuscular inhibition technique (INIT), which is described briefly earlier in this chapter, and fully in Chapter 9.

Chapman (Owen 1977) suggests a vibratory treatment, lasting 10–15 seconds, on neuro-lymphatic reflexes. He used fingertip pressure to impart the required energy, although thumb pressure of varying intensity is just as effective. This can be applied as a gradually intensifying pressure building up over 5–8 seconds, easing for 2–3 seconds, and then repeated. Altogether, this should not take more than 1/2 minute. These points can be overtreated, and the optimal time would seem to be 15–30 seconds, with the pressure (or squeeze) of a variable nature.

It is important to realise that the objective 'feel' of local soft tissue contractions involving fibrosis is unlikely to change much during such treatment, whereas taut bands in which triggers lie frequently do 'release' (Baldry 1993).

The main changes resulting from the treatment of fibrotic tissue will occur later, when homeostatic self-regulating mechanisms have come into operation. While the author believes that use of a variable degree of pressure during trigger point treatment is more desirable than a constantly held degree of pressure (which may irritate and exacerbate the condition), this view is not universally held, with researchers such as Simons et al (1999) urging a sustained compression/pressure until change is noted or reported.

All the methods described in this chapter may be incorporated into general neuromuscular technique treatment.

REFERENCES

Abrams A 1922 New concepts in diagnosis and treatment. Physicoclinical Co., San Francisco

Acolet D 1993 Changes in plasma cortisol and catecholamine concentrations on response to massage in preterm infants. Archives of Disease in Childhood 68:29–31

Arbuckle B 1977 The selected writings of Beryl Arbuckle. National Osteopathic Institute and Cerebral Palsy Foundation

Baldry P 1993 Acupuncture, trigger points and musculoskeletal pain. Churchill Livingstone, Edinburgh

Castlio Y 1955 Effect of direct splenic stimulation in infectious diseases. American Academy of Osteopathy Yearbook 1955:121

Chaitow L 1990 Beat fatigue workbook. Thorsons, London

Chaitow L 1994 INIT in treatment of pain and trigger points. British Journal of Osteopathy XIII:17–21

Chaitow L 2001 Muscle energy techniques. 2nd edn. Churchill Livingstone, Edinburgh

Chaitow L 2002 Positional release techniques. 2nd edn. Churchill Livingstone, Edinburgh

Chengnan S, ed. 1990 Chinese bodywork. Pacific View Press, Berkeley, California

D'Ambrogio K, Roth G 1997 Positional release therapy. Mosby, St Louis, Missouri

Deig D 2001 Positional release technique. Butterworth Heinemann, Boston

Ferel-Torey A 1993 Use of therapeutic massage as a nursing intervention to modify anxiety and perceptions of cancer pain. Cancer Nursing 16(2):93–101

Field T 2000 Touch therapy. Churchill Livingstone, Edinburgh

Fielder S, Pyott W 1955 The science and art of Manipulative Surgery. American Institute of Manipulative Surgery, Salt Lake City, Utah

Fielding S 1983 Journal of Alternative Medicine December:10–11

Hoag J 1969 Osteopathic medicine. McGraw Hill, New York

Hovind H, Nielson SL 1974 Effects of massage on blood flow in skeletal muscle. Scandinavian Journal of Rehabilitation Medicine 6:74–77

Ironson G et al 1993 Relaxation through massage associated with decreased distress and increased serotonin levels. Touch Research Institute, University of Miami School of Medicine, Miami

Janda V 1990 Muscle function testing. Butterworths, London

Janda V 1992 Muscle and back pain. Physical Medicine Research Foundation presentation, Vancouver, British Columbia, October 1992

Johnson A 1939 Principles and practice of drugless therapeutics. W Straube, Los Angeles

Jones L 1963 Foot treatment without hand trauma. Journal of the American Osteopathic Association January

Jones L 1977 Strain and counterstrain. Academy of Applied Osteopathy, Colorado Springs

Kuchera M, Kuchera W 1994 Considerations in systemic dysfunction. Greyden Press, Columbus, Ohio

Lederman E 1997 Fundamentals of manual therapy. Churchill Livingstone, Edinburgh

Lewit K 1985 Manipulative therapy in rehabilitation of the motor system. Butterworths, London

Lewit K 1992 Manipulative therapy in rehabilitation of the locomotor system. 2nd edn. Butterworths, London

Lewit K 1996 Role of manipulation in spinal rehabilitation. In: Liebenson C, ed. Rehabilitation of the spine. Williams & Wilkins, Baltimore

Lewit K 1999 Manipulative therapy in rehabilitation of the locomotor system. 3rd edn. Butterworths, London

Liebenson C 2001 Manual resistance techniques in rehabilitation. In: Chaitow L, ed. Muscle energy technique. 2nd edn. Churchill Livingstone, Edinburgh

Mennell J 1969 Joint pain. Little Brown, Boston

Mennell J 1975 The therapeutic use of cold. Journal of the American Osteopathic Association 74(12):1146–1158

Morrison M 1969 Lecture notes. Charing Cross Hotel, London

Nimmo R 1969 Lecture notes. British College of Naturopathy and Osteopathy, London

Norris C 1999 Functional load abdominal training (part 1). Journal of Bodywork and Movement Therapies 3(3):150–158

Owen C 1977 An endocrine interpretation of Chapman's reflexes. Academy of Applied Osteopathy, Newark, Ohio

Polstein B 1991 In: DiGiovanna E, ed. Osteopathic approach to diagnosis and treatment. JB Lippincott, Philadelphia

Puustjarvi K et al 1990 Effects of massage in patients with chronic tension headaches. Acupuncture and Electrotherapeutics Research 15:159–162

Rathbun J, MacNab I 1970 Microvascular pattern of rotator cuff. Journal of Bone and Joint Surgery 52:540–553

Retzlaff EW, Bemy AH, Haight AS et al 1974 The piriformis muscle syndrome. Journal of American Osteopathic Association 73:799–807

Sandler S 1983 The physiology of soft tissue massage. British Osteopathic Journal 15:1–6

Simons D, Travell J, Simons L 1999 Myofascial pain and dysfunction: the trigger point manual. Vol. 1: upper half of body. 2nd edn. Williams & Wilkins, Baltimore

Sleszynski SL, Kelso AF 1993 Comparison of thoracic manipulation and incentive spirometry in preventing postoperative atelactesis. Journal of American Osteopathic Association 93:834–838, 843–845

Stoddard A 1969 Manual of osteopathic practice. Hutchinson Medical, London

Te Poorten B 1969 The piriformis muscle. Journal of American Osteopathic Association 69:150–160

Travell J 1952 Ethyl chloride spray for painful muscle spasm. Archives of Physical Medicine and Rehabilitation 33:291–298

Travell J, Simons D 1983 Myofascial pain and dysfunction. vol. 1. Williams & Wilkins, Baltimore

Travell J, Simons D 1992 Myofascial pain and dysfunction. vol. 2. Williams & Wilkins, Baltimore

Wallace E, McPartland J, Jones J, Kuchera W, Buser B 1997 Lymphatic manipulative techniques. In: Ward R, ed. Foundations for osteopathic medicine. Williams & Wilkins, Baltimore

Walther D 1988 Applied kinesiology. SDC Systems, Pueblo

Weinrich S, Weinrich M 1990 Effect of massage on pain in cancer patients. Applied Nursing Research 3:140–145

Xujian S 1990 Effects of massage and temperature on permeability of initial lymphatics. Lymphology 23:48–50

Zhao-Pu W 1991 Acupressure therapy. Churchill Livingstone, Edinburgh

Zink G, Lawson W 1979 An osteopathic structural examination and functional interpretation of the soma. Osteopathic Annals 12(7):433–440

9

NMT in clinical use (including integrated neuromuscular inhibition technique)

Wherever possible, statements made in this text up to this point have carried citation references. Those statements not referenced represent the personal opinion of the author, based on 40 years of clinical experience as an osteopathic and naturopathic practitioner, in both private and National Health Service settings, in office practice, residential clinic and academic settings, in Britain, Greece and the USA. It is therefore suggested that any 'unsubstantiated' (by citations) statements are seen as demanding personal evaluation, by the reader, before being used clinically.

CONTEXTUAL THINKING AND SYNCHRONICITY

Contextual thinking is a valuable approach when confronted by symptoms that are other than obvious (sprained ankle, whiplash injury, etc.). The tendency in clinical practice to consider symptoms in a linear manner, in which cause and effect are plotted almost mathematically, is often flawed. It is possible to learn to see the patient's symptoms in terms of the tip of an iceberg. It is obvious that the bulk of the iceberg is invisible, as are the interacting systemic, constitutional, inherited and acquired, biochemical, biomechanical and psychosocial influences operating within the individual (the remainder of the iceberg). To that needs to be added the influence of the ocean in which the iceberg floats, which, in this metaphor, incorporates the entire physical and psychological environment in which the individual lives and functions. Unless we take these additional factors into account, we are doomed to see symptoms as arising from simplistic backgrounds, which in the case of chronic problems is seldom the case.

Another way of expressing the idea of context is to speak of synchronicity. There are linear and spatial ways of interpreting what happens in life in general, and to the body in particular. Cause and effect represent the way many people in the West understand the relationships between events (causality). One thing causes, or is caused – or at least strongly influenced – by another.

A different way of viewing two events is to see them as being part of a complex continuum, each being part of the same (larger) process, but with neither event dependent on the other, linked by a synchronistic connective principle. The words synchronicity or 'simultaneity' have been used to describe this way of viewing patterns and events. Such spatial thinking may represent the most effective way of evaluating health problems, avoiding simplistic cause and effect approaches (Jung 1973).

Three examples of contextual thinking

1. Hyperventilation and anxiety: which 'causes' which?

Hyperventilation is commonly associated with anxiety. Therefore, if we think in simple terms of cause and effect, we might assume that hyperventilation 'causes' anxiety. However, anxiety commonly leads to hyperventilation; therefore, again, if thinking simplistically, we might assume that anxiety 'causes' hyperventilation. Or, if thinking more contextually, we might observe (more accurately) that anxiety and hyperventilation not only 'feed' each other, but can be triggered and/or aggravated by: low blood sugar levels, increased progesterone levels, sympathetic arousal ('stress'), adrenal stimulation, metabolic acidosis, climatic conditions, altitude, emotional stimuli, allergic reactions, extreme fatigue, and so on. Therefore, we might conclude that anxiety and hyper-

ventilation are part of a continuum, involving all or any of these (and numerous other) factors, interacting with the unique genetic and acquired biochemical, biomechanical and psychological individuality of the person affected. And we might reflect that treatment that takes account of the broader context is more likely to succeed than a simple, linear, 'cause and effect' assessment.

2. Possible 'usefulness' of trigger points

Clinical experience suggests that myofascial trigger points may at times form part of a functional system for sustaining tension, where this is required by the body – for instance in posturally affected tissues, as repositioners (i.e. for the mandible due to forward head posture), or for sustaining tension across the sacroiliac joint when it is unstable, by strategically increasing hamstring tone (Vleeming et al 1997).

In such a situation the tissue is doing exactly what it was set up to do, as changes occur leading to trigger point development. Simons et al (1999) have shown that, in the absence of adequate levels of adenosine triphosphate (ATP), and in the presence of calcium, the actin and myosin elements of muscles are designed to lock in a shortened position. Trigger points function effectively in the absence of ATP (therefore displaying an economy of resources), and are often strategically located in tissues that are straining to accommodate dysfunctional posture, or habits of use, and often clear up spontaneously when the posture (or other stressors such as dietary imbalance strain, breathing dysfunction, dehydration, etc.) is corrected (Chaitow & DeLany 2002).

Trigger points also appear to demonstrate a built-in, silent (latent) and non-silent (active) alarm mechanism, when being abused. Therefore, to release trigger points without regard to correcting the underlying causes, to which they are responding, may result in a less than ideal outcome, not least of which could be a rapid, or chronic, return of the trigger point activity.

Rather than always being seen as dysfunctional entities, trigger points might be considered as low-energy-consuming contractile devices, established by the absence of available ATP, to maintain a structural or localised tensional element, for immediate or long-term adaptational/compensational purposes, until no longer required. Additionally they may be seen as alarm signals when tissues are being overloaded and abused.

In this way of thinking, it is the individual's posture, patterns of use or lifestyle that are dysfunctional, not the tissues housing the trigger point, which may be doing exactly what they were designed to do. When this is true – and when we can recognise the causes – it is the context from which trigger points emerge that requires attention, not the trigger points.

3. Assessment of sacroiliac dysfunction

Lee (2002) reports that Hungerford & Gilleard (1998) have shown that normal individuals, performing a one-legged, standing, hip flexion ('stork') test, vary their motor control strategy *each time they perform the test*, implying that different muscles can be used to perform the same osteokinematic motion. This will vary the amount of compression each time they lift the leg, and thus vary the range of motion. Lee (2002) has written:

Unless trials are repeated and motions averaged, reliability is impossible – not because the tester can't feel what's happening, but because the subject keeps changing from moment to moment . . . Unless the specific muscle activation pattern is noted during whatever range of motion test (active or passive) is being evaluated for reliability – there is no way of knowing what amount of compression the SIJ is under (at that moment) and therefore what the available range of motion should be.

As if this is not enough to create hesitation as to the validity of such tests, a range of other possible influences has been noted. For example, what if:

• the patient's head was slightly turned toward the side being tested, causing increased tension in the hip extensors (i.e. hamstrings) (Murphy 2000)?

• the patient's eyes were turned one way or the other, or were looking slightly up or down, changing markedly the tone in hip flexors, extensors and rotators (Janda 1988, Lewit 1999)?

• the patient's suboccipital muscles had recently been stretched, altering tone in the extensors of the leg (Pollard & Ward 1997)?

• the patient was anxious, hyperventilating (Garland 1994), suffering an allergic reaction (Randolph 1976), or had fallen arches (Myers 2001)?

There are multiple influences, only some of which can be controlled, during tests of this sort, suggesting that clinical reasoning as to what single tests 'mean' is essential.

A single test result cannot define dysfunction, offering at best a shadowy indication, and becoming more relevant only when other assessment findings and the patient's symptom picture and history are added. Assessment is therefore a spatial exercise, not a linear one, seeking synchronous pieces of evidence that, together, lead to a working hypothesis as to what is happening – and what to do.

Conclusion

Hopefully these three examples, hyperventilation, trigger points and sacroiliac joint assessment, offer sufficient evidence to point towards a need to think contextually, to look for synchronicity, and to be cautious regarding linear thinking, especially when dealing with the complexity of the human body.

EVALUATION BEFORE TREATMENT

If therapeutic intervention is to be structured and organised, and something other than hit-and-miss, there is an absolute requirement for sound evaluation and assessment as to the causes, extent and possible influences on other areas and tissues, of patterns of pain and restriction, such as myofascial trigger points, locally traumatised areas, shortened and/or weakened muscles, joint restrictions and/or general/systemic factors (such as exist in arthritic conditions).

As discussed above, the contexts in which symptoms exist, and out of which they emerge, are of profound importance in arriving at a stage where a programme of intervention and therapeutic modification can be formulated.

NMT provides one such diagnostic/assessment tool and also offers, by switching from its assessment to its actively therapeutic mode, a means whereby precisely focused and modulated degrees of force can be directed towards influencing restricted tissues, directly or reflexively. Myofascial release techniques, as well as ischaemic compression (osteopathic inhibitory technique), can be applied to precise targets via the contacting thumb or finger in NMT.

Perhaps NMT's greatest usefulness in assessment relates to the opportunity it offers for the identification of local soft tissue dysfunction in a gentle, non-invasive manner.

In the USA, as well as in the UK, the focus of many therapists utilising NMT is primarily on myofascial trigger points (and the often widespread musculoskeletal and other dysfunctional patterns that produce them). To utilise NMT to its full advantage, it is useful to have a clear understanding of the process of facilitation that can occur paraspinally or locally in muscle and fascia (trigger points), as described in detail in Chapter 3.

By learning how to use NMT diagnostically and therapeutically, a good deal of information can be obtained regarding the patterns of dysfunction that are operating.

It is important to stress, once more, that NMT may be used in both a diagnostic mode and a therapeutic mode, and that to some extent these overlap, and may be carried out simultaneously. Having identified the structures and tissues that require greater attention, NMT is available as a tool with which to make contact and give direct localised treatment to areas that are contracted or tightened. Specific associated and complementary techniques exist to deal with reflex activity, as is noted in trigger points. Muscle energy methods, as described by Lewit (1999), and elaborations on these derived from a variety of sources, provide a further array of techniques that can be brought into operation, depending on the particular indi-cations. Many of these associated techniques were described in Chapter 8.

What about joints?
(Chaitow 1983, 1991a,b, Jones 1981, Mitchell et al 1979)

Soft tissue manipulation, which includes positional release methods ('strain/counterstrain'), NMT and MET, is capable of normalising a great many joint problems, without recourse to active manipulative effort. MET and NMT are symbiotic, and it is possible to achieve more by combining their repertoire of useful techniques than either can achieve individually. By adding the knowledge of suitable techniques by which to influence reflex activity, demonstrated by the presence of localised areas of soft tissue dysfunction (trigger points, Chapman's points, localised fibrosis, etc.), as well as by using the tender points described by Jones, in gentle functional techniques, the scope of soft tissue manipulation methods should become apparent.

Employment of these approaches does not necessarily preclude the need for active joint mobilisation and/or manipulation in correcting restriction, but can make for a lesser need to utilise high-velocity thrusts or long lever techniques, while making such manipulation simpler and far less likely to traumatise the local tissues, or the patient.

Avoiding trauma

By combining MET and NMT, some degree of the potential problem of tissue damage is likely to be solved. NMT, applied to a region containing fibrotic change, will allow for subsequent use of 'normal' MET, or of an isolytic contraction, with less discomfort or likelihood of microtrauma (see Ch. 8).

Are some musculoskeletal problems best left untreated?

The enormous privilege that the patient allows in permitting the practitioner to make physical contact also grants a degree of 'power' to the practitioner. Defences are lowered, and the patient is likely to be amenable to discussing areas of their emotions and thoughts, which they might resist in other situations. This presents opportunities for therapeutic intervention on levels other than the physical. The practitioner should be aware of the potent 'placebo' effect that such a situation allows. Suggestions, and positive guidance, can have powerful influences on the patient, and so care should be exercised, and diligent application of healing techniques undertaken, knowing that the recipient is commonly receptive and highly suggestible.

When considering treatment of soft tissue changes, which relate to an emotional or psychogenic background, it is important to realise the need for an adequate ability on the part of the practitioner/therapist to handle any emotional repercussions resulting from 'releasing' (or attempting to release) the soft tissue manifestations of emotional turmoil, as well as there being a need to have an adequate referral system in place to support the patient in times of crisis.

If the patient is not capable of processing whatever emotional baggage is attached to a particular pattern of soft tissue dysfunction, then it is probably best left intact, until the patient is ready and equipped to process the issues that are submerged in the soma.

A scenario is conceivable in which a patient with obvious musculoskeletal dysfunction, but without obvious mento-emotional problems, could be left in a fragile and vulnerable state following apparently appropriate bodywork. The oft-quoted phenomenon of 'emotional release', which occurs during or following treatment, may be something that therapists could usefully reflect upon and possibly re-evaluate. Just how beneficial – or how dangerous – is such a reaction without further support such as counselling or psychotherapy?

Additionally, there are times when apparently purely physical symptoms, such as active trigger points in a tight hamstring, as in the example given earlier in this chapter, may best be left untreated until underlying, contextual, causes have been evaluated and dealt with.

A FOCUS ON TRIGGER POINTS

Travell & Simons (1983) have demonstrated the clear connection between myofascial trigger point activity and a wide range of pain problems and sympathetic nervous system aberrations. Wall and Melzack confirm that there are few chronic pain problems that do not have myofascial trigger point activity as a component, with these acting, in many instances, as prime maintaining factors of the pain (Melzack & Wall 1988, Wall & Melzack 1989).

Trigger (and other non-referring pain) points commonly lie in muscles that have been stressed in a variety of ways, including postural imbalances (Barlow 1959, Goldthwaite 1949, Simons et al 1999), congenital factors such as warping of fascia via cranial distortions (Upledger 1983), short leg problems, small hemipelvis (Travell & Simons 1992), occupational or leisure overuse patterns (Rolf 1977), emotional states reflecting into the soft tissues (Latey 1986), referred/reflex involvement of the viscera producing facilitated segments paraspinally (Beal 1983, Korr 1977), and trauma.

The repercussions of trigger point activity go far beyond simple musculoskeletal pain, however distressing that may be. Take, for example, the involvement of trigger points in cases of hyperventilation, chronic fatigue and apparent pelvic inflammatory disease. Trigger point activity is particularly prevalent in the muscles of the neck/shoulder region, which also act as accessory breathing muscles (scalenes, upper trapezius, etc.). In situations of increased anxiety the incidence of borderline or frank hyperventilation is frequent (Bass & Gardner 1985) and may be associated with chronic fatigue. Clinically these muscles palpate as tense, and often fibrotic, with active trigger points being common (Garland 1994, Roll & Theorell 1987). Successful breathing retraining and normalisation of diminished energy levels seem in such cases to be accelerated and enhanced, following initial normalisation of the functional integrity of the involved muscles (Chaitow et al 2002).

Trigger points and pelvic pain

Slocumb (1984) has shown that in a large proportion of chronic pelvic pain problems in women, often destined for surgical intervention, the prime cause involves trigger point activity in muscles of the lower abdomen, perineum, inner thigh and even on the walls of the vagina:

The search for common pathological processes such as endometriosis, active inflammation, or pelvic adhesions is the primary objective in assessing the patient with chronic pelvic pain. However, the frustration of finding normal pelvic structures too often results in the conviction that psychiatric causes must somehow account for the pain . . . What is probably the most alarming aspect of the inadequacy of gynecologic management of chronic pelvic pain is the frequent recourse by the physician to operative exploration and removal of pelvic structures for normal physiologic variations . . . As a result of concentrating patients with pelvic pain in a single clinic I have identified a neurological syndrome that can be shown to account for the majority of those patients with chronic abdominal pain . . . Several unusual and unexplained phenomena were repeatedly observed. First, the same pain sensation was reproduced by pressure over localized points in several different tissues seemingly anatomically unrelated. These hyperpathic points are consistent with the term trigger points described by Travell and Simons and appear to cause referred pain symptoms as well as sharp pain.

Slocumb describes how the following areas can all produce the identical referred pain:

1. Pinching the skin over the lower abdominal wall
2. Single-finger pressure in one abdominal wall location
3. Single-finger pressure on tissue overlying the pubic bone
4. Lateral pressure with single finger over one or both levator muscles
5. Single-finger or cotton-tip applicator pressure lateral to the cervix
6. Single-finger or cotton-tip applicator pressure over vaginal cuff scar tissue more than 3 months after hysterectomy
7. Single-finger pressure over the dorsal sacrum.

Slocumb demonstrated, in one research study involving 130 patients, that he was able to remove chronic pelvic pain in nearly 90% of cases by deactivating such triggers.

The significance of this and other studies is that trigger points are the cause of serious levels of suffering (see Box 7.1 for evidence relating to trigger point influence on the painful symptoms associated with interstitial cystitis and urgency), and that we need to have an array of tools with which to deal with their activities (Weiss 2001).

Local facilitation

According to Korr (1977), a trigger point is a localised area of somatic dysfunction that behaves in a facilitated manner, i.e. it will amplify and be affected by any form of stress imposed on the individual whether this is physical, chemical or emotional. A trigger point is palpable as an indurated, localised, painful entity with a reference (target) area to which pain or other symptoms are referred (Chaitow 1991a).

Muscles housing trigger points can frequently be identified as being unable to achieve their normal resting length using standard muscle evaluation procedures (Janda 1983). The trigger point itself commonly lies in fibrotic tissue, which has evolved as a result of exposure of the tissues to diverse forms of stress.

Treatment methods

A wide variety of methods has been advocated for treating trigger points, including inhibitory (ischaemic compression) pressure methods (Lief 1989, Nimmo 1966), acupuncture and/or ultrasound (Kleyhans & Aarons 1974), chilling and stretching of the muscle in which the trigger lies (Simons et al 1999), procaine or xylocaine injections (Slocumb 1984), active or passive stretching (Lewit 1992) and even surgical excision (Dittrich 1954).

Clinical experience, confirmed by the diligent research of Travell & Simons (1992), has shown that, while all or any of these methods can successfully inhibit trigger point activity in the short term, more is often needed to eliminate the noxious activity of the structure completely.

Common sense, as well as clinical experience, dictates that the next stage of correction of such problems should involve re-education (postural, breathing, relaxation, etc.) or the elimination of factors that contributed to the problem's evolution. This might well involve ergonomic evaluation of home and workplace, as well as the re-education methods mentioned above.

Travell & Simons (1992) have also shown that, whatever initial treatment is offered to inhibit the neurological overactivity of the trigger point, the muscle in which it lies has to be made capable of reaching its normal resting length following such treatment, or the trigger point will rapidly reactivate.

In treating trigger points, the method of chilling the offending muscle (housing the trigger) while holding it at stretch in order to achieve this end was advocated by Travell & Simons (1992), whereas Lewit (1999) has espoused the muscle energy method of a physiologically induced post-isometric relaxation (or reciprocal inhibition) response, before passive stretching. Both methods are commonly successful, although a sufficient degree of failure occurs (trigger points may rapidly reactivate, or fail to 'switch off' completely) to require investigation of more successful approaches.

One reason for failure may relate to the possibility of the tissues that are being stretched not being the very fibres housing the trigger point. A popular method for achieving tonus release in a muscle, prior to stretching, involves the introduction of an isometric contraction to the affected muscle (producing post-isometric relaxation) or to its antagonist (producing reciprocal inhibition). See discussion of muscle energy technique in Chapter 8 (Chaitow 1991b, 2001).

The original use of isometric contractions before stretching was in proprioceptive neuromuscular facilitation (PNF) techniques which emerged from physical medicine in the early part of the 20th century. In most forms of muscle energy technique (MET) methodology, derived from osteopathic research and clinical experience, a partial (not full strength) isometric contraction is performed before the stretch in order to preclude tissue damage or stress to the patient and/or therapist, which PNF quite frequently produces (Greenman 1989, Hartman 1985).

An integrated combination of methods designed to deactivate trigger points effectively, known as integrated neuromuscular inhibition, will be described later in this chapter.

Lief's methods

Stanley Lief, the prime developer of NMT, employed few specific manipulative techniques. His main concern was to attempt to normalise mobility and function (circulation, drainage, nerve function, etc.) and, to this end, his neuromuscular treatment was often accompanied by no more than general mobilisation of the cervical and lumbar areas, together with a degree of 'springing' or stretching of the dorsal region. Derision on the part of the 'specific' manipulators should be tempered by the fact that this general, 'constitutional' treatment approach (some would call it 'engine wiping') achieved phenomenal results in terms of improvement in general well-being, and the alleviation of many specific dysfunctional patterns.

Undoubtedly there exist specific spinal and joint problems that require an individual approach; however, the correction of the supporting mechanisms (muscles, fascia, ligaments, tendons) via NMT on its own, or together with general mobilising techniques offered by soft tissue manipulation, is able frequently to obviate the need for any more detailed technique. Indeed, it is strongly suggested that specific 'adjusting' of joints, which pays no heed to the soft tissue component, is far more likely to fail (in the sense that symptoms speedily return) than the Lief method.

Speransky and Selye: common findings
(Selye 1984, Speransky 1943)

The final conclusion, which Speransky offers us, and which is pertinent to acupuncture as well as all methods of physical treatment, is the following: 'Hence we obtain the rule that only weak degrees of irritation can have a useful significance; strong ones inevitably do damage.'

These words should be locked in the minds of all therapists, of whatever school. The term 'irritation' is used by Speransky, and this is of interest, as a little thought will indicate that whatever is being done to a patient, in terms of therapy, involves to a greater or lesser extent an element of stress (or irritation) – stress, in this sense, being defined as any stimulus, pleasant or unpleasant, that calls upon the body to respond, or adapt, in some manner.

Manipulation, acupuncture, pressure techniques, use of heat and cold, hydrotherapy, electrical and mechanical therapies, surgery, and indeed the whole gamut of medications, whether they be drugs or homeopathic dilutions of herbal substances, all call for a response on the part of the body. All are, therefore, to a degree, 'stress' factors. Speransky insists that only mild irritants can have a useful role to play in evoking a positive (i.e. healing) response.

Selye shows stress can be helpful

Hans Selye (1976) has come to precisely the same conclusion in his important research into stress. In experiments carried out in his extensive studies, Selye produced subcutaneous sacs in experimental animals by injecting a given volume of air under the skin. This was followed by the insertion of an irritant of some sort. He first demonstrated that the amount of exudate, and the thickness of the sac wall, varied, as one might anticipate, with the strength and concentration of the irritant substance. He followed this by introducing a form of stress, such as intense cold, heat or forced immobilisation.

The response of the animals varied greatly. In those that had been injected initially with a weak irritant, the stress that was then added seemed to aid the recovery, as evidenced by resolution of the irritated area and inhibition of tissue fibrosis. Those animals, however, that had had strong irritants injected into the subcutaneous sacs responded to the subsequent stress factor by showing an increase in inflammation, widespread necrosis, and often death. Selye concluded with these words: 'This was the crucial experiment, showing that stress can either cure or aggravate a disease, depending upon whether the inflammatory response to a local irritant is necessary or superfluous.'

We now have Speransky's and Selye's combined evidence, that what we do to a patient, in terms of therapy, can be beneficial or harmful, and that this to a great extent will depend upon the degree of the irritation involved in the treatment, whatever form it takes.

Speransky's work further teaches us that Mann's words are true (see Ch. 4): any part of the surface of the body can be an initiator of a process involving neurological changes, which can be pathological or therapeutic. The classification of certain points as being trigger points, others as being acupuncture alarm points, and yet others as being neurolymphatic or neurovascular – or any other – points, is merely a matter of convenience. It helps us to make a degree of sense out of the enormous amount of information available to us. That, to an extent, these points may be interchangeable is obvious, for many are patently found in the self-same position, on different 'maps' of points. There are subtle variations in the behaviour of some points, such as has already been described with trigger points having a reference area (target area) and other points being found in pairs, etc. This is a matter of practical classification and interpretation of the characteristics of different points. They are all to some extent interchangeable, however, and a latent trigger point, which may be identified as sensitive but with no referral capabilities, might become an active trigger by the simple introduction of a chill, or a strain, to that area.

Bearing in mind, therefore, that the distinction between the variously classified points discussed in this book is man-made, we will continue to classify them in these ways as a matter of convenience. It should also be borne in mind that, whenever acupuncture points are mentioned, the availability of these for manual treatment (pressure, chilling, heating, etc.) remains. There is some evidence that needling can achieve particular effects, not available to pressure techniques, but this is equivocal and, for the purposes of soft tissue manipulation, pressure can usually be shown to be as effective as needling, with the one major drawback, that only a limited number of points can be contacted by hand at any one time, compared with the multiple needling that is possible in acupuncture.

Lewit's view

We are in the midst of a change in the concepts of manipulative therapy that has far-reaching implications. One of the major changes is the restoration of the soft tissue component to centre stage, rather than the peripheral role to which it has been assigned in the past. Lewit (1985) discusses aspects of this. He describes the 'no man's land' that lies between neurology, orthopaedics and rheumatology, which, he says, is the home of the vast majority of patients with pain derived from the locomotor system, and in whom no definite pathomorphological changes are found. He makes the suggestion that these be termed cases of 'functional pathology of the locomotor system'. These include most of the patients attending osteopathic, chiropractic and physiotherapy practitioners.

The most frequent symptom of individuals involved in this area of dysfunction is pain, which may be reflected clinically by reflex changes such as muscle spasm, myofascial trigger points, hyperalgesic skin zones, periosteal pain points, or a wide variety of other sensitive areas that have no obvious pathological origin. It is a major part of the role of NMT to help in both identifying such areas and offering some help in differential diagnosis. NMT and other soft tissue methods are then capable of normalising many of the causative aspects of these myriad and mysterious sources of pain and disability.

Selye's local adaptation progression

Selye has described the progression of changes in tissue that is being locally stressed. There is an initial alarm (acute inflammatory) stage followed by a stage of adaptation or resistance when stress factors are continuous or repetitive, at which time muscular tissue becomes progressively fibrotic, and, if this change is taking place in muscle that has a postural rather than a phasic function, the entire muscle structure will shorten (Janda 1985, Selye 1984).

Clearly such fibrotic tissue, lying in altered (shortened) muscle, cannot simply 'release' itself in order to allow the muscle to achieve its normal resting length (as we have seen, this is a prerequisite of normalisation of trigger point activity). Along with various forms of stretch (passive, active, MET, PNF, etc.), it has been noted above that inhibitory pressure is commonly employed in treatment of trigger points. Such pressure technique methods (analogous to acupressure or shiatsu methodology), which are often successful in achieving at least short-term reduction in trigger point activity, may be considered as 'neuromuscular techniques' (Chaitow 1991b).

IDEALS

The holistic, total, approach to the problems of human health is one that looks to the causes of dysfunction and disease and, by removing these, allows the homeostatic, self-regulating, efforts of the body to restore normality. This ideal is not always attainable but it should remain the aim of the therapist. Each individual has an optimum degree of biomechanical (structural, postural, functional), biochemical and psychological efficiency that can be realised. It is this optimum that is being aimed for in all therapies that fall into the broad net of holistic healing methods.

NMT takes its place amongst these methods, because its objective is to help to restore the structural, functional and postural integrity of the body, by removing restrictions and aiding in the normalisation of dysfunction. NMT aids the economy and functional ability of the body further by reducing self-perpetuating stress factors such as contractions, spasms and tensions in the soft tissue components of the system. By improving function, removing pain, reducing energy loss, improving posture, etc., the effect on psychologically negative states is a positive one.

In itself NMT is only a tool, a useful method or technique, which can be of immense use in a variety of conditions. It possesses one further criterion that places it firmly in the holistic 'tool box': it does nothing to the body that is harmful to its overall state of health (i.e. it has no side-effects). Indeed, by normalising the soft tissues, NMT often saves the individual from techniques of a more 'violent' nature, such as surgery, traction and immobilisation, which might well produce outward reactions, and from techniques that, while not usually harmful, can be painful, such as manipulative joint techniques.

NMT has an immense capability for diagnostic application and, because this can take place at the same time as its therapeutic application, it shows economy in the use of time and energy. As NMT is entirely a manual technique, it is not wasteful of resources such as heat, power, etc., and is applicable under almost any circumstance or condition.

NMT AND SPORTS INJURIES: MOULE'S METHODS

One practitioner who has achieved outstanding success in applying NMT to athletic injuries of marked severity is osteopath Terry Moule, son of Tom Moule, a one-time associate and assistant to Stanley Lief. In the 1970s Terry Moule restored the former captain of England's soccer team, Gerry Francis, to playing fitness. Surgery to the lumbar spine was the only prospect left for Francis after months of agony under orthopaedic investigation. In desperation, Moule was consulted and within a few weeks Francis was playing again. He remains fit and continues to be involved in professional soccer as a manager.

A similar return to full function was achieved in the case of the then captain of England's rugby football team, Roger Uttley, whose career appeared to be over following a back injury. Treatment, consisting largely of NMT, resulted in Uttley returning to the England squad in its successful 1980 season.

An even more startling result of the application of NMT to a spinal injury involved then world mile and 1500-metre record-holder Sebastian Coe. He stated in late 1979: 'Last winter I had a back problem. I was having trouble getting a diagnosis, let alone treatment.' Within a few treatments incorporating NMT he was running again and setting world record times.

At the time of writing (2002), Moule continues to treat sporting injuries using NMT as a primary tool. He has described NMT as follows (T. Moule, personal communication):

The principle of NMT is that it is of prime importance to treat connective tissue lesions and abnormalities, prior to any manipulative treatment of the bony structures. If more orthodox and less penetrating soft tissue techniques are used, whilst the bony abnormality may be corrected by the application of a specific adjustment, because the soft tissues remain in a similar state to that existing prior to the manipulation, there is a strong likelihood of a recurrence of the lesion. NMT tends to dispense with specific adjustment, for, subsequent to using these specialised soft tissue measures, a generalised mobilisation adjustment will allow the muscular and connective tissues to encourage the bony structures to return to their normal alignment. This may take a little longer to produce relief from discomfort, but in the long run it means that the correction is more permanent and there is less danger of any damage to the muscular and connective tissues from forceful manipulation.

The great advantage of NMT is that it may be applied to any part of the body. It is particularly effective in dealing with problems related to interference with nerve supply; to any form of muscular or connective tissue lesion; to treatment of the abdominal and pelvic organs etc. It is applied mainly by use of the thumb. It may take some years to develop an adequate 'feel' in the hands in general and the thumbs in particular, to effectively diagnose and treat lesions. It is the ability to diagnose through the thumb which is so helpful in the rapid and efficient treatment of all forms of dysfunction. Correctly used it precludes a large number of more conventional techniques and saves a considerable amount of time.

NMT has proved invaluable in the treatment of sports injuries, particularly for the diagnostic reasons outlined above and for the fact that it produces a rapid response as compared to orthodox soft tissue and physiotherapy techniques. With sports injuries one of the major problems is to get the player back in action as soon as possible, particularly where the injury is to a professional sportsman. NMT has been used very effectively on a large number of sportsmen and women following all types of sports.

One of the most common injuries one encounters is hamstring problems. These are particularly prevalent amongst footballers, who in many cases develop the injury through overdevelopment of the quadriceps without adequate attention to the maintenance and mobility (i.e. lengthening and stretching) of the hamstrings at the same time. The normal treatment of hamstring injuries is ultra-sonic and massage. These techniques are not particularly rapid and the resultant loss of overall muscle tone, due to the inability of the leg to be used normally, retards a return to normal function. With NMT a lesion can be accurately and rapidly detected and, by the use of deep thumb manipulation, the soft tissue lesion can be dealt with rapidly and effectively. Where there is muscular fibre damage this can be felt and literally ironed out. The effect of the technique is to stimulate circulation in the area thus encouraging healing. Where there is inflammation and swelling the technique promotes drainage and the restoration of normal tone. With acute lesions the technique is unfortunately painful, but where speed is the prime order in recovery this is a small price to pay.

NMT is also beneficial in the treatment of knee lesions, particularly ligamentous problems and the subsequent inflammation in the joint itself. Correct application of NMT to these lesions will improve drainage from the knee and encourages healing to take place far more rapidly than through orthodox techniques. Where there is knee misalignments or dislocation, reduction of spasm is most important as a prerequisite to satisfactory manipulation of the joint. In many cases injury occurs when the legs become anchored due to studs in the boots. If rotation of the trunk is superimposed onto this static lower limb situation the stress imposed on the knee joint is enormous. The application of NMT prior to attempting correction not only makes the correction less painful but ensures that the result is lasting.

NMT is also beneficial in the treatment of prepatellar bursitis, and any synovial inflammatory problems.

A problem which plagues many sportsmen, particularly footballers, basketball players and volleyball players, is pain in the groin and down the inside of the leg. This is commonly treated as a sacroiliac or a lumbar problem when, in many cases, it is due to a lesion of the symphysis-pubis. There are a number of techniques for dealing with problems of this joint but none so dramatically successful as the application of NMT.

The technique's effectiveness in producing long-term benefits is perhaps best underlined by the results with sportsmen such as Roger Uttley and Gerry Francis, who had both received short-term benefit from manipulative treatment. The application of NMT, without any change in the manipulative

techniques being employed, except to make them less specific, produced long-term improvement which allowed a return to active participation in their respective sports. In both cases the main problem was an imbalance in muscle tone with excessive tension causing persistence of the joint dysfunction. The removal of these soft tissue factors restored balance and encouraged the body to return to normal function, as it always tries to do.

In summary, the benefits of NMT in general are

(1) It is a technique which removes causes rather than dealing with symptoms.
(2) It removes the necessity for the bulk of specific manipulation, instead it encourages the body to normalise itself.
(3) It is applicable to any part of the body.

From the specific sports injury point of view the main advantage of NMT is that it provides (a) a more rapid recovery rate and (b) a more permanent one.

The author's own experience confirms the validity of Terry Moule's comments. NMT, apart from all the myriad applications discussed in earlier chapters, is the finest soft tissue system for helping to normalise acute and chronic injuries. The successful use of NMT calls for the applied thought of the practitioner. The body responds rapidly to the help this technique offers. Its limitations are almost always related to the limitations of the practitioner. Its success is in direct proportion to the dedication and intelligence with which it is applied.

WHEN IS NMT USEFUL?

NMT may be universally applied to any patient of any age suffering from any condition. This is not to say that it will be curative, or even of marked value, in all conditions. However, it will be of some diagnostic and therapeutic value in every condition, and of enormous value in others, because no one is free from some degree of dysfunction, affecting the overall efficiency and economy of the body.

In general terms, NMT may be applied to all cases of musculoskeletal dysfunction and mento-emotional dysfunction with benefit. The basic spinal and basic abdominal techniques are used as diagnostic and therapeutic tools in the majority of cases. The more specific techniques, such as psoas, piriformis, tensor fascia lata and abdominal release techniques, are used as and when indicated. A general, full-body NMT treatment may be applied as part of a programme of postural reintegration.

In specific terms, NMT is applied as follows. All conditions of the spine and conditions that involve the arms or legs would receive general spinal technique as well as consideration of local areas, in the limbs affected. Such treatments would be repeated once or twice weekly until a degree of normality had been achieved. As should be obvious, other modalities and techniques would and should be used if called for. NMT combines with anything of a supportive nature that is aimed at the restoration of normal function, such as (in appropriate conditions) ultrasound therapy, diathermy, manipulation, etc.

At the outset, the aim of general treatment is to remove the more obvious areas of contraction and stasis. All active trigger points should be neutralised by pressure techniques, if possible and if appropriate, or, if found stubborn, by chill and stretch, MET or infiltration methods. As therapy progresses, individual patterns of dysfunction will become clearer, and more specific NMT would be applied to spinal, abdominal, intercostal and pelvic areas that may be slow to improve.

Manipulative techniques of a non-specific type are often useful in the normalisation of spinal integrity, once the initial soft tissue rigidity or dysfunction has been improved. NMT may be applied with infinite gentleness or with robust enthusiasm, as it is possible to use the same techniques with a marked difference in the degree of force employed. This enables its application to areas of acute sensitivity as well as in fragile (osteoporotic) and tender areas. As long as the practitioner is thinking about the task in hand and not applying the techniques in a mechanical, repetitive manner, there is no danger of injury or harm.

If treatment is aimed at the removal of symptoms stemming from trigger points, it is essential to normalise all the structures related to the local area of dysfunction. Simply to neutralise

the trigger that is causing, say, a headache will produce short-term benefits. If the particular trigger lies in the trapezius muscle, then not only must the trigger be normalised and the trapezius treated, but the entire cervical and spinal musculature and soft tissues must receive attention, as should the patterns of posture and use that provoked the tissues to the state where headaches became a natural consequence.

A general rule should be that no part of the whole should be considered without the whole also being considered. Thus, even if the spinal areas are receiving the main attention of the therapist on any one visit, the muscles of the lower limb and associated structures should be given some consideration to assess their involvement and possible requirements. The treatment of the back, therefore, calls for the treatment of the front, and this calls for the whole to be considered and treated. The condition in the context of the body, and the body in the context of its (total) environment, are the appropriate areas of investigation and care.

General abdominal technique is useful in all cases of digestive and intestinal dysfunction of a non-pathological nature. NMT is applicable to all cases of respiratory dysfunction. It is also applicable to all genitourinary conditions of a non-pathological nature. NMT applied to the abdomen will reduce many tension states emerging out of mento-emotional backgrounds. General abdominal technique improves circulatory efficiency through the pelvis and abdominal regions, and it enhances respiratory function. The reflex points and zones in the spinal area should always be treated prior to thoracic and abdominal technique, as indicated. In a case of spastic constipation, for example, NMT to the lower spinal areas and the use of neurolymphatic points followed by general abdominal technique would be the pattern recommended. This could be followed by specific abdominal release techniques if areas of marked contractions or 'adhesion' were elicited during the general treatment. In the author's experience, such an approach, combined with general health measures such as nutritional reform, together with appropriate exercise and relaxation programmes, will promote a return to normal. If the body is being given those factors required for normality, its self-healing tendency (homeostasis), which is constantly acting, will respond positively to the removal of obstacles to recovery (structural, mechanical, dietary).

In dealing with tension and stress of psychic origin, it is as well to recall that the mind will not be calm or relaxed as long as neuromuscular tensions are present. In applying any form of psychotherapy, the use of NMT, applied to the spine and abdomen, will increasingly improve the patient's ability to relax. NMT is not seen as an end in itself in this regard, but to be a catalyst to the removal or easing of the physical component of a vicious circle. In some cases this physical release of tension, especially when applied to the solar plexus, can produce a sudden emotional release in which the patient may cry and sob. The body becomes a solid mass of tensions and contractions for many individuals. The tensions of life are mirrored by layers of muscular 'armour'. The posture and tensions thus created all carry specific emotional charges and memories and, as the physical components are eased, so do the emotional memories and feelings associated with their origins come to the surface. Just how appropriate it is to initiate such 'releases' was discussed earlier in this chapter.

In restoring total structural and postural integrity to the body, it is necessary to apply NMT to all the supporting structures. This might involve the spinal, thoracic and abdominal soft tissues and the limbs, including the feet. NMT and manipulation, where appropriate, will lay the foundations for a return to normal (or to the patient's individual optimal norm).

Specific and general exercise, as well as postural re-education, may then follow. It is possible, via such systems as the Alexander technique, to achieve postural and functional normality. It is contended, however, that with the judicious use of NMT and soft tissue and, if necessary, osseous manipulation, such re-education becomes much easier and less arduous. It must be easier to learn to use a machine correctly if that machine is capable of functioning correctly!

The same proviso applies to breathing retraining. Unless the thoracic and diaphragmatic structures are to some extent made pliable by therapeutic interventions, such as those detailed in earlier chapters, such retraining will of necessity involve struggling against great odds.

In attempting to achieve postural and functional normality, a fairly long-term view is required. Some workers assert that a series of eight to ten treatment sessions will produce this result. It is the author's experience that, whilst the basic groundwork can be done in eight to ten treatments, the majority of cases require weekly or fortnightly treatment for 12–18 months if they are to achieve optimum improvement. This should be followed by maintenance visits at intervals of not less than 3 months.

Just as retraining (posture, breathing) without appropriate bodywork is doomed to partial success at best, so bodywork methods that ignore retraining and re-education will have only short-term benefits, since much of any chronic dysfunctional pattern of use will be firmly locked into habitual neural and behavioural patterns.

Structural and functional changes are interdependent: they follow each other causally as well as therapeutically. NMT is universally applicable. It has no side-effects. It combines with all other methods of positive health care. In itself it is capable of improving general function, releasing tension and removing noxious triggers, which may be responsible for myriad symptoms. NMT has limits, but within the framework of its own area of application its only limits lie in the ability of the practitioner.

THE INIT HYPOTHESIS
(Chaitow 1994)

The author hypothesises that a partial isometric contraction (using no more than 20–30% of patient strength, as is the norm in MET procedures) may sometimes fail to achieve activation of the fibres housing the trigger point being treated, because light contractions of this sort fail to recruit more than a small percentage of the muscle's potential.

Subsequent stretching of the muscle may therefore involve only marginally the critical tissues surrounding and enveloping the myofascial trigger point (or may not involve them at all!).

Failure actively to lengthen the muscle fibres in which the trigger is housed may account for the not infrequent recurrence of trigger point activity in the same site following treatment. Repetition of the stress factors that produced it in the first place could undoubtedly also be a factor in such recurrence – which emphasises the need for re-education in rehabilitation. A method that achieved precise targeting of these tissues (in terms of tonus release and subsequent stretching) would be advantageous.

Clinical experience indicates that, by combining the methods of direct inhibition (pressure mildly applied, continuously or in a 'make and break' pattern) along with the concept of strain/counterstrain and MET, a specific targeting of dysfunctional soft tissues can be achieved.

Strain/counterstrain (SCS) explained briefly

Jones (1981) has shown that particular painful 'points' relating to joint or muscular strain, chronic or acute, can be used as 'monitors' – pressure being applied to them as the body or body part is carefully positioned in such a way as to remove or reduce the pain felt in the palpated point.

When the position of ease is attained (using what is known as 'fine tuning' in SCS jargon), in which pain vanishes from the palpated monitoring tender point, the stressed tissues are felt to be at their most relaxed – and clinical experience indicates that this is so because they palpate as 'easy' rather than having a sense of being 'bound' or tense.

SCS is thought to achieve its benefits by means of an automatic resetting of muscle spindles – which help to dictate the length and tone in the tissues. This resetting apparently occurs only when the muscle housing the spindle is at ease, and usually results in a reduction in excessive tone and release of spasm. When positioning the body (part) in SCS methodology, a sense

of 'ease' is noted as the tissues reach the position in which pain vanishes from the palpated point.

 ## INIT methods

Method 1 (Fig. 9.1)

It is reasonable to assume, and palpation confirms, that when a trigger point is being palpated by direct finger or thumb pressure, and when the very tissue in which the trigger point lies is positioned in such a way as to take away the pain (entirely or at least to a great extent), the most (dis)stressed fibres in which the trigger point is housed are in a position of relative ease.

We would then have a trigger point under direct inhibitory pressure (mild or perhaps intermittent) which had been positioned so that the tissues housing it are relaxed (relatively or completely).

Following a period of 20–30 seconds of this position of ease and inhibitory pressure – if the patient is asked to introduce an isometric contraction into the tissues and to hold this for 7–10 second – involving the very fibres

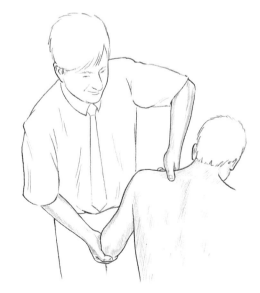

Figure 9.1A First stage of INIT in which a tender/pain/trigger point in supraspinatus is located and compressed ischaemically, either intermittently or persistently.

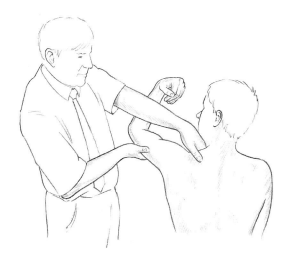

Figure 9.1B   The pain is removed from the tender/pain/trigger point by finding a position of ease which is held for at least 20 seconds, after which an isometric contraction is achieved involving the tissues that house the tender/pain/trigger point.

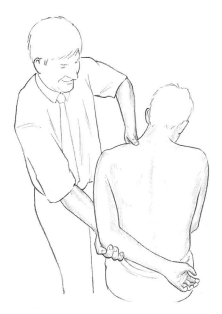

Figure 9.1C   After holding the isometric contraction for an appropriate period, the muscle housing the point of local soft tissue dysfunction is stretched. This completes the INIT sequence.

that had been repositioned to obtain the strain/counterstrain release – there would subsequently occur a degree of reduction in tone

in these tissues (post-isometric relaxation). These could then be gently stretched (locally) as in any muscle energy procedure, with the strong likelihood that specifically involved fibres would be stretched.

Subsequently the whole muscle could be stretched following a further isometric contraction.

Method 2

There is another possibility – a variation in which, instead of an isometric contraction followed by stretch being commenced following the period of ease (strain/counterstrain position), an isolytic (isotonic eccentric) approach could be used.

The muscle receiving attention is actively contracted by the patient at the same time as a stretch is introduced, resulting in mild trauma to the muscle and the breakdown of fibrous adhesions between it and its interface and within its structures (Mitchell et al 1979).

To introduce this method into trigger point treatment, following the application of inhibitory pressure and SCS release, the patient is asked to contract the muscles around the palpating thumb or finger (lying on the now inhibited pain point) with the request that the contraction should not be a full-strength effort because the practitioner intends to stretch the tissues gently while the contraction is taking place.

This isotonic eccentric effort – designed to reduce contractions and break down fibrotic tissue – should target precisely the tissues in which the trigger point being treated lies buried. Following the isolytic stretch the tissues could benefit from effleurage and/or hot and cold applications to ease local congestion. An instruction should be given to avoid active use of the area for a day or so.

Summary and comment

The integrated use of inhibitory pressure, strain/counterstrain and a form of muscle energy technique – applied to a trigger point or other area of soft tissue dysfunction involving pain or restriction of range of motion (of soft tissue origin) – is a logical approach, because it has the advantage of allowing precise targeting of the culprit tissues.

Clearly, the use of an isolytic approach as part of this sequence will be more easily achieved in some regions than in others – upper trapezius posing less of a problem in terms of positioning and application, perhaps, than quadratus lumborum.

After either INIT method, it has been found to be useful to instruct the patient to learn a method of gentle activation of the antagonist muscles to the muscle housing the trigger point that has been treated. The patient is asked to reproduce this activity a number of times daily for the days immediately after treatment. This activation of antagonists produces a reciprocal inhibition of the previously hypertonic muscle, and assists in maintaining the deactivation.

REFERENCES

Barlow W 1959 Anxiety and muscle tension pain. British Journal of Clinical Practice 13(5)

Bass C, Gardner WN 1985 Respiratory and psychiatric abnormalities in chronic symptomatic hyperventilation. British Medical Journal 290:1387–1390

Beal MC 1983 Palpatory testing for somatic dysfunction in patients with cardiovascular disease. Journal of the American Osteopathic Association 82:822–831

Chaitow L 1983 Neuromuscular technique. Thorsons, Wellingborough, UK

Chaitow L 1991a Palpatory literacy. Thorsons, London

Chaitow L 1991b Soft tissue manipulation. Healing Arts Press, Rochester, Vermont

Chaitow L 1994 INIT in treatment of pain and trigger points. British Journal of Osteopathy XIII:17–21

Chaitow L 2001 Muscle energy technique. 2nd edn. Churchill Livingstone, Edinburgh

Chaitow L, DeLany J 2002 Clinical applications of neuromuscular technique. Vol. 2. Churchill Livingstone, Edinburgh (in press)

Chaitow L, Bradley D, Gilbert C 2002 Multidisciplinary approaches to breathing pattern disorders. Churchill Livingstone, Edinburgh

Dittrich R 1954 Somatic pain and autonomic concomitants. American Journal of Surgery

Garland W 1994 Somatic changes in hyperventilating subject. Presentation at Respiratory Function Congress, Paris

Goldthwaite J 1949 Essentials of body mechanics. JB Lippincott, Philadelphia

Greenman P 1989 Manual medicine. Williams & Wilkins, Baltimore

Hartman L 1985 Handbook of osteopathic technique. Hutchinson, London

Hungerford B, Gilleard W 1998 SIJ angular rotation during the stork and hip drop tests in normal subjects: pilot study results. Third Interdisciplinary World Congress on Low Back and Pelvic Pain, Vienna: 332–334

Janda V 1983 Muscle function testing. Butterworths, London

Janda V 1985 In: Glasgow E, ed. Aspects of manipulative therapy. Churchill Livingstone, Edinburgh

Janda V 1988 In: Grant R, ed. Physical therapy in the cervical and thoracic spine. Churchill Livingstone, New York

Jones L 1981 Strain/counterstrain. Academy of Applied Osteopathy, Colorado Springs

Jones L 1981 Strain and counterstrain. Academy of Applied Osteopathy, Colorado Springs

Jung C-G 1973 Synchronicity: an acausal connecting principle. Princeton University Press, Princeton, New Jersey

Kleyhans & Aarons 1974 Digest of Chiropractic Economics September

Korr I 1977 Spinal cord as organiser of the disease process. 1976 Yearbook of the Academy of Applied Osteopathy, Colorado Springs

Latey P 1986 Muscular manifesto. Published privately, London

Lee D 2002 Palpation issues. Journal of Bodywork and Movement Therapies 6(1):26–27

Lewit K 1985 Manipulative therapy in rehabilitation of the motor system. Butterworths, London

Lewit K 1992 Manipulation in rehabilitation of the locomotor system. 2nd edn. Butterworths, London

Lewit K 1999 Manipulation in rehabilitation of the locomotor system. 3rd edn. Butterworths, London

Lief S 1989 Cited in: Chaitow L, ed. Neuro-muscular technique/soft tissue manipulation. Thorsons, Wellingborough, UK

Melzack R, Wall P 1988 The challenge of pain. Penguin, London

Mitchell F, Moran P, Pruzzo N 1979 Evaluation of osteopathic muscle energy procedure. Pruzzo, Valley Park, Illinois

Murphy D, ed. 2000 Conservative management of cervical spine syndromes. McGraw Hill, New York

Myers T 2001 Anatomy trains. Churchill Livingstone, Edinburgh

Nimmo R 1966 Receptor tonus technique. Lecture notes, British College of Naturopathy and Osteopathy, London

Pollard H, Ward G 1997 A study of two stretching techniques for improving hip flexion range of motion. Journal of Manipulative and Physiological Therapeutics 20:443–447

Randolph T 1976 Stimulatory withdrawal and the alternations of allergic manifestations. In: Dickey L, ed. Clinical ecology, pp 156–175. Charles C. Thomas, Springfield, Illinois

Rolf I 1977 The integration of human structures. Harper & Row, USA

Roll M, Thorell T 1987 Acute chest pain without obvious cause before age 40 – personality and recent life events. Journal of Psychosomatic Research 31(2):215–221

Sandler S 1983 The physiology of soft tissue massage. British Osteopathic Journal 15:1–6

Selye H 1984 The stress of life. McGraw-Hill, New York

Simons D, Travell J, Simons L 1999 Myofascial pain and dysfunction: the trigger point manual. Vol. 1: Upper half of body 2nd edn. Williams & Wilkins, Baltimore

Slocumb J 1984 Neurological factors in chronic pelvic pain, trigger points and abdominal pelvic pain. American Journal of Obstetrics and Gynecology 49:536

Speransky 1943 A basis for the theory of medicine. International Publishers, New York

Travell J, Simons D 1983 Myofascial pain and dysfunction: the trigger point manual. Vol. 1. Williams & Wilkins, Baltimore

Travell J, Simons D 1992 Myofascial pain and dysfunction: the trigger point manual. Vol. 2: The lower extremities. Williams & Wilkins, Baltimore

Upledger J 1983 Craniosacral therapy. Eastland Press, USA

Vleeming A, Mooney V, Dorman T, Snijders C, Stoeckart R, eds. 1997 Movement, stability and low back pain. Churchill Livingstone, Edinburgh

Wall PD, Melzack R, eds. 1989 Textbook of pain. 2nd edn. Churchill Livingstone, Edinburgh

Weiss J 2001 Pelvic floor myofascial trigger points: manual therapy for interstitial cystitis and the urgency–frequency syndrome. Journal of Urology 166:2226–2231

10

American neuromuscular therapy

Judith DeLany

HISTORY

As detailed in Chapter 2, neuromuscular therapy (NMT) evolved out of the work of a number of clinicians working in both Europe and the USA.[1] The 'evolutionary' development of American protocols of NMT (neuromuscular 'therapy' rather than neuromuscular 'technique', the preferred term in Europe) was based largely on the methods devised and taught by the late Raymond Nimmo (DeLany 1999). Nimmo's research into the pathological influences and relevance, as well as the therapeutic implications of treating, 'noxious pain points' mirrors closely that of his contemporary, Janet Travell, in relation to her research into myofascial trigger points. Nimmo's protocols were subsequently modified and expanded by Paul St John, who studied with Nimmo, and then by St John and Judith (Walker) DeLany, who worked together in the 1980s. Both St John and DeLany have continued expanding their separate NMT programmes over the last decade.

While the American protocols of NMT were initially based on that of Nimmo, they were strongly influenced by the writings and research of Travell & Simons (1983, 1992), Vannerson & Nimmo (1971), Cailliet (1977), Chaitow (1980)

---

[1] Variations existing between the European and American versions of NMT are highlighted in this chapter by brief comments, given in footnotes. The European version is commonly known as 'Lief's NMT', which is how it is described in these notes.

and others. Both St John's and DeLany's variations on Nimmo's protocols resulted in revisions of previous concepts and methodology, leading to significant changes in recommended treatment techniques. St John currently incorporates structural homeostasis of the body and cranium as the basis of his St John Method™, while DeLany takes a broader view in NMT American version™ (Chaitow & DeLany 2000), where she incorporates a systematic approach, which involves attention to biochemical, biomechanical and psychosocial factors.

In 2000, DeLany and co-author Leon Chaitow, published the first of two volumes that present NMT American version™ alongside the European NMT protocols, positional release, muscle energy techniques and other modalities that can be used as adjuncts to its application. *Clinical Application of Neuromuscular Techniques*, volumes 1 & 2, distinguish NMT American version™ as a practical, systematic approach for training palpation and assessment skills, as well as for clinical application.

The following introduction to NMT American version™ will concentrate on the basic techniques and examples of application to selected muscles. There is no substitute for supervised hands-on instruction, which is highly recommended as the safest means of acquiring NMT skills.

PLATFORM OF NMT AMERICAN VERSION™

Homeostasis incorporates the processes through which the various functions of the body, including everything from postural adjustments to the chemical compositions of the body's fluids, are maintained in balance (Stedman 1998). It is through this goal of equilibrium that the body deals with the many stresses and demands placed upon it in daily life, accomplishing this through adaptation and compensation. If stresses are excessive, or if compensation mechanisms have been compromised or overloaded, the adverse effects of decompensation, where frank disease and degeneration occur, are likely to emerge.

Categories

The broad foundation of NMT American version™ is based on the assessment of three categories capable of adaptation that, on a constant basis, modify, adjust to and compensate for the stresses of life. Within the three categories – biomechanical, biochemical and psychosocial – are to be found subdivisions of most of the major influences on health, with a number of these features being commonly involved in causing or intensifying pain (Chaitow 1996, Chaitow & DeLany 2000). In addressing these categories, it is acknowledged that there can be local and/or global causes of pain and dysfunction, as well as perpetuating factors, that, if left untreated, may cause 'mysterious' recurrence of the condition (Simons et al 1999). Local, global and perpetuating factors should all be considered in a thorough recovery programme. These include (Chaitow & DeLany 2000), amongst others, locally dysfunctional states such as:

- hypertonia
- ischaemia
- prolonged inflammation
- trigger points
- neural compression or entrapment

as well as the following global factors that affect the whole body systemically:

- genetic predisposition (e.g. connective tissue factors leading to hypermobility) and inborn anomalies (e.g. short leg)
- nutritional deficiencies and imbalances
- toxicity (exogenous and endogenous)
- infections (chronic or acute)
- endocrine imbalances and deficiencies (hormonal, including thyroid)
- stress (physical or psychological)
- trauma
- posture (including patterns of misuse)
- hyperventilation tendencies.

Although the entire list should be kept in mind, NMT American version™ focuses largely on six 'subdivisions' from this list. NMT practitioners particularly address ischaemia, trigger points, neural entrapments/compressions, postural imbalance, nutritional components/deficiencies and emotional factors. In clinical application, any of these (or others from the above list) that lie outside the scope of practice and licence of the practitioner should be considered for referral.

It should be kept in mind that the influences of a *biomechanical*, *biochemical* and *psychosocial* nature do not produce single changes. Their interaction with one another is profound, and intervention in one category can affect the others remarkably. The practitioner's role may be to alleviate the stress burden or simply to lighten the load. At times, all that may be accomplished is to work towards more efficient handling of the adaptive load by teaching and encouraging the individual to alter daily habits. While it is important to remove or modify as many aetiological and perpetuating influences as can be identified, this must be done without creating further distress or a requirement for excessive adaptation. For each therapeutic intervention applied, adaptation will probably also be required. It is important that the adaptive mechanisms are not overloaded in the healing process.

The six factors of NMT

When working with a person in chronic pain, the six subdivisions derived from the local and global lists above should be addressed systematically to assess for and, hopefully, reduce underlying causes of discomfort and/or dysfunction. If assessment of one or more of these factors is omitted, the person may plateau or regress in his or her recovery. These particular six factors should be considered and clinically addressed by the practitioner in all patients (Chaitow & DeLany 2000). If the practitioner is without skill or licence in one or more of these, it is suggested that the patient be referred to another practitioner who is suitably trained and licensed in the subject. If progress is not seen within a few treatments, or if pain, fatigue, or other primary symptoms return, other factors (hormonal, organ or bone health, toxicity, etc.) should be considered. The six factors, as noted by DeLany (2002), are:

Ischaemia – A state in which the current oxygen supply is inadequate for the current physiological needs of tissue. Causes of ischaemia can be pathological (narrowed artery or thrombus), biochemical (vasoconstriction by the body to reduce flow to a particular area), anatomical (tendon obstruction of blood flow) or as a result of overuse or facilitation. Ischaemia reduces the level of oxygen, nutrients and waste removal and the tension produced by the resultant muscle shortening can alter joint mechanics and/or entrap neural structures. Ischaemia, and its resultant local energy crisis, can also lead to the production of trigger points (Simons et al 1999).

Trigger points (TrPs) – localized areas within muscle bellies (central TrPs) or at myotendinous or periosteal attachments (attachment TrPs) which, when sufficiently provoked, produce a referral pattern to a target zone. The referral pattern may include pain, tingling, numbness, itching, burning or other sensations. In addition to its location (central or attachment), a TrP can be classified as to its state of activity (active or latent) as well as whether it is primary, key or satellite. (See also trigger point formation theories, described in detail in Ch. 3.)

Neural interferences – compression (by osseous structures) or entrapment (by myofascial tissues) of neural structures may result in muscle contraction disturbances, vasomotion, pain impulses, reflex mechanisms and disturbances in sympathetic activity

Postural and biomechanical dysfunctions – repeated postural and biomechanical insults over a period of time, combined with the somatic effects of emotional and psychological origin, will often present altered patterns of tense, shortened, bunched, fatigued and, ultimately, fibrotic tissues with resultant alterations from healthy postural positioning

Nutritional factors – nutritional deficiencies/imbalances, sensitivities, allergies and stimulants all play roles in myofascial health as well as hormonal, emotional and mental health

Emotional well-being – the degree and type of the emotional and stress loads the individual is carrying can influence various systems of the body. Ultimately, if excessive or prolonged, these factors can result in distress and disease.

APPLICATION OF NMT

Effective application of NMT techniques may be achieved more easily by applying the following guidelines. As knowledge of anatomy is enhanced and the necessary skills are attained, each practitioner will develop his or her own style by blending NMT knowledge with that acquired from other disciplines studied.

Note: In the USA, laws regarding scope of practice vary from state to state and among the many healthcare professions. Most states require a 'licence to touch' in order to treat patients. It is suggested that each practitioner perform within the scope of his or her own licence regardless of what is presented within this text. NMT is practised in multiple disciplines in many different states and countries, and this text may contain techniques or concepts that lie outside of the scope of a particular licence. It is each practitioner's responsibility to know his or her scope of practice and to work within the boundaries of licensure.

Order of the routine

What should be treated first? Where should treatment begin? Sequencing is an important element in bodywork and, to some extent, is a matter of experience and preference. However, in many instances protocols and prescriptions based on clinical experience – and sometimes research – can be offered.

NMT is written about and usually applied as a sequence of steps. Each step of the 'routine' is performed in the initial examination to assure maximum results, as skipping some steps may cause a significant detail to be missed and result in less than optimal outcomes. In subsequent treatment sessions some of the steps may be omitted if particular tissues are not involved.

The techniques are applied to the muscles in a suggested order that is designed to enter the tissues by layers, to treat the proximal portion of an extremity before the distal portion, and to best manage the therapy time. When the order of the routine needs to be altered, two rules should always be applied:

1. *Superficial tissues are treated before deeper layers.*
2. *The proximal portion of any extremity is addressed before the distal.*

Clinical application of NMT

The clinical examination that uses NMT moves almost seamlessly from the gathering of information into application of treatment. The process of discovery leads to therapeutic action as the practitioner searches for evidence of tissue dysfunction, and then applies the technique to turn 'finding into fixing'. This transition from examination to treatment and back to examination is a characteristic of NMT and will become habitual as the methods and objectives of NMT and its associated modalities become more familiar. NMT palpation techniques can be blended with the application of muscle energy techniques and positional or myofascial release methods by moving from one modality to the other and back to examination without delay.

A variety of techniques is used in NMT, the choice of which depends on the practitioner's skills and what is discovered in examination, as well as the desired effect on the tissues. The use of skin lubrication will vary from step to step depending upon the technique being applied. Dry techniques, such as connective tissue work or tissue lifting techniques, should be applied before lubrication, because some muscles become difficult to palpate when oiled. Generally, gliding procedures require lubrication, while friction and tissue lifting techniques do not.

Application of dry techniques is generally followed by manipulation or lightly lubricated gliding, which is aimed at increasing blood flow and 'flushing' tissues while simultaneously evaluating for ischaemic bands and/or trigger points. Static digital pressure is subsequently employed in order to release ischaemic bands and for treatment of trigger points, and is usually applied after several repetitions of gliding have been completed. Pressure bars may be used instead of (or in addition to) finger or thumb compression (Fig. 10.1B,C) in certain areas; however, precautions apply and proper training is suggested. Manually applied gliding strokes are usually repeated after applications of compression, friction or pressure bar techniques.

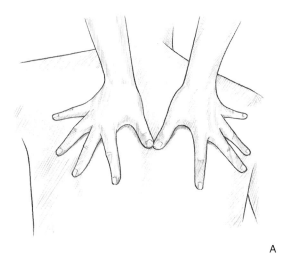

Figure 10.1A The fingers lead and steady the thumbs, which are the primary tools used in most of the gliding techniques.

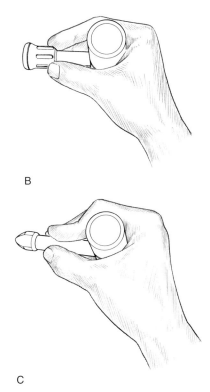

B

C

Figure 10.1B,C Pressure bars, held properly, are excellent treatment tools that relieve stress on the practitioner's thumbs and fingers.

NMT TECHNIQUES

The choice of NMT technique depends upon what is discovered in examination as well as the desired effect on the tissues.

● *Skin rolling and tissue lifting techniques* can be applied to soften the fascia associated with the skin and underlying muscles. The skin can be grasped and lifted, thereby creating mechanical tension on the subcutaneous fascia, which assists in changing the state of the fascia's ground substance from a 'gel' to a 'sol' (Oschman 1997) due to its thixotropic properties (DeLany 2000a). The tissue can also be rolled between the fingers and thumb. Subcutaneous tissue layers and/or muscle bellies may be grasped and lifted, then manipulated between the fingers and thumb, if tolerable, thereby stretching fascia and separating fascial layers. Any of these may result in increased blood and/or lymph flow.

● *Effleurage (gliding stroke)* is an important and powerful component of the NMT American version™. It warms the fascia, flushes blood through the tissues, and therefore increases oxygenation and perfusion of nutrients while simultaneously eliminating waste products from the tissues (Yates 1989). During the gliding process, the practitioner will discover contracted bands, nodules and tender points unique to that individual. Gliding repeatedly on these bands often reduces their size and tenacity, lessening the time and effort needed to modify or eliminate them. Clinical experience indicates that the best results tend to come from gliding on the tissues several times, then working somewhere else and returning to glide again. The direction of application of glides may be either with or across the direction of the muscle fibres, and usually involves a combination of both. Unless contraindicated, a moist hot pack can be placed on the tissues between gliding repetitions to enhance the effects further. A short time of rest of the tissues is usual before additional gliding. This allows circulatory and drainage functions to flush the tissues further. Tenderness and ischaemia are commonly reduced rapidly in this way.

● To glide on the tissues most effectively, the practitioner's hands are held with the fingers spread slightly and 'leading' the thumbs (Fig. 10.1A). The thumbs become the treatment tools, while the fingers support and stabilise the hands. The hand and forearm move as a unit, with the wrist being stable. Little or no motion is allowed in the wrist joints or the thumb joints. Excessive movement in the wrist or thumb may lead to joint problems and inflammation of the practitioner's forearms, wrists and hands. A proper and stable hand position helps avoid practitioner injury. When two-handed glides are used, the thumbs are side by side, or one ahead of the other.[2]

• When dealing with tissue that is not excessively tender or sensitive, the 'glide' should cover 3–4 inches per second (speed of application is reduced for comfort if tissues are sensitive), which is significantly faster than the thumb stroke used in Lief's NMT. It is important to develop a moderate gliding speed in order to ensure adequate opportunity for simultaneous palpation of muscles. Too rapid a movement may cause unnecessary discomfort and may also skim over congestion in the tissues, missing vital information sources. Movement that is too slow may displace the tissues, making identification of an individual muscle difficult. A moderate speed will allow for repetitions that significantly increase blood flow and, at the same time, palpate bands or nodules of ischaemia within the tissues.[3]

• *Compression techniques* can be used to press soft tissues against a bone or underlying muscle (*flat compression*), or the non-lubricated tissues may be lifted and grasped between the finger(s) and thumb (*pincer compression*). Pincer compression can be broadly applied with flattened fingers (like a clothespeg; see Fig. 10.2B) or pre-

cisely applied with curved fingers (resembling a 'C' clamp; see Fig. 10.2D).

• *Static compression* (also called TrP pressure release, ischaemic compression or sustained pressure) applies pressure to tissues without movement of the fingers or thumb. Tissues that are ischaemic, extremely tender or contain TrPs usually respond well to static compression (see below regarding use of static pressure).

• *Compression with manipulation* can be applied by lifting the tissues and then rolling or twisting them between the fingers and thumb. It is an effective way of mechanically distressing the connective tissue and altering its ground substance from a gel to a sol (DeLany 2000b), and may also help to separate the fibres and increase blood flow. Generally, this technique is used after the tissue tenderness has been decreased by the use of gliding strokes and static compression. It can follow those techniques or be used before TrP pressure release.

• *Friction techniques* can usually be applied to myofascial tissues with variations, depending on the condition of the tissues and the desired results. Friction techniques may include those applied transversely (cross-fibre friction, strumming or transverse friction) or those applied with the fibre direction (longitudinal friction). If tissues are tender, caution should be exercised as tenderness may be indicative of inflammation. If significant tenderness is present or if application of friction results in tenderness, ice may be applied for 10–15 minutes (see Ch. 8). Friction on that particular tissue should then be avoided until no evidence of inflammation is present.

Pressure considerations

After gliding and manipulation of tissues, the muscles may be compressed with static (ischaemic compression) pressure. Pressure should be constant and could even be mildly increased as the tissues relax and release. The length of time for which pressure is maintained will vary, although, as a rule, it is found that tissue contraction begins to ease within 8–12 seconds when the ideal pressure is being used. The practitioner should feel the tissues 'melting

---

[2] The American NMT glide is seen in this description to vary from the European hand application in which, while placed ahead of the thumbs, the fingers remain static so that only the thumb moves during the assessment/treatment 'glide'. In the American version the whole hand moves.

[3] As noted in the text, NMT in Europe is usually significantly more deliberate and slow than the American version, especially in the assessment mode.

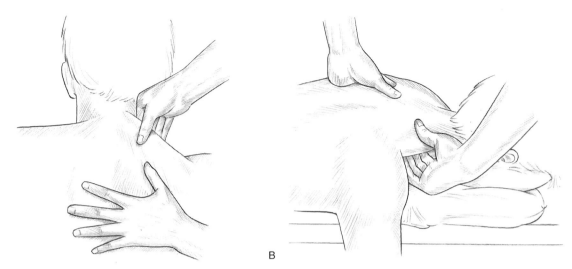

A   B

Figure 10.2A,B   Fingers should curl completely around the upper trapezius to touch the anterior surface of the muscle under the forward 'lip'.

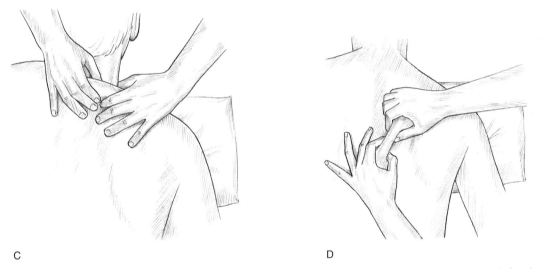

C   D

Figure 10.2C,D   Middle and lower portions of trapezius may be effectively lifted and compressed on most people by elevating the head of the humerus to shorten the fibres.

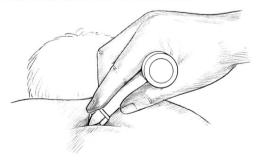

E

Figure 10.2E   A bevelled-tip pressure bar may be used in grooves and under bony ledges not easily reached with the thumbs, such as here in the spinal lamina groove.

and softening' under the pressure. The patient frequently reports that they believe the practitioner is reducing the degree of applied pressure.[4]

Pain reduction not always an adequate guide

While a reduction of pain may be achieved via static compression that is sustained for longer than suggested, this is usually of only short-term benefit. Increased pain and a reduction in local mobility may result from the irritation caused by sustained or excessive pressure. A greater, longer-lasting, beneficial effect will usually be gained when the practitioner goes back to an area four or five times for 8–12 seconds, rather than once for 40–60 seconds. If release of palpated contractions has not commenced within 8–12 seconds, the pressure may be too heavy or too light and should probably be altered.

Degree of pressure

The appropriate degree of pressure utilised in static compression varies with the individual (and even from one part of the body to another); however, it usually matches the tension palpated in the tissues. Pressure that is too light may not produce a tissue response, whereas heavy pressure may result in reflexive spasms. Age, oxygenation, past trauma, exercise status, previous therapies, hydration, nutritional and hormonal imbalances/deficiencies, tissue toxicity and dysfunctional postures all appear to influence the amount of pressure most appropriately applied.

How does one determine the amount of pressure to use? In addition to matching the tension within the tissues, a 1–10 scale of patient discomfort in the tissues being treated can be established and may be used to help guide the practitioner, where 1 = no discomfort and

10 = extreme pain. Only enough pressure to elicit mild to moderate discomfort is used, with a score of 5, 6 or 7 representing an ideal report. A score of 9 or 10 has no place in therapy! 'Biting the bullet' and 'digging it out' has no advantage – and offers real disadvantages – in NMT. Pressure should be adjusted routinely until the ideal level is found *for that particular tissue.*

Application of static pressure

Static pressure can be applied to soft tissues as an effective means of reducing spasm and contractures as well as for deactivating TrPs. While the blanching effects of applied compression may enhance blood flow when pressure is subsequently released, restriction of blood flow can produce an ischaemic state if held for too long. Additionally, the patient may not tolerate long applications of pressure if the tissue is extremely tender or inflamed. The amount and duration of pressure appropriate for an individual can vary greatly – even from one muscle to the next.

It is important to be specific when applying pressure to dysfunctional soft tissues. To treat TrPs most successfully, the practitioner should be directly on the TrP rather than next to it. When the patient keeps asking for more pressure, moving the point of pressure slightly, in one direction or another, may reveal that the practitioner was close to but not right on, the desired spot.

The length of time for which static pressure should be applied will vary; however, the practitioner should feel the tissue begin to soften within 8–12 seconds. The pressure can, however, be maintained for up to 20 seconds. The patient may feel a tissue 'melting' sensation and report that it feels as if the practitioner is lightening the pressure. A reduction of discomfort may be achieved with pressure that lasts longer than suggested, although clinical experience suggests that increased pain and decreased mobility often result when overly sustained or heavy pressure is used. Pressure should be constant and may be mildly increased as the tissues begin to soften. (See Box 3.6. and further discussion in Ch. 3 for details of algometer usage.)

---

[4] The pressure applied in Lief's NMT has two distinct modes: the assessment mode 'meets and matches' tissue tension, whereas the pressure applied in NMT treatment mode is largely in accord with that described for American NMT.

Use of pressure bars

Pressure bars may be used as valuable treatment tools to protect the practitioner's thumbs from excessive pressure and to access crevices that the thumbs may not be able to reach. These classical tools for NMT are constructed of lightweight wood and comprise a 1-inch dowel horizontal cross-bar and smaller vertical dowel shaft. Each has either a flat rubber tip or a bevelled rubber tip at the end of the vertical shaft (see Fig. 10.1B,C). The large flat tip is used to press into large muscle bellies, such as in the gluteal region, or to glide on flat broad muscles, such as the tibialis anterior. The bevelled tip is useful in the lamina groove, under the spine of the scapula, and to friction certain tendons that are difficult to reach with the thumb. The bevelled end of a flat typewriter eraser can also be used. The pressure bars are never used on extremely tender tissues, at vulnerable nerve areas such as the clavicle, or to 'dig' into tissues. Contracted tissues, fibrosis and bony surfaces may be 'felt' through the bars – just as a grain of sand or a crack in the table under writing paper may be felt through a pencil when writing.

The pressure bar is held securely on the shaft while wrapping the hand around the horizontal dowel, as shown in Fig. 10.1B,C. The practitioner's wrist is kept relatively straight so as to avoid strain. The pressure bar and the practitioner's hand and forearm move as a unit, with no ulnar and radial deviation at the wrist being allowed.

Pressure bar tips and handles should be cleaned after each use and can be scrubbed as the hands would be, using an antibacterial soap and scrub-brush. The use of alcohol on the rubber tips is not recommended because it may cause them to become dry and brittle. If the tip contacts oil, the rubber may begin to break down, causing it to split open. Scrubbing the oil off the rubber tip should help prevent this.

The pressure bars should *not* be used on the face, in the cervical region, under the posterior base of the cranium, or on arteries or veins. Avoid placing the pressure bar tip on a bony surface where nerves are exposed (such as the head of the fibula), above or under the clavicle, behind the knee, or on any other vulnerable part of the body, such as in the abdomen.

The use of pressure bars to treat myofascial tissues is considered to be an advanced massage technique, the use of which requires experience and training to determine when the technique may be used safely and effectively, and to prevent injury or strain of the practitioner's hands. The author suggests that the practitioner seek training in the proper use and handling of pressure bars before attempting to use them.

NMT METHODS

The following descriptions and illustrations of NMT American version™ are not meant to be fully comprehensive; they do, however, provide accurate examples of the way in which NMT would be used if restriction were being addressed and/or trigger points were being sought and treated in these structures. A more thorough discussion of NMT routines, as well as regional anatomy, dysfunctional conditions and precautions, is offered by Chaitow & DeLany (2000, 2002).

These protocols are described for the right side of the body. All steps should be repeated on the left side. It is particularly important to treat both sides of muscles that attach to the spine, because release of one side only could result in reflexive shortening of the muscles of the untreated side and resultant postural distortions.

Trapezius

The patient lies prone with the arm hanging off the side of the table or with the ipsilateral hand placed near the head.

1. Grasp the upper trapezius between the thumb and first three fingers with the thumb on the posterior surface and the fingers wrapping all the way around and up underneath the anterior fibres (Fig. 10.2A,B). This 'pincer' grip is suitable for this muscle as well as (with slight variations) the sternocleidomastoid and other muscles.

'Uncoil' the fibres of the outermost portion of the upper trapezius by dragging three fingers over the anterior surface against posteriorly applied thumb pressure. Do not allow the fingers to flip over the uppermost edge of the trapezius as this area can be very tender and often houses violent trigger points. Keep the wrist low to angle the fingers around the most anterior fibres. Thoroughly examine the toothpick size strands of the outermost edge; these often contain trigger points that induce noxious referrals into the face and eyes.[5]

2. Place the prone patient's arm on the table at his or her side. To define the middle trapezius, draw parallel lines from the two ends of the spine of the scapula to form right angles with the spinous processes. The fibres of middle trapezius lie between these two lines. Elevation of the humeral head 3–6 inches by use of a rolled-up towel, wedge, etc. will usually shorten the middle and lower trapezius, which allows it to be treated more easily.

Grasp the middle trapezius with both hands and compress and/or manipulate the belly of the middle portion (Fig. 10.2C). Repeat the grasping manipulation to the outer (diagonal) edge of the lower trapezius (Fig. 10.2D). This manipulation is similar to skin rolling techniques (see Ch. 8 for details of skin rolling) but includes more than the skin: lifting, evaluating and stretching the fibres of the muscle itself. If trigger points are found, static pincer-like compression is used to treat them.

3. Place the bevelled tip of the pressure bar against the lateral aspect of the spinous process of C7 (in the lamina groove) and at a 45° angle. Friction cephalad to caudad at tip-width intervals all the way down to L1 to treat the trapezius attachments on the spinous processes as well as deeper attachments (Fig. 10.2E).[6] When tissues are excessively tender, thumb or finger gliding

strokes or friction can be substituted for the pressure bar frictional techniques.

4. The bevelled pressure bar may be used on the scapular and acromial attachments of the trapezius. Gliding strokes with the thumb may be substituted for the pressure bar frictional techniques if tissue tenderness warrants a gentler approach. Thumb glides may be used with caution on the clavicular attachments where the pressure bar is *not* used.

Caution: It is suggested that the pressure bar not be used on clavicular attachments of the trapezius due to the proximity of the brachial plexus.

5. Gliding strokes can be used to soothe the tissues that have been treated with the pressure bar and with the manipulation techniques. Unless contraindicated, moist hot packs can be placed on the trapezius to increase blood flow. A cold pack or lymphatic drainage should follow the hot pack to enhance fluid drainage.

Levator scapula

The patient is prone.

1. Grasp the lower angle of the scapula and ease it toward the patient's ear to elevate the upper angle of the scapula away from the torso. The practitioner's lower hand is used to increase and secure this elevation at the lower angle of the scapula (Fig. 10.3).

2. The practitioner's fingers of the cephalad hand are passed around the anterior fibres of the trapezius and directly on to the anterior surface of the upper angle of the scapula. It is necessary to ensure that the trapezius fibres are bypassed, because trying to access levator scapula by pressing through the trapezius fibres will fail to achieve optimal results. Friction should be applied gently as these fibres are often extremely tender and referral patterns can produce a dull to moderate ache in the shoulder or trapezius area. The cephalad ends of these fibres attach to the atlas transverse process and are therefore involved in its stability. Gliding strokes may be applied to the remainder of the muscle, and cross-fibre friction can be used carefully at its

---

[5] Lief's NMT would access these structures from a position in which the practitioner is at the head of the table; see position 3 of spinal NMT application in Chapter 6.

[6] Lief's NMT would use thumb pressure to achieve the same effect.

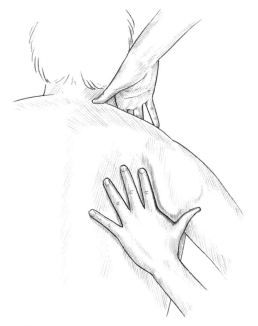

Figure 10.3 Fingers are wrapped around the anterior trapezius and placed directly on the upper angle of the manually elevated scapula to access the bony surface where levator scapula attaches.

attachments on the transverse processes of C1–C4.

Posterior mid-thorax

The patient is prone.

1. Gliding strokes are applied repeatedly to the interscapular region, which lies between the two vertebral borders of the scapulae. Avoid pressing on the spinous processes. Unless contraindicated, moist hot packs can be placed on the rhomboid region between repetitions of gliding strokes.

2. Place the patient's hand behind the small of the back, if possible, so distracting the vertebral border of the scapula from the rib-cage wall; this will allow additional access and deeper palpation. The following steps may be performed more easily if the practitioner stands on the contralateral side and reaches across to apply treatment.

3. Place the thumbs on the medial anterior surface of the scapula and introduce a glide or

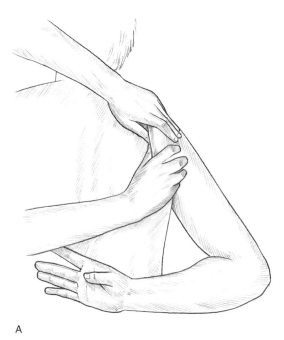

A

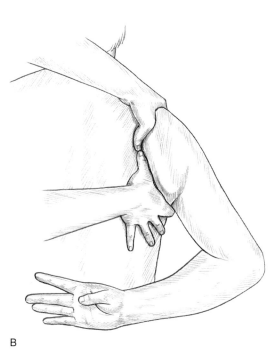

B

Figure 10.4A,B 'Hidden' trigger points in serratus posterior superior may be accessed under the vertebral border of the scapula.

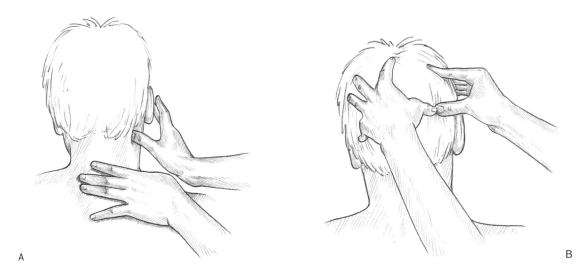

A   B

Figure 10.5A,B (A) Attachments of several muscles may be treated at the transverse process of the atlas. (B) The thin, flat, occipitalis muscle refers strongly into the eye region.

use cranial/caudal friction to examine the attachments of the serratus anterior and the subscapularis along the entire anterior vertebral border of the scapula (Fig. 10.4A).

4. With the scapula still elevated, rotate the thumbs so that the thumb pads press on to the thorax. Apply pressure anteriorly, deep to the vertebral border of the scapula, and glide or friction while pressing down on to the rib-cage (Fig. 10.4B). This step will address the 'hidden' tendinous attachments of the serratus posterior superior and its associated trigger point. Trigger points in this area refer significantly into the chest and down the arm, duplicating anginal pain. They may be hidden from palpation unless the scapula is sufficiently elevated.[7]

5. Apply gliding strokes in all directions between the scapulae while avoiding the spinous processes to treat several layers of muscles, including (from superficial to deep) trapezius, rhomboid major and minor, serratus posterior superior, erector spinae and possibly portions of the intercostal group.

---

[7] Lief's NMT would access these areas from positions 4 and 5 of the spinal sequence as described in Chapter 6.

Posterior cranium

The patient is prone.

1. Carefully examine the attachments on the transverse process of C1 of obliquus capitis superior and inferior, levator scapula and splenius cervicis muscles (Fig. 10.5A). The sternocleidomastoid (SCM) may need to be displaced laterally in order to palpate the muscles that attach to the transverse process of C1. The remainder of the posterior cranial attachments and the bellies of the suboccipital muscles may be treated with transverse friction from midline to the transverse process between C1 and the occiput, and between C1 and C2. This suboccipital region is often involved in forward head posture and chronic headache patterns.

Caution: The vertebral artery courses through the suboccipital triangle, which is formed by the rectus capitis posterior major, obliquus capitis superior and obliquus capitis inferior. Avoid excessive pressure or friction on the artery.

2. Use combination friction to examine the belly of the thin, flat, occipitalis muscle which is located about 1.5–2 inches lateral to the occipital protuberance (Fig. 10.5B). Movement of this muscle may be palpated on some individuals when the eyebrows are raised repeatedly, as it

merges with the cranial aponeurosis and connects with the frontalis muscle. Trigger points in this muscle may refer strongly into the eye and into the frontal sinus area.[8]

Cervical lamina supine

The patient is supine.

1. Lubricate the lamina groove from the occiput to T1. The left hand lifts and supports the head. The fingers of the right hand lie across the back of the neck at the occipital ridge with the thumb placed next to the lateral surface of the spinous process of C1 (Fig. 10.6A). Glide from C1 to T1 while simultaneously pressing toward the ceiling. Repeat the gliding movements five or six times, increasing pressure slightly with each repetition, if appropriate. The practitioner's elbow should remain low and the treating arm should remain in the same plane as the spine. Observe the chin moving in extension as the gliding movements of the thumb help to restore flexibility to the posterior cervical muscles.

2. Rotate the patient's head contralaterally (away from the side being treated). Move the right thumb laterally one thumb's width (about 1 inch) and repeat the gliding movements five or six times (Fig. 10.6B). The chin will not move while gliding on the lateral strips.

Caution: Extreme head rotation is not recommended for the elderly as it may induce stress to the vertebral artery, which lies within the transverse processes.

3. Continue a series of caudad glides with the thumb, moving laterally in strips until the entire lamina groove has been treated (Fig. 10.6C). The treating thumb should remain posterior to the transverse processes. The muscles being treated include trapezius, semispinalis capitis, semispinalis cervicis, splenius capitis, splenius cervicis, levator scapula, rotatores and multifidus.

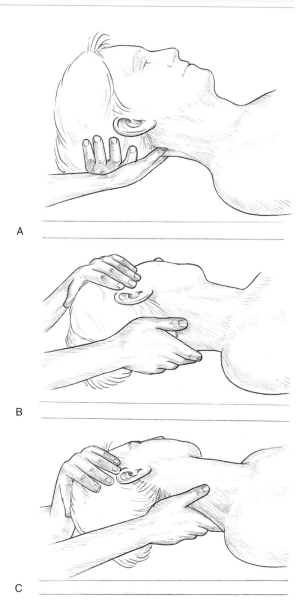

A

B

C

Figure 10.6A,B,C Gliding techniques may be applied to the cervical lamina from the occiput to the thorax as far laterally as the transverse processes.

Caution: It is necessary to ensure that the gliding strokes remain posterior to the transverse processes because the brachial plexus exits the vertebrae on the anterior aspect of the transverse processes. The foraminal gutters, which cradle the nerves, are sharp and, if placed anteriorly, pressure from the gliding thumb could press the nerves against the sharp processes.

---

[8] The position 3 of NMT spinal sequence as described in Chapter 6 would effectively assess and treat these structures working from the head of the table.

4. Return to any ischaemic bands or trigger points found and treat with static compression.[9]

Splenii tendons

The patient is supine.

Caution: Use no pressure until the thumb is securely in place, as described below.

1. To treat the right-side splenius capitis, the patient is supine and the practitioner's right-hand fingers cup across the back of the neck like a shirt collar. Place the right thumb anterior to the trapezius and posterior to the transverse processes, while pointing the thumb towards the patient's feet. Use the left hand to rotate the head towards the side being treated (Fig. 10.7A).

2. The right hand should rotate with the neck as if moulded to the back of the neck. This rotation will open a 'pocket' anterior to the trapezius, allowing room for the thumb to slide into position. The thumb is angled towards the nipple of the opposite breast and is pressed lightly against the lateral surface of the spinous processes (Fig. 10.7B,C). This hand position will rotate the thumb so that the thumb pad faces toward the ceiling. Slide the right thumb into the 'pocket' formed by the trapezius. If the 'pocket' does not allow penetration of the thumb due to excessive tension, or if pressure of the thumb produces more than moderate discomfort, press lightly at the 'mouth' of the pocket until the tissues relax enough to allow the thumb to slide in further.

3. Apply pressure toward the lateral surface of the spinous processes and simultaneously toward the ceiling for 8–12 seconds. The thumb will press into the tendons of the splenius capitis

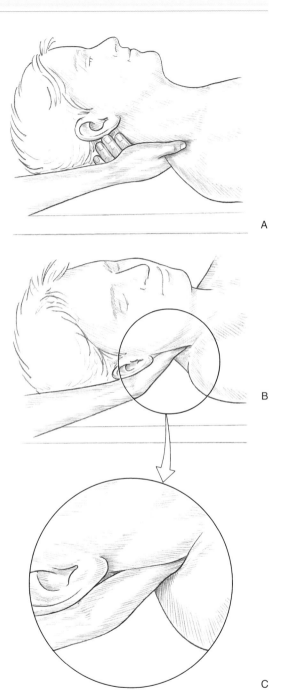

A

B

C

Figure 10.7A,B,C Originally called the corkscrew technique by Dr Nimmo, treatment of the spleni tendons from C7–T4 is applied 'in the pocket' anterior to the trapezius.

[9] Lief's NMT would have accessed these areas alongside the cervical spine with the patient prone, in positions 1, 2, 3, 4 and 5 of the spinal sequence as described in Chapter 6. Direct strokes over the tips of the spinous processes are included in this sequence, but caution is suggested so that pressure remains light. The interspinous spaces commonly house trigger points, and the attachments to the spinous processes themselves may manifest as periosteal pain points, indicating a need for attention from the muscles that are producing the stress.

and splenius cervicis, as well as the deeper muscles (rotatores and multifidus). After the initial application of pressure, allow the tissues to rest for a few seconds and then press the thumb into the pocket a little deeper to repeat the manoeuvre. When the tissues prevent any further caudad movement of the thumb, mild to moderate static pressure that is sustained for a few seconds may produce more opening of the pocket and allow the thumb to slide a little further down the spinal column.

4. If tender, repeat the entire process three or four times during a session. This step will usually help restore cervical rotation as well as reduce tilting pull on the transverse processes of C1–3. Trigger points in the splenii tendons can refer strongly into the eye, causing eye (pressure-like) discomfort. Practitioners should rule out glaucoma or other serious eye conditions as a cause of such discomfort, in addition to treating these tissues.

Sternocleidomastoid

The patient is supine.

The release of the SCM muscle is important because of its propensity to distract the head anteriorly. Compensating postural distortions relating to such forward head positions can include anterior rotation of the pelvis and changes in cervical, thoracic and/or lumbar curvature. Trigger points in SCM can cause severe eye pain, temporomandibular joint pain, sore throat, hearing loss or ear pain, and can mimic migraine headaches.

1. Grasp the tendon of the non-lubricated SCM lightly between the thumb and first two fingers as close to the mastoid process as possible. Rotate the head toward the side being treated to rotate the SCM away from the carotid artery. Passively tilt (side-bend) the head toward the side being treated to grasp the SCM more easily and so lift it away from the deeper tissues (Fig. 10.8A). Both heads of the SCM can be grasped in the cephalad half of SCM, although they separate into two distinct bellies in the caudad half. A paper tissue placed between the treating hand and the patient's skin may help to prevent slippage if the area is oily.

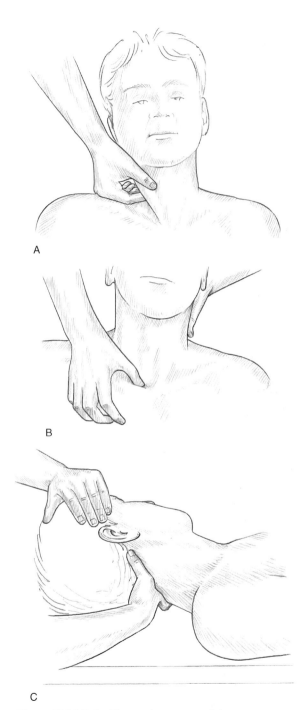

A

B

C

Figure 10.8A,B,C Thorough treatment of the sternocleidomastoid often relieves symptoms associated with migraine headaches, temporomandibular joint dysfunction and hearing problems. (C) Longissimus capitis and splenius capitis may be reached under the posterior aspect of the mastoid attachment of the SCM.

Caution: If a pulse from the carotid artery is noted while compressing the SCM, release the muscle immediately and reposition the fingers to ensure the artery is not compressed.

2. Compress the SCM for 8–12 seconds at 1-inch intervals from the mastoid process to the sternal and clavicular attachments. Each head can be treated separately. Medial to lateral friction may be used on the sternal and clavicular attachments (Fig. 10.8B).

3. Support the head at 45° of flexion and rotate it away from the side being treated. Glide inferiorly on the upper 1 inch of the mastoid attachment of the SCM, while being careful to avoid the styloid process located anterior to it. Do not glide further down the SCM as gliding pressure across the carotid sinus may stimulate baro-receptors, resulting in a rapid drop in the patient's blood pressure.

4. Place the thumb posterior to the SCM tendon at the mastoid process and displace the tendon anteriorly while simultaneously pressing on to the mastoid attachment of the longissimus capitis (erector spinae) and the splenius capitis. Use static pressure or combination friction to treat them (Fig. 10.8C).[10]

Spinal lamina groove

The patient is prone.

Trigger points lying close to the lamina of the spinal column often refer pain across the back, wrapping around the rib-cage and/or anteriorly into the chest or abdomen, and frequently refer 'itching' patterns. The treatment technique described below is particularly useful if scoliosis is evident as it addresses the many layers of muscular attachment to the posterior aspect of the spine.

1. Angle the bevelled tip of a pressure bar at 45° against the lateral surface of the spinous processes (Fig. 10.9A,B). Use caudad/cephalad

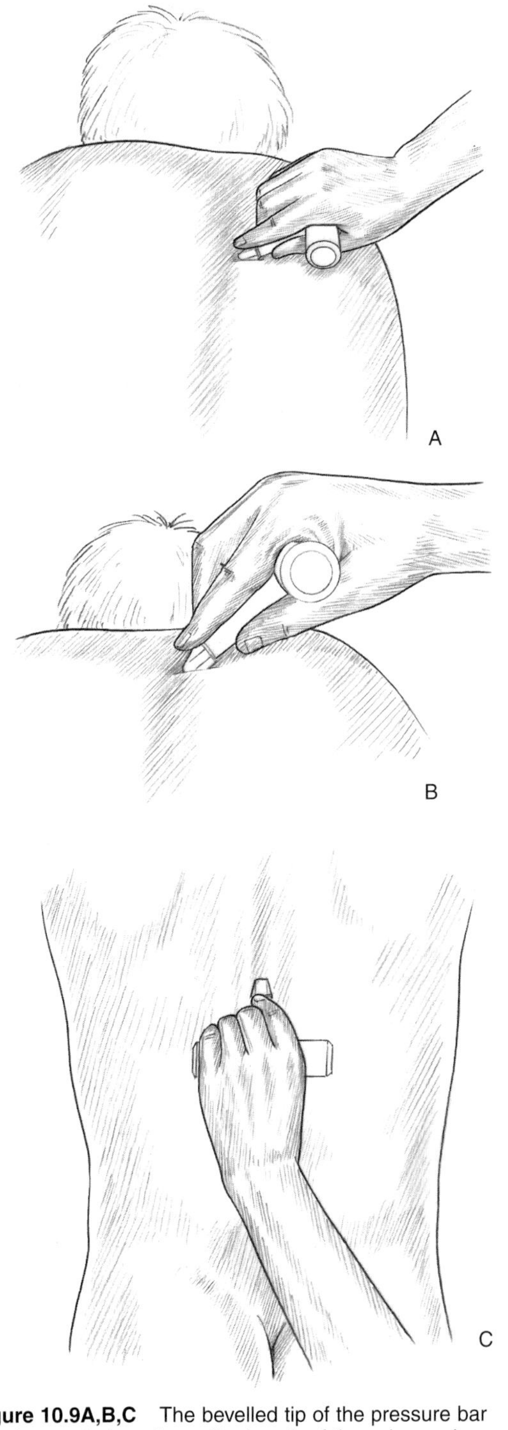

A

B

C

Figure 10.9A,B,C The bevelled tip of the pressure bar may be used along the entire length of the spine and sacrum, both in the lamina (A,B) and between the spinous processes (C). The cervical region should not be treated with the tool.

---

[10] Lief's NMT would access and treat dysfunction in these structures with the patient prone, from positions 1, 2, 3 of the sequence described in Chapter 6.

friction at tip-width intervals from C7 to the coccyx on each side of the spine. Avoid pressing on the coccyx.

2. When moving the pressure bar, lift it and place it at the next site to avoid gliding it as the bevelled tip may cause tissue irritation. Avoid treating the cervical lamina with the pressure bar as the cervical vertebrae are less stable than those below C7. (See Cervical lamina supine (above) for procedures used in the cervical region.)

3. Friction may also be performed between spinous processes with the bevelled tip in order to treat interspinalis muscles and the supraspinous ligament (Fig. 10.9C).[11]

Intercostal muscles

The patient is treated in supine, side-lying and prone positions in order to access as many of the intercostal spaces as possible.

Caution: When use of the pressure bar as described produces excessive discomfort, the tip of an index finger should be substituted for the pressure bar tip in the frictional work. Should this procedure also produce moderate discomfort, single-digit gliding strokes can be applied repeatedly with the index finger in each intercostal space and the frictional work delayed until a subsequent treatment session.

1. Place the bevelled tip of the pressure bar inferior to the clavicle of the supine patient, just lateral to the sternum, in the first intercostal space (Fig. 10.10A). The bevelled tip should lie between the ribs and parallel with them. Using medial/lateral friction at each application site, move the bar laterally at tip intervals until pectoralis minor is reached.

2. Return to the sternum, move down one rib space and repeat the tip-width examination while using frictional pressure as described in step 1, until pectoralis minor is reached. Avoid pressure into pectoralis minor because of sensitive neural structures in the area.

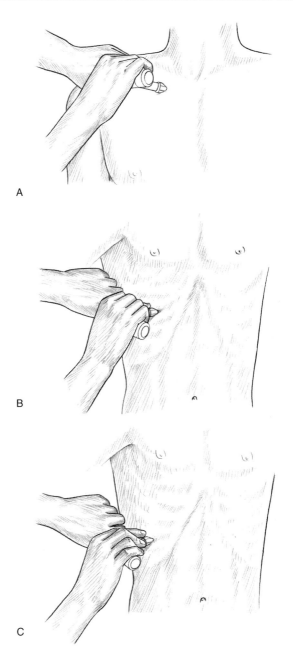

A

B

C

Figure 10.10A,B,C The bevelled tip of the pressure bar may be used at tip-width intervals throughout each intercostal space, especially on people with respiratory ailments. Avoid pressing on the brachial plexus or breast tissue. Friction with a fingertip (or a fingertip gliding stroke) should be substituted when tissue is excessively tender.

3. Avoid contact with breast tissue. When working around the breast, use the patient's hand to displace the breast away from the treat-

---

[11] Lief's spinal NMT application addresses these tissues with thumb and/or finger contacts, as described in Chapter 6.

ment site inferiorly, laterally, superiorly and medially, as appropriate, in order to allow access for the pressure bar to treat the muscles that lie deep to the margins of the breast.

4. Continue the intercostal work as far caudad and laterally as possible. The patient can also be placed in a side-lying position, which allows access to the more lateral aspects of the inter-costal spaces (Fig. 10.10B,C).

5. With the patient prone, place the pressure bar into the intercostal space lateral to the first thoracic vertebra. With the bevelled tip placed parallel to the ribs and in the rib space, use medial/lateral friction at tip-width intervals in the same manner as that applied on the anterior surface. Continue the treatment in all intercostal spaces as far caudad and laterally as possible.[12] Distinction of the rib spaces may be difficult in the upper posterior thorax where superficial tissue is thicker. The rib spaces will be more distinct in the lower posterior thorax, but cau-tion should be exercised regarding pressure on the last two 'floating' ribs.

Iliolumbar ligament and sacroiliac ligament

1. In order to locate the iliolumbar ligament, one of the practitioner's thumbs is placed on the posterior superior iliac spine (PSIS) and the index finger of the same hand is placed on the spinous process of L5 (Fig. 10.11A). The practi-tioner's other hand holds the flat pressure bar as indicated in Fig. 10.11B. The flat tip of the pres-sure bar is pressed directly towards the floor into the tissue between the two contact digits. The bony surface of the sacrum will be felt deep

---

[12] Lief's NMT would access the intercostal spaces from the mid-axillary line to the spine, using fingertip pressure while treating the prone patient, as described in Chapter 6 (positions 4, 5, 6 and 7). Anterior intercostal evaluation and treatment would be performed as appropriate, with the patient supine as illustrated in Chapter 7 (lower intercostal only described and illustrated) relating to abdominal application of NMT. The same cautions discussed in the text in this chapter would be issued for manual as for pressure bar applications in the intercostal tissues.

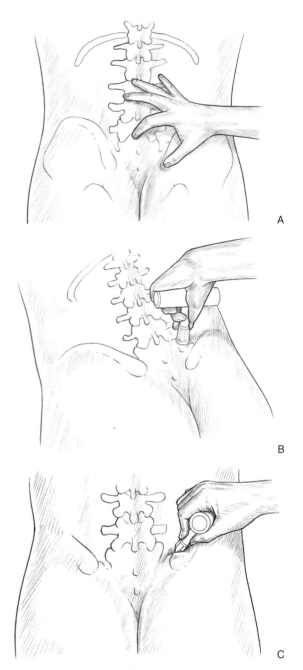

A

B

C

Figure 10.11A,B,C The iliolumbar ligament located between the spinous process of L5 and the posterior superior iliac spine and just above the sacrum can be treated through the erector spinae (B) or under its lateral edge (C).

to the overlying tissues. The pressure bar is then moved cephalad a tip width and pressed towards the floor. This position should place the pressure bar on the tissue superficial to the ligament, and osseous contact of the sacrum should not be felt. If the sacrum is still palpable, the pressure bar tip should be moved slightly cephalad until it is in contact with soft tissue only and is felt to 'sink in' the soft tissue. The pressure is held for 8–12 seconds in order to apply ischaemic compression to the overlying muscles and influence the iliolumbar ligament itself.

2. The same contact should then be re-examined with the bevelled tip of the pressure bar, with the bevel held parallel to the crest of the ilium. To contact the iliolumbar ligament most directly, the tip is placed lateral to the erector spinae and under that muscle's lateral edge. A cross-fibre movement is used with the bevelled tip while it is angled in this described manner in order to access the tissues anterior to the lateral edge of the erector spinae muscles (Fig. 10.11C), which includes the iliolumbar ligament.

3. In order to treat the sacroiliac ligament using NMT, the bevelled tip of the pressure bar is placed at a 45° angle on to the lateral aspect of the sacral tubercles (Fig. 10.12A) with the edge of the bevelled tip being parallel to the tubercles. This position is similar to that previously described for the lamina groove. Commencing at the cephalad aspect of the sacrum, a cephalad/caudad frictional movement is introduced in order to examine the tissues that lie superficial to the sacrum. The pressure bar is then moved one tip-width caudad and the friction is repeated. This continues to the cephalad edge of the coccyx, which should not itself receive any treatment of this sort.

4. Returning to the sacral base, the pressure bar is applied into the soft tissues one tip-width lateral to the initial contact, at 90° to the surface (i.e. to the dorsum of the sacrum) (Fig. 10.12B). The procedure as above is then repeated until the coccyx is reached. In this way the entire sacral dorsal surface should be treated in 'strips'. No pressure should be applied on to the sacroiliac joint or to the tissues lateral to the border of the sacrum.

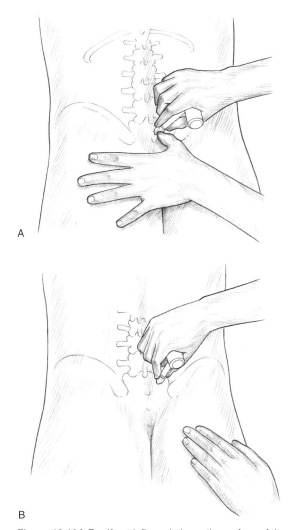

A

B

Figure 10.12A,B If not inflamed, the entire surface of the sacrum can be treated to address sacroiliac ligaments as well as multifidus and erector spinae attachments. Trigger points here will refer sciatica-like pain.

A uniform pattern should be visible with no gaps between the prints left by the tip pressure applications. All the strips of prints should be parallel to the sacral tubercles.

Erector spinae

The patient is prone.

1. The erector spinae muscles are lubricated from C7 to the sacrum. The thumbs or palm are used to glide along this pathway (C7 to sacrum)

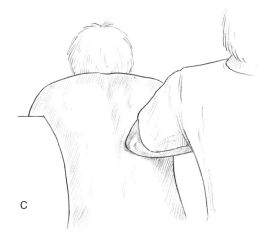

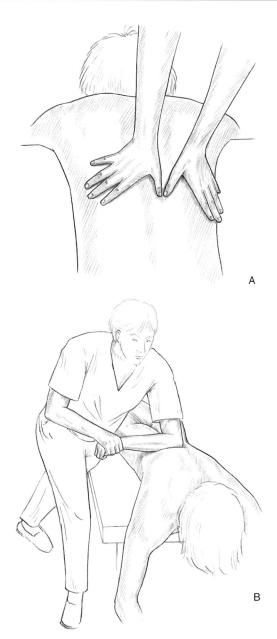

A

B

Figure 10.13A,B Long gliding strips, applied with the thumbs, palms, fists or forearm, lengthen thoracic fascia while treating several layers of muscle.

Figure 10.13C When working near the spine, avoid pressing on spinous processes.

flexed. The olecranon process of the practitioner's table-side elbow is placed against, but not on to, the spinous processes at the level of L5 (Fig. 10.13B). With a moderate pressure and speed, the entire length of the paraspinal tissues, including the erector spinae, receives the benefit of a glide from this contact. The pressure should be moderated when the thoracic region is being traversed. Modification of the angle of contact will be necessary when covering the erector spinae medial to the scapulae. Care should be taken not to apply pressure on to the spinous processes themselves (Fig. 10.13C). The stroke ceases at C7, and the thumbs are used in the cervical region.

3. Turn to face the feet. Apply forearm contact in a similar manner as described in step 2 to the erector spinae as a series of glides is performed from C7 to the iliac crest. No pressure should be applied in this way on to the iliac crest itself or the sacrum or spinous processes.

4. The thumbs, knuckles or large pressure bar may be used cautiously to cross-fibre the long tendons of the erectors; however, the spinous processes should not be involved in these contacts.[13]

repeatedly, then alternating from side to side while gradually increasing pressure in order to relax and warm the tissues (Fig. 10.13A).

2. Standing at waist level with the forward foot at shoulder level and the back foot at waist level, face towards the head with knees slightly

---

[13] Lief's NMT attention to these same tissues forms a major element of the approach described in Chapter 6, most notably in relation to positions 3, 4, 5, 6, 7, 8 and 9 where thumb and/or finger strokes would be the main means of contact.

Quadratus lumborum

The patient is prone.

1. After application of a lubricant, a glide up quadratus lumborum is made using both thumbs, from the crest of the ilium to the 12th rib. The initial contact remains just lateral to the erector spinae as four or five repetitious glides are applied to the medial aspect of the muscle (Fig. 10.14A). The thumbs are then placed approximately 1 inch laterally and the glides are repeated. A series of glides is then performed, in 'strips', moving laterally until the entire muscle has been treated. If necessary, by moving more laterally, the obliques can be treated as well.

2. While standing at chest level and facing the feet of the prone patient, glide caudad from the 12th rib to the crest of the ilium, ensuring that contact is lateral to the erector spinae. A series of glides moving laterally is then performed (Fig. 10.14B).

3. Facing the head, and with the fingers of the lateral hand moulded around the curve of the trunk and the thumb angled at 45° to the spine, the thumb is glided medially on the inferior surface of the 12th rib until it reaches the lateral aspect of the erector spinae. Apply static pressure or friction on posterior aspect of the transverse process of L1. In order to avoid trauma, no pressure should be applied on to the lateral aspect of the tip of the transverse process, which is located just lateral to the lateral border of the erector spinae. Follow this with similar applications of friction or pressure on to the lumbar transverse processes at 1–2-inch intervals down to the level of L4 (Fig. 10.14C).[14]

OVERVIEW OF DIFFERENCES

The key variations existing between the European (Lief's) and NMT American version™ – which emerge from these examples – seem to

---

[14] Lief's NMT would access these tissues from positions 8 and 9 of the spinal application described in Chapter 6.

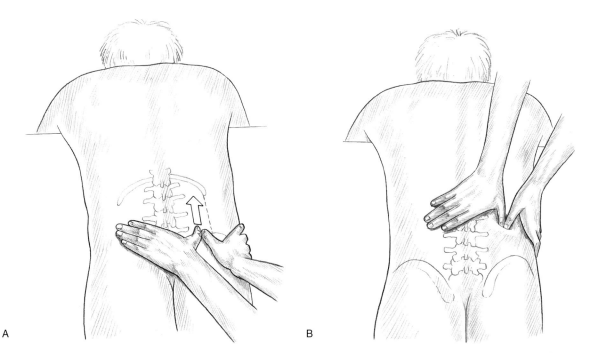

A   B

Figure 10.14A,B   The quadratus lumborum will be treated lateral to the erector spinae by gliding between the crest of the ilium and the last rib.

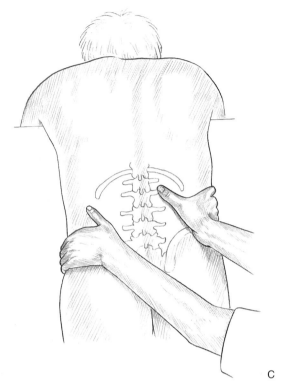

Figure 10.14C Quadratus lumborum's transverse process attachments may be felt on some people just lateral to the erector spinae. L2 and L3 are palpable on most people. L1 and L4 may be more difficult to locate.

relate to a far more structured and prescriptive approach in American NMT, with a variety of additional 'tools' being used, including elbows and pressure bars. While Lief's version also has a (different) structured outline, it seems to require fewer 'strokes' or 'glides', while remaining in assessment mode until something is discovered that calls for therapeutic input. In therapeutic mode, the way in which tissues are addressed (ischaemic compression and frictional or cross-fibre methods) seems very similar to the American method, apart from the more restricted variety of contacts (European relies almost solely on finger or thumb contact).

NMT American version™ seems to move directly into a therapeutic 'glide' which has assessment potential, whereas Lief's approach separates assessment from therapeutic input more definitively. Both approaches have proven to be successful training systems for those who are learning NMT techniques as well as reliable clinical protocols, which can be used as primary modalities for treating chronic pain and soft tissue dysfunction.

REFERENCES

Cailliet R 1977 Soft tissue pain and disability. FA Davis, Philadelphia
Chaitow L 1980 Soft tissue manipulation: a practitioner's guide to the diagnosis and treatment of soft tissue dysfunction and reflex activities. Healing Arts Press, Rochester
Chaitow L 1996 Modern neuromuscular techniques. 1st edn. Churchill Livingstone, Edinburgh
Chaitow L, DeLany J 2000 Clinical application of neuromuscular techniques, vol. 1: The upper body. Churchill Livingstone, Edinburgh
Chaitow L, DeLany J 2002 Clinical application of neuromuscular techniques, vol. 2: The lower body. Churchill Livingstone, Edinburgh
DeLany J 1999 The roots and branches of neuromuscular therapy, no. 11, pp 16–17. American Massage Therapy Association, Florida
DeLany J 2000a Connective tissue perspectives: introduction. Journal of Bodywork and Movement Therapies 4(4):273–275
DeLany J 2000b Connective tissue perspectives: neuromuscular therapy. Journal of Bodywork and Movement Therapies 4(4):276–277

DeLany J 2002 Neuromuscular therapy: care of soft tissue pain and dysfunction. Applications pack. NMT Center, St Petersburg, Florida
Oschman JL 1997 What is healing energy? Pt 5: gravity, structure, and emotions. Journal of Bodywork and Movement Therapies 1(5):307–308
Simons D, Travell J, Simons L 1999 Myofascial pain and dysfunction: the trigger point manual. vol. 1: The upper body. 2nd edn. Williams & Wilkins, Baltimore
Stedman's electronic medical dictionary 1998. Version 4.0. Online. Available: http://www.stedmans.com
Travell J, Simons D 1983 Myofascial pain and dysfunction: the trigger point manual. vol. 1: The upper body. Williams & Wilkins, Baltimore
Travell J, Simons D 1992 Myofascial pain and dysfunction: the trigger point manual. vol. 2: The lower body. Williams & Wilkins, Baltimore
Vannerson J, Nimmo R 1971 Specificity and the law of facilitation in the nervous system. Reprinted in: Schneider M, Cohen J, Laws S 2001 The collected writings of Nimmo & Vannerson, pioneers of chiropractic trigger point therapy. Self-published, Pittsburgh, Pennsylvania
Yates J 1989 Physiological effects of therapeutic massage and their application to treatment. Massage Therapy Association of British Columbia, Vancouver

11

Progressive inhibition of neuromuscular structures (PINS) technique

Dennis J. Dowling

Progressive inhibition of neuromuscular structures (PINS) is a manipulative medicine technique that, when properly utilised, can be included in the treatment regimen of patients with musculoskeletal dysfunction. Knowledge of anatomy and neuromuscular physiology, as well as reliance on standard forms of palpatory diagnosis and treatment, are necessary.

As a variant of a technique known as 'inhibition', PINS bears some resemblance to other manual medicine techniques. The practitioner must determine any alteration of the related soft tissues due to dysfunction. Then he or she must gauge the direction and amount of treatment based on palpatory evaluation and patient feedback.

Initially, two related sensitive points are located. One is usually in the immediate region of the patient's symptoms, and the other is sometimes at the other end of a soft tissue structure, such as a muscle, nerve, fascial link or ligament. The practitioner exerts a mild amount of pressure progressively from one to the other.

Other similar techniques are also discussed. Some theoretical as well as selected practical applications are presented.

Parts of this chapter that appear in the case study component were used in preparation for application to Fellowship of the American Academy of Osteopathy (FAAO).

NEUROMUSCULAR TECHNIQUES

Manipulative treatments have been used throughout history, although the aetiology of musculoskeletal dysfunction, as well as the processes by which dysfunctions are maintained, have been poorly undertood until recently. What is obvious to anyone who practises palpation is that the soft tissues, including the skin, muscles, fascia and ligaments, may be involved. With knowledge of anatomy, separate hypertonic individual muscles, as well as groups of muscles, can usually be discerned in association with somatic dysfunction. While many skeletal muscles are capable of being activated by conscious initiation, many muscular actions operate via reflexive mechanisms.

Clinical experience shows that injured muscles may remain in a state of hyper-alertness, as evidenced by their hypertonicity, due to unconscious mechanisms that maintain them in a dysfunctional state. Looking past the usual concepts associated with intent and activity, attention most logically turns towards reflex activity as a maintaining factor. With the capability of being enhanced or inhibited by higher neurological functions, the stimuli that maintain undesirable hypertonicity operate at a spinal cord level. Oftentimes, a reflex that seems to be programmed for the purpose of protection is inappropriately maintained afterwards. Muscles innervated by segmental nerves may become activated consciously or reflexively. When the latter occurs, possibly following injury, there can be maintenance of a dysfunctional hypertonic state. The potential for the central nervous system to inhibit or eliminate such activity may have been overridden reflexively.

Understanding this process suggests that the process of manipulative treatment should involve more than the 'prodding', 'kneading' or 'folding-and-holding' of dysfunctional tissues. Through a combination of observation, assessment and diagnosis, the manipulative specialist may postulate the causes as well as the the most appropriate treatment choices. Appreciation of the connection between the musculoskeletal and the neurological influences involved in somatic dysfunction allows for the therapeutic manual interventions that follow to be designated as neuromuscular techniques.

Many neuromuscular modalities have been developed. Some practitioners and physicians apply these in a narrow regional manner involving localised dysfunction. Others learn to apply the concepts and principles behind any particular technique more widely, involving global appreciation of the interactions between body regions and systems. Jones' strain/counterstrain system, for example, started as a form of treatment for low back pain in an individual patient (Jones et al 1995). It is almost certain that in treating low back pain, others had practised locating a local tender point and then holding the region until it dissipated. The crucial leap beyond these limitations occurred when Jones postulated the underlying principles involved, and then developed the practical methods that flowed from this hypothesis, to locate tender points throughout the body in a similar way. Similarly, as later discussion in this chapter will elaborate, understanding the basic principles involved in manual methods, such as applied pressure, allows for a variety of different methods of application, all of which are neuromuscular, by definition.

BACKGROUND

Osteopathy has been practised since the late 1800s. Many osteopathic treatment modalities have been developed in the 100 or more years of the profession. Several are adaptations of other methods. There are many other modalities developed before or since in other related fields of manual medicine. Sometimes, the similarities are greater than the differences. Appropriate clinical selection of any one depends upon experience, skill, suitability, efficacy, ease of use and expected outcome. As a new technique, PINS is a variation of the technique known as inhibition.

Having suffered from headaches over 20 years ago, the author was frustrated with the treatments that were available. Having little knowledge of anatomy, early attempts involved the application of pressure on various portions of his scalp. The related symptoms involved pain at and near the right eye, increased lacrimation (tearing), facial pain, nasal stuffiness and scalp pain. There were also suboccipital symptoms, which appeared to be related to the periorbital pain. As the symptoms appeared to progress following a great deal of reading, eyestrain was a typical initiating condition. Exposure to bright sunlight without the benefit of sunglasses could also precipitate the cephalgia. Each of the symptoms could occur independently and was worsened by stress.

By trial and error, manual pressure was exerted at several sensitive points. There appeared to be a temporary effect when any point was pressed singly, but sometimes, within seconds, secondary adjacent regions of the scalp developed pain. When these secondary points were likewise pressured, patterns seemed to appear.

Treatment of these patterns as a succession of points was the most successful approach – more so than addressing any individual point or pair of points. When similar symptoms of headache that developed in others were likewise treated, the results were equivalently successful.

Later, after beginning osteopathic medical education at the New York College of Osteopathic Medicine, the author began to integrate knowledge of osteopathic manipulative medicine theory along with clinical observations. As it was utilised more and more, and taught to others, the rationale as well as further expansion of use of this inhibitory technique beyond just headache was determined. During this exploration, similarities and differences were noted in relationship to other methods of 'point therapy'.

INHIBITION

PINS is related to the osteopathic modality of inhibition. According to the *Glossary of Osteopathic Terminology* (American Osteopathic Association 1998), inhibition is 'a term that describes steady pressure to soft tissues to effect relaxation and normalize reflex activity.' Inhibition, or this use of 'steady pressure to soft tissues', is perhaps one of the oldest methods of

manual treatment, regardless of the name applied. Typically, inhibition is performed by pressing the fingers or other body parts at a constant mild-to-moderate amount of force on regions of inappropriately hypertonic muscle. Even though the patient may complain of pain or decreased function, the object of the treatment is to decrease the tonicity of the muscles. The symptoms that the patient has are directly related to this increased dysfunctional muscular tone (Dowling & Scariati 1997).

Large superficial muscles are most easily identified in both the normal relaxed and hypertonic states. A series of regional muscles can be identified and treated in pairs or individually. The supine or prone positions may facilitate the process as the patient will not need to use some of these muscles for positional support of the trunk and neck. With the patient in the supine position a muscle, such as the trapezius, can easily be located in the cervical, shoulder and upper thoracic regions. The body of the muscle can be grasped, pressed or pinched. A hypertonic muscle is usually found to be firmer than its counterpart on the other side. An initial response of the tissue to pressure may be an increase in tonus and perhaps greater sensitivity. Gradually, with sustained pressure, the structures relax.

Another consideration is the relationship between musculoskeletal structures and the underlying organs. The viscera receive innervation from the spinal cord via nerves that originate from the same segments as the nerves that service the more superficial structures. As the sympathetic chain lies just anterior to the rib heads, dysfunction of the vertebra result in increased sympathetic activity, or stimulation, to the innervated visceral target organs and the segmental musculoskeletal region (Ehrenfeuchter 1997).

The sympathetic system is often referred to as the 'flight or fight' response mechanism. It allows for rapid response to perceived danger or injury. The organism's reactions are channelled towards self-preservation. The heart rate increases, pupils dilate, blood is shunted to the skeletal muscles and away from the internal organs, and respiratory rate increases. Gastro-intestinal activity, among other visceral concerns, effectively shuts down. This normal reaction to stresses becomes abnormal when it does not abate. Inhibition also has a specialised purpose in the thoracic region. In theory, constant pressure on to an area, which is the source of increased sympathetic activity, will result in reduction of the autonomic activity. Raised blood pressure, ischaemic changes, arrhythmias, tachycardias or myocardial infarction secondary to vasospasm of a congested coronary artery may result from the effect of the stimulation on a visceral organ such as the heart. Musculoskeletal response includes spasm, decreased circulation due to vasoconstriction, impaired drainage of waste products, sensitivity changes and trophic alterations. Acute responses to this activity are the same as those to any new injury: redness (rubor), pain (dolor), swelling (tumour), heat (calor) and decreased function (functio laesa) (Robbins et al 1984).

- The skin and subcutaneous tissue may have a 'doughy' consistency and the pain sharp and throbbing.
- As the state persists without relief, the alterations reflect the chronicity of the dysfunction. Muscles and the surrounding fascia become more fibrotic ('ropy').
- The skin is thinner, paler and cooler.
- Pain responses may be more variable from insensitivity ('anaesthetic') to altered sensitivity ('paraesthesia') to hypersensitivity.

External pressure, such as is provided by inhibition, may initially result in a transitory increase in spasm or sensitivity. However, subsequent reduction of some or all of these components can be readily appreciated. Research regarding the visceral responses has indicated reduction of the undesirable autonomic responses (Hermann 1965). However, the persistence may be more dependent on the aetiology. If the visceral organ's structure or function were somehow altered, either primarily or secondarily, then the results of surface inhibition might be short lived. The more observable musculoskeletal signs and symptoms might represent a viscerosomatic reflex. When a musculoskeletal injury is the origin, a somatovisceral reflex may occur. Manipulative treatment of the musculoskeletal structures may result in a more persistent reduction of all elements.

In the suboccipital and sacral regions, the intention switches from the sympathetic half of the autonomic system towards resetting parasympathetic activity, the other half of the autonomic nervous system. Rather than being reactive to external danger like the sympathetic system, the parasympathetics comprise nerves affecting the modifying reconstructive processes. Upgrading of parasympathetic activity coordinates increased gastrointestinal motility, decreased sphincter closure, reduction of heart rate, constriction of pupils, and sleepiness, to name just a few of the reactions.

Parasympathetic fibres travel only to the head and trunk, not to the extremities. Any region that has a visceral organ will have parasympathetic innervation. Although there are other cranial nerves (III, V, VII and IX) with some parasympathetic fibres, the vagus nerve (cranial nerve X) is the major influence to the head, neck, and thoracic and abdominal cavities. The origin of the vagus nerve is in the upper spinal cord and lower brainstem. The pelvic organs and the terminal portions of the gastrointestinal system are influenced by branches of nerves originating from the terminus of the spinal cord and exiting from foramen in the sacrum (S2, S3 and S4). The parasympathetic centres also receive sensory information from the target organs.

Persistent conditions such as nausea, vomiting, diarrhoea, dysmenorrhoea and dyspepsia are parasympathetic in nature. Dysfunction of the upper cervical, occipital and sacral regions may reflect or result in inappropriate parasympathetic activity. Inhibitory treatment results in reduction of the more superficial representation, increased musculoskeletal tone and congestion, and theoretically downregulates the more internal mechanisms. A thorough understanding of the structure and function of all of the factors related to dysfunction should guide accurate treatment.

Andrew Taylor Still first developed the concepts of osteopathy in 1874. An American practitioner primarily trained through apprenticeship with his father, a Methodist missionary and itinerant practitioner, AT Still practised what could be called conventional medicine until he suffered personal loss as a result of its inadequacy. Despite calling in other practitioners to assist, he watched as members of his family succumbed to meningitis. Realising that the heroic approaches, which were the primary tools of the allopathic profession at that time, were oftentimes more dangerous than the diseases they were meant to combat, and seeking other means, Still began using manipulative treatments. These, he found, were quite effective in managing or facilitating his patients' health.

Theorising that the body was a unit, structure and function were interrelated, and the body had the ability to heal and defend itself, he set about reorganising medical theory. In 1892, he established the first school of osteopathy in Kirksville, Missouri. As a rural institution, osteopathy spread slowly and experienced much prejudice. In the United States, there are currently 19 medical schools of osteopathy and approximately 47 000 osteopathic practitioners with full medical practice rights. Brought to England at the turn of the century by J. Martin Littlejohn, osteopathy spread to the rest of Europe, and the Empire (now Commonwealth).

The origins of some of Still's treatments apparently predate his professional separation from his allopathic colleagues. When he was a young man suffering from chronic headaches, Still treated himself with a rope-swing. He lowered the rope to a few inches above the ground and slung a blanket across it. Lying on the ground, he positioned himself with the contraption supporting his neck at the base of the skull, and subsequently fell asleep. He awakened refreshed and pain-free. This method may represent inhibition as well as a positional intervention (Still 1908). Some descriptions of both inhibition and stimulation methods were included in Still's early writings (Still 1902).

Some of Still's early students likewise described inhibitory techniques as well as their rationale. Eduard Goetz, one of Still's earliest students, described and illustrated inhibition for various conditions, both somatic and visceral, in his book *A Manual of Osteopathy* (Goetz 1905). Selected photographs in this small handbook clearly demonstrate and detail inhibitory treatment of several regions. Two such areas are the orbital and suboccipital regions of the head. Pressure is applied individually to each of these areas for a few minutes.

Dain L. Tasker delivers a more extensive description in *Principles of Osteopathy* (Tasker 1916). Tasker describes a rationale as to the effectiveness of inhibition and that it is a natural phenomenon. Activities such as defaecation and urination could not come under conscious and unconscious control without the ability of the individual to perform inhibition. In discussing the ability of externally applied inhibitory pressure, applied by a practitioner of manual medicine, to lessen hyperactivity, Tasker states that it is not the palpation itself but the initiation or alteration of the reflex arc that occurs. Observation reveals that placing a pressure should be a form of stimulation because it is impacting on the soft tissue. The effect of inhibitory pressure is to produce neural resetting of tone, modification of the dysfunction, and a beneficial modulation of distant or deeper reflexively linked structures. In citing Hilton's law 'that the skin, muscles and synovial membrane of a joint, or the skin, muscles of the abdomen and contents covered by peritoneum, are innervated from the same segment of the cord', Tasker states that the 'over-stimulation' caused by inhibition brings about a diminution or elimination of the over-reactivity.

OSTEOPATHIC POINT AND/OR PRESSURE TECHNIQUES

Strain/counterstrain (see also p. 199)

Several passive direct and indirect systems of osteopathic treatment of somatic dysfunction exist. Standard points and diagnoses are used as fulcrums, or monitoring locations, in practically all. Monitoring by constant palpation at the points allows both practitioner and patient to experience feedback as to the success of the treatment when performing Jones' strain/counterstrain treatment (Glover & Yates 1997, Jones 1981, Jones et al 1995).

The practitioner determines a tender point, such as those that have been identified and mapped by Laurence Jones and his followers. The pressure on the point is designed to create a degree of discomfort, which the patient reports on as the tissues are positioned to remove the discomfort. The positioning of the region or the whole patient into a direction of ease is the actual therapeutic intervention. Although the diagnostic points are named for spinal segments, bony landmarks, ligaments or muscles, it appears that the treatment positions bring about shortening, and therefore relaxation of the muscles and ligaments.

In theory, during the period in a position of ease muscle spindle resetting occurs. The muscle spindle apparatus is a sensory organ embedded into the larger muscle. Small, almost primitive, fibres exist in parallel within the larger extrafusal muscle. Two distinct shapes of the muscular fibres, as well as two of the sensory ends of the nerve fibres, exist. The nuclear bag muscle spindle fibre has all the nuclei collected in the centre. Nuclear chain fibres have the nuclei set almost in line. The sensory fibre ends to the first nuclear bag appear almost like a coiled spring, and are termed annulospiral. The descriptive name 'flower spray' is applied to the endings of the fibres to the nuclear bag fibres. The muscle spindle fibres, unlike the other muscle fibres, do not have a great deal of contractile ability.

The sensory ends to these fibres are stimulated by stretch of any kind. One is more responsive to rate of stretch, and the other to constant stretch. This assists in the regulation of muscle tonicity as stretch brings about contraction. Ordinarily, this is short in duration and recovery is quick. Sometimes, the reflex persists longer than is appropriate. The signals from the spindle continue as if the tissue were being stretched too rapidly, or overstretched, even though the length may be normal.

Increased neural activity is evidenced by increased sensitivity of a 'tender point'. Applied pressure elicits a report of tenderness. The positioning process during application of strain/counterstrain technique shortens the whole muscle, allowing the spindle reflex mechanism to be reset. The position that relieves the tenderness in the palpated point is typically held for 90 seconds and is then slowly returned to neutral. When successful, the previously hypertonic muscles relax and the sensitivity disappears.

Facilitated positional release

Facilitated positional release (FPR) (Schiowitz 1997) is similar in many respects to strain/counterstrain. It differs in its use of an activating force, usually compression or torsion, after initially positioning the region in neutral (ease). By comparison, strain/counterstrain is a form of positional release, whereas FPR utilises an additional facilitating force. As with most manipulative techniques, the efficacy is directly proportional to the accuracy of diagnosis. The diagnosis includes relative motion freedom in the sagittal plane (flexion/extension), coronal plane (lateral flexion/abduction/adduction) and horizontal plane (rotation). Any increase in tissue tension in the surrounding tissue is also noted by means of palpation.

Initially, at least with spinal dysfunctions, the region is brought into a neutral position relative to the sagittal (anterior–posterior) plane. The lordosis of the cervical spine and the kyphosis of the thoracic spine are flattened. The practitioner then further brings the somatic dysfunction into the directions of relative ease. A facilitating force, usually compression and/or torsion, follows this. Release of the dysfunction and localised tension is noted almost immediately, as shown by the practitioner's monitoring finger.

Both strain/counterstrain and FPR theoretically utilise the same neurophysiological mechanism. However, because of an inverse myotactic reflex caused by the facilitating force, a release occurs within seconds instead of in 1.5 minutes. The muscle spindle has a specialised motor nerve known as the γ motor neuron. Even though the nuclear chain and bag fibres are weakly contractile, increased γ activity causes the ends to contract and the central regions become stretched. Regardless of whether the whole muscle is stretched or not, the spindle will react as if it were. The reaction results in overall protective contraction. The γ gain, as it is known, tends to persist longer than is necessary and is modified by many factors including stress, pain, anxiety, endocrine alterations, medications and food substances. FPR, with its initial manoeuvres to flatten curves and adding a facilitating force, addresses the γ-activity component as well as the spindle stretch response. Diagnosis for FPR is less reliant on the localisation of a tender point, but when such a point is found it is used solely for the purpose of monitoring.

The recently described Still technique (van Buskirk 1996) shares many similar applications with these two previously described techniques. Richard van Buskirk attributes the writings of Charles Hazzard (Hazzard 1905), as well as those of Still himself, as the sources for the method. The descriptions revolve around the palpatory diagnosis of dysfunctions followed by motion into the directions of freedom/ease, and finally by movement past the neutral point into the barrier directions. A low-velocity, relatively low-amplitude articulatory movement towards the barriers follows positional treatment and the utilisation of forces into the directions of ease (freedoms).

Functional technique

Functional technique (Johnston 1997) utilises the diagnostic tender points to define the somatic dysfunction that exists at that level relative to the two adjoining vertebrae, the one above and the one below. Detection is typically made by percussion testing to scan and screen the regions. Once an anomaly is determined, the practitioner tests the dysfunction more specifically. The practitioner guides the region into a compound position of freedom ('ease', comfort) along various axes. Fine tuning to

achieve release of the dysfunction includes side-bending and lateral translation, flexion/extension together with anterior or posterior translation, as well as rotation combined with compression or distraction. The breath is then held in either exhalation or inhalation, dependent upon which phase is associated with greatest sense of tissue freedom.

Additional osteopathic methods using palpated points

Monitoring points as sites where some form of pressure is exerted to relieve dysfunction is used in other osteopathic techniques. The intent goes beyond monitoring.

Elaine Wallace developed Torque unwinding (Dowling 1997) and has taught this on a limited basis. She advises that the body can be imagined as a collection of adjacent or overlapping cubes. Injuries place forces into a whole 'cube'. Even though the vector force may be straight initially, entry rarely remains so fixed. The pathway, because of bodily composition, motion or twists, becomes arced or more twisted. The tissues, especially the fascia, maintain memory for these injurious forces. In theory, the cubes are imagined as superimposed on to regions of the body. The practitioner's fingers direct rhythmic, balancing, pressures centrally from two opposing cube faces. Placed on the contralateral sides of the head, trunk or extremity, the therapeutic forces negate the residual traumatic ones. A light percussive test on one side that is monitored on the other yields a sense of resonance that confirms the correct selection of the connected points.

Osteopathic literature is filled with many other variations of myofascial or fascial release techniques (Chila 1997, Ward 1997) that utilize point contacts as references, contact points and/or diagnostic reflections. Steven Typaldos (1994) has written about trigger band technique – a method intended to change the pathological cross-linkages of fascial bands. Using an instrument or fingers, the practitioner exerts significant pressure along certain connective pathways. This occurs along involved tissue in a basically linear fashion from an area of relative dysfunction towards the more involved region. Leon Chaitow (Chaitow 1980, 1996) describes the development of neuromuscular technique by two of his relatives, Stanley Lief and Boris Chaitow. Consisting mostly of point localisation, reflected dysfunctions are treated by pressure followed by deep stroking and/or rolling of the tissue.

Standardised patterns of Chapman's point treatment (Owens 1937) reflect a neurological/endocrine/lymphatic internal alteration to the surface. The palpatory finding has been described as a lenticular (bean-shaped) subcutaneous structure. Although they may not be tender or sensitive to pressure, clinical correlation should raise suspicion either to locate Chapman's points or possibly to search for a latent visceral correlate. Apparently developed independently, some of the specific points are similar to those of acupuncture. Circular pressures are applied rhythmically by the pad of the manipulator's finger(s) to the nodular findings that are related to visceral conditions.

NON-OSTEOPATHIC POINT AND/OR PRESSURE SYSTEMS

There are some similarities between typical inhibition technique and some other manual medicine systems of treatment. These include the Cyriax method (Cyriax 1959), triggerpoint therapy (Chaitow 1990, Travell & Simons 1983), acupressure (Kenyon 1988, Cerney 1974), reflexology, rolfing and shiatsu (Schultz 1976, Weil 1995). Some of the common elements include the practitioner providing the treatment by pressing the patient's soft tissue with the intent of bringing about a persistent alteration. Another similarity is the reliance upon a system of diagnosis and/or treatment points.

James Cyriax was most noted as a medical orthopaedist who practised joint mobilisation and massage. He discussed the use of a 'pinching' technique on several locations (Cyriax 1959). The end goal was relaxation and stretching of tissue, as well as a relative hyperaemia. Triggerpoint therapy, developed by Janet

Travell, recognises the relationship between a remote referral point and a damaged myofascial nexus. Manual pressure can be used, but more commonly dry needling, vapocoolant spray, or a combination of anaesthetic and/or steroid agents are injected into the trigger point. By these means the practitioner locates and interrupts the aberrant patterns. Regardless of the method, theoretically restricted soft tissue is released by means of deep pressure applied to the selected points. Another manual version of the triggerpoint concept, Bonnie Prudden myotherapy, consists of primary points, as well as satellite points. Both are treated for short intervals several times a day over several sessions (Burton Goldberg Group 1994, Prudden 1980). After the treatment, stretching is also incorporated.

Like the better-known acupuncture, acupressure utilises similar surface points that represent reflections of visceral changes. Traditional oriental concept meridians align the specific point locations. Generally, one or two points are treated at any given time and the technique generally involves the application of pressure as well as circular motions.

Injured in a horse-riding accident as a young girl and treated by an osteopathic practitioner, Ida Rolf developed the eponymous system, Rolfing (Burton Goldberg Group 1994). She proposed utilising deeply applied pressure on regions of the body as the tool to re-establish symmetry and more normal function. The actual force of deeply applied pressure used in this modality exceeds that which is commonly applied in inhibition. Some initial discomfort to the patient usually results. There is a great deal of emphasis placed on approximating ideal symmetry and alignment. Modifications to this basic theme were made by followers of Rolf, and integrated into other modalities involving movement patterns (Hellerwork, Aston-patterning).

One of the oldest forms of manual therapy, shiatsu, usually involves relatively heavier pressures applied for short intervals. Increases in 'the circulation of vital energy' (Schultz 1976) is reflected by a reduction of the tissue tension. The amount of force, especially in the hands of a traditional practitioner, is intense and brief (10 lbs for 10 seconds), as opposed to the lower, steady force used in inhibition. Specific conditions dictate the sequencing of points based on energy flows throughout the body. Some points are adjacent, and others are quite distant to the primary location.

Reflexology correlates treatment points with certain visceral organs that are hypothesised as reflecting on to resonant areas located on the hands, feet and ear. In theory, the name has more to do with the functional contribution to the integrity or energy component of the organ than to the actual physical structure.

PROGRESSIVE INHIBITION OF NEUROMUSCULAR STRUCTURES (PINS) METHOD

There is no doubt that practically all modalities of manual pressure treatment have merit, given the appropriate circumstances. PINS shares some commonality with several of these, including the localisation of points and the application of pressure. The PINS system allows for versatility that is based on the practitioner's ability to utilise anatomical and clinical knowledge to determine treatment. A thorough knowledge of the typical and variant courses of nerves, fascial bands and muscles must be augmented by clinical decision-making skills for efficacy and accuracy. Treatment of contiguous muscles, which is modified by an understanding of 'watershed' areas of innervation (the overlapping zones where more than one nerve can be contributing to sensory and motor innervation), leads to the sequencing of PINS treatment.

Anyone can locate a sensitive point. The practitioner must also be fully aware of anatomically normal, as well as variable, connections. For example, shoulder pain invites attention to the glenohumeral joint, and when treatment is successful, as evidenced by increasing mobility and decreasing discomfort, investigation can end. However, when localised attention is unsuccessful, more of the same treatment is not the answer. This will prove frustrating to both the patient and the practitioner. Restriction of

motion of the shoulder into flexion, abduction and external rotation, as well as reduction of scapulothoracic motion, should instigate investigation further afield. For example, latissimus dorsi, originating from the mid to lower back and attaching at the bicipital groove of the humerus, would merit assessment. Expanding the focus, in this example, might also incorporate treatment of the upper ribs, pectoralis muscles, lower cervical spine, clavicle, thoracic spine, lumbar spine, pelvis and lower extremity. Fascial planes – and therefore fascial stresses – overlap and influence one another.

In PINS, patients participate in the treatment by describing the amount of pain or other sensitivity. As the treatment proceeds, changes that occur, as well as the comparison of symptom intensity, are evaluated. Frequently, PINS is not the only treatment modality employed. It can be used before or after other methods of treatment, manipulative or otherwise.

Procedure

The development of an appropriate and specific diagnostic and treatment protocol using PINS requires:

1. In examining the patient, any relationship between the presenting symptoms, somatic dysfunctions and soft tissue findings should be determined.
2. The components comprising a somatic dysfunction must be determined. The mnemonic 'S-T-A-R' (Dowling 1998) can be used to track the different aspects:

    S – Sensitivity changes are the patient's subjective experiences at the sites of dysfunction, in response to the palpation performed by the practitioner. These sensations include tenderness, numbness, radiation, warmth, irritation, throbbing, etc.

    T – Tissue texture changes are the soft tissue conditions as found by palpation by the practitioner. They can be *chronic* (prolonged blanching of the skin, ropy or fibrous texture of the muscles and fascia, coolness, dryness, vascular changes) or *acute* (increased redness, swelling and oedema, moist and/or increased temperature). The findings may worsen with palpation, to a slight degree.

A – Asymmetry is the utilisation of the non-dysfunctional side of the patient in comparison with the dysfunctional side. An area of dysfunction should be compared to the analogous structure on the other side of the body. An imaginary line down the middle of the body should reveal an almost mirrored functional symmetry of one side to the other in a non-dysfunctional person.

R – Restriction of motion is the most important determinant of dysfunction, especially when range of motion shows asymmetry. The restriction can be by quantity (number of degrees of motion) and quality (stiffness, tremors, cogwheel rigidity, extraneous movement, etc.). Although one or more elements may be present, and the patient may or may not complain of a decrease in available motion, abnormal movement is perhaps the most important determinant of somatic dysfunction (see also p. 54).

3. Complaints of pain can be deceptive and may not help in the localisation of the patient's true problem. They are, however, a very good indication that there is a problem. Often, tight muscles on one side may be relatively pain free while the contralateral muscles that are being stretched are more 'attention seeking'. Exclusive attention to the symptoms may distract treatment from the more needy locations. Pain, or any other symptom, suggests that there is a problem, although the site of pain may or may not correlate with the site of dysfunction.

4. A 'primary sensitive' point is determined by examination of the tissue in the region of the patient's complaint. If a significant one is not found, the practitioner utilises knowledge of anatomical relationships and widens the search to contiguous areas.

5. Using knowledge of anatomical structures, another point, designated as the 'end point', is located distal or proximal to the primary point. Knowledge and understanding of muscle and ligamentous origins and insertions is a good beginning concept in determining this pair of points. If the primary point is at the origin, the end point may be at the insertion. The reverse can also be true.

Sometimes the primary point is located in the belly of the muscle. In that case, exploration of both ends of the attachments to bone may reveal the location of an end point. Ligaments, which are generally shorter and more fibrous, have points that are probably also fairly close to one another. Fascia encompasses all structures, and the path between one point and another may seem to cross other structures. Generally, the more specialised the fascia, the more palpable and tendinous it is.

Tracing superficial and deep pathways of nerves is useful when determining paths that do not correlate with the other structures. Primary and end points may be found where a nerve passes out of a foramen, between or through muscles, or around bony protrusions. Sometimes, if more than one nerve innervates a region, the primary point can be found at the beginning of one nerve and the end point at the beginning of the other. In the case of nerve distribution of an extremity, one point will be found closer to the body while the other will be closer to the end of the extremity.

There is no substitution for an excellent working knowledge of typical anatomy. Regardless of the aetiology, the chosen primary point will probably be nearer to the patient's symptoms. The end point may also elicit symptoms, but to a lesser extent. As the two ends of the same problem, both (and all intervening) points must be addressed. In any case, the practitioner makes the determination of the two ends of the pattern. Sometimes the clue for the practitioner is that the patient relates what appears to them as unrelated complaints. Assuming patient knowledge of anatomy is

Table 11.1   Examples of primary and end points

Primary point	End point	Connection
Supraorbital notch	Suboccipital region	Frontalis–occipitalis muscles Trigeminal–greater occipital nerves
Medial elbow epicondyle	Scaphoid wrist region Pisiform at wrist	Flexor carpi radialis muscle Ulnar nerve
Greater trochanter of femur	Fibular head	Iliotibial band
Sternum at 2nd rib	Upper humerus	Pectoralis major
Temporomandibular joint	Side of head	Temporalis muscle
Gluteal region	Greater trochanter Popliteal region	Piriformis muscle Sciatic nerve
Xiphoid process	Public ramus	Rectus abdominis
Maxillary	Angle of mouth	Trigeminal nerve
Temporomandibular joint	Maxillary region	Facial nerve

small, it is left to the practitioner to draw the conclusions necessary to begin treatment. For the purpose of proceeding in a logical fashion, the point that is more sensitive is designated as the initial 'primary'. The other point, which is found distant from it but on a structure that links the points, is considered as the 'end point'.

A few examples of primary and end points are shown in Table 11.1.

6. A muscular, fascial and/or neurological pathway is drawn between the primary sensitive point and the end point. The line may be curved rather than straight. The direction of treatment may be from distal to proximal, or vice versa.

7. The physical connection between the two points may involve:
    (a) *Nerve innervation*:
        (i) Direct connections (The connection of a point near the medial epicondyle at the elbow to a point along the medial arm near the wrist – ulnar nerve.)
        (ii) Overlap or 'watershed regions' of innervation – The ophthalmic division of the trigeminal nerve travels from the supraorbital notch over the frontal region and to the top of the head. The greater occipital nerve exits the infraorbital region in the occipital sulcus and travels over the occiput to the top of the head. Rather than have a region of nerve free scalp, there is an area at the top of the head that is innervated by both the trigeminal and greater occipital nerves.

    (b) *Muscle origins and insertions*
        (i) Typical – A sensitive point may be found at the medial aspect of the clavicle and another at the mastoid process representing involvement of the sternocleidomastoid muscle.
        (ii) Overlap – The location of a sensitive point medial to the scapula and another in the upper cervical spine might represent splenii, levator scapula and/or trapezius muscles.
        (iii) Contiguity – The tensor fascia lata and iliotibial band actually form a continuity for two possible tender points located, respectively, at the greater trochanter and the fibular head. If a terminal point were actually found near the lateral malleolus instead of the fibular head, there might be a tensor facia

lata, iliotibial band, peroneal muscle connection.

(c) *Fascia* (see Ch. 1; Figs 1.3, 1.4)

(i) The interosseous ligaments are actually specialised fascia connecting the radius and ulna in the arm, in the same way that the fibula and tibia are connected. These ligaments should be suspected when the pattern appears to overly their locations. When analysing the line of connection between the two points, there are no obvious neural, muscular or ligamentous analogues.

(ii) Septa – Although it represents muscular components to a greater extent, the central tendon and crus of the thoracoabdominal diaphragm are fascial in nature. The diaphragm supports the thoracic viscera, and separates the abdominal cavities. Points found around the lower costal cartilage, the 12th rib and T10–T12 may represent a diaphragmatic involvement.

(iii) Overlaps – The fascia in the lumbar region acts as an attachment for muscles such as the latissimus dorsi and overlaps muscles such as the quadratus lumborum, iliocostalis and other erector spinae muscles. Points may be found anywhere within the region and may extend to the lateral edge of the 12th rib (quadratus lumborum) or even to the bicipital groove of the humerus (latissimus dorsi).

(d) *Ligamentous attachments*

(i) Typical – Points can be found at the attachments of either end of the collateral ligaments in the elbow and knee.

(ii) Relationships to muscles – Surface of the points found on the superior C7 spinous process and the base of the occiput may represent spinalis muscles or the nuchal ligament.

(iii) Relationships to nerves – The flexor retinaculum and palmar aponeurosis are key components to treat when the median nerve in the forearm is involved. There may actually be a need to treat the articular relationships of the four carpal attachments (pisiform, hamate, scaphoid and trapezium) of the retinaculum as well.

(e) *Bones* – Although the bones are the deepest of the musculoskeletal structures, they and their components should be considered as connective tissue as well.

(i) Construction of joints – The joint capsules represent encompassing connections of two or more bones. At joints such as the elbow and the knee, the capsules are stronger and reinforced on their medial and lateral surfaces by collateral ligaments. The anterior and posterior surfaces tend to be more flaccid in one direction of motion or the other. Points may occur in the middle of the capsule and at the bony attachments.

(ii) Lever action – More of a concern for the analysis of the aetiology of strains and somatic dysfunctions. The bony prominences are relatively strong extensions of the bones. Muscle tendons and ligaments attach to bone and, as a result of frequent usage, lead to the development of enlargements including tubercles, trochanters and other processes. Points theoretically located at tendinous insertions may also represent a contribution from the periosteal anchors.

8. Both the primary point and the end point are pressed simultaneously using the pad region of a finger on each hand (for the sake

of simplicity the practitioner can identify the primary point as the 'first point' for the patient). The pressure exerted is a few ounces, enough to elicit the patient's symptoms, and should be of equal degree on both points. The patient may experience a mild to moderate increase in sensitivity. The practitioner should also determine the soft tissue response to pressure by sensing changes in the tissues:

(a) Dysfunctions that are acute may be more sensitive than chronic ones. A muscle that has been hypertonic will usually be more sensitive to pressure than the same muscle on the contralateral side.

(b) Muscles that are used excessively will hypertrophy and be bulkier than their contralateral pair.

Larger muscles do not necessarily indicate dysfunction. When muscles have been subjected to increased usage or there is preference to one side being used more, such as in sports activities that preferentially utilise muscles in an asymmetrical manner (e.g. bowling, archery), the dominant side will typically be larger, but not necessarily dysfunctional.

Whether dysfunctional or not, hypertonic muscles that have been so for some time may not be quite so sensitive to pressure. This may be due to the chronicity of usage. A more sensitive, but less hypertonic, muscle indicates a problem. This does not necessarily indicate the laterality of the problem. Both sides can be dysfunctional. One may be more symptomatic than the other, but to varying degrees. Given a choice of examined findings versus symptoms, the findings take precedence. The practitioner should initially treat the more dysfunctional tissue, re-examine, and treat the less involved side as well.

(c) Whenever possible, the patient should be in a comfortable position, which generally means one where the muscle is not actively being utilized. Because postural muscles do not fully relax while the patient is seated or standing, a supine or prone position is preferred.

(d) The pressure exerted on both the primary point and the end point should be equal:

(i) Patients may assume that the more sensitive location is receiving more pressure. They should be reassured that the reason for the asymmetrical degree of sensitivity is because of the dysfunctional state of the involved tissue.

(ii) Occasionally, patients will direct the practitioner to apply greater pressure. Increased pressure does not accelerate the treatment. It is not necessary to increase the pressure, and doing so may be counterproductive.

(iii) Pain or tenderness may not be the only sensations experienced as a result of the applied pressure. The chronic nature of some dysfunctions may result in the patient reporting other sensations such as paraesthesia, which may occur alone or in combination with pain.

(e) Maintain constant pressure on the end point throughout the treatment (this can be identified as the 'end point' or 'final point' for the patient).

9. Initiate pressure on the point that produces the greatest sensitivity (primary point). A series of points will be located for application of inhibitory pressure between this 'primary' (i.e. the most sensitive) point and the end point during the course of the treatment.

10. Request that the patient report the initial amount and type of sensitivity. Feedback should be given if the sensation at any sensitive point decreases or increases. When inhibition is utilised properly, the sensitivity

will usually have a transient initial increase. Also usual is a typical subsequent decrease in sensitivity as the tissue accommodates to the irritation of the inhibition. Ultimately sensitivity may totally disappear. The duration can vary from several seconds to minutes.

11. The practitioner maintains contact with the two points for 20–30 seconds and then seeks another point:
    (a) A finger of the same hand that has a finger applying pressure to the primary point is used to locate a 'secondary point'. If the index finger is on the primary point, then the middle finger can be used to palpate for the secondary point.
    (b) Usually the secondary point will be approximately 2–3 cm (about 1 inch) away from the primary point in the direction of the end point. (The practitioner can identify the secondary point as the 'second point' for the patient.) This will typically follow the predicted course of an anatomical structure (innervating nerve, along the direction of the muscle fibres, or following fascial planes).

12. Equal pressure is exerted on to both the primary and secondary points while maintaining pressure on the end point.

13. The patient is requested to determine which of the two points (primary versus secondary or 'first versus second') is more sensitive. The practitioner can state: 'I am pressing on two points that are close together. Please tell me which of the two, the "first" (practitioner may move the finger slightly) or the "second" is more sensitive.'
    (a) If the second point is more or equally sensitive than the first:
        (i) pressure is relieved and removed from the first point (primary)
        (ii) and then constant pressure is maintained on the second (secondary) sensitive point for 20–30 seconds.

(iii) The sensitivity at any point does not have to abate completely before moving on to the next point. It is important that the next point is more sensitive.
(iv) The initial pressure on a new 'secondary' point will usually cause a response of both increased tension and sensitivity. This usually returns to a baseline after a few seconds, as noted above; the amount of time depends on the soft tissue response.
(b) There are a few considerations if the primary point persists as the more sensitive of the two contiguous points:
    (i)   Maintain pressure at the location of the primary point.
    (ii) The practitioner moves the finger pressing on the secondary point more laterally or medially. A point may be found that has more or the same sensitivity as the primary point by searching slightly out of line with the targeted end point. (The anatomical structure, which is being inhibited, may have slight variations in the specific course in this individual.)
    (iii) Once a secondary point that is equally or more sensitive (compared with the primary point) is located, pressure is released from the primary point and maintained on the new secondary point, as described above.
    (iv) The secondary point then becomes the new 'first' point in the continuing sequence of treatment towards the end point.

14. Before searching or inhibiting any subsequent points, the practitioner should wait approximately 20–30 seconds.

15. If no secondary point can be located despite searching in a 2-cm radius from the primary point, the clinician maintains pressure on

the primary point (or the new 'primary' point) for an additional 30 seconds. Sometimes certain points require further inhibition before progress can be made. After doing so, a new secondary point may be located where previously there was less sensitivity.

16. The end point will have received inhibitory pressure throughout. Often the patient will forget that this point is being inhibited and it may lose all sensitivity.

17. The process is continued successively until the ultimate 'second' point is 2 cm from the end point.

18. Once there are the two final points being inhibited, the practitioner determines the amount of dysfunction that persists at the end and secondary point locations. The dysfunction may have reduced or disappeared totally.

19. If the dysfunction, including the end point, remains persistent, the practitioner can choose to treat the dysfunction with whatever additional modality is deemed necessary and appropriate. The end point and dysfunction, having been recalcitrant to treatment previously, may now be more amenable. Strain/counterstrain, facilitated positional release, muscle energy technique, balanced tension techniques or some other modality may be used. Single-segment somatic dysfunctions that were difficult to position or resistant to thrust technique may now be more responsive to articulatory techniques such as high-velocity, low-amplitude thrust.

20. PINS technique can be the sole approach to the somatic dysfunctions that were found, or may be used in conjunction with any other modality of manual treatment. Determining this is:
    (a) The persistence of the dysfunction or related components after treatment.
    (b) The ability of the practitioner to perform other modalities of treatment.
    (c) The need or capability of the patient to accept additional treatment.

   (i) After any treatment, some soreness or other symptom may persist despite sufficient treatment. The practitioner should determine termination of treatment based on the findings for the individual; it should not be based on the patient's subjective complaints. Overtreatment can cause as many problems as undertreatment.
   (ii) Based on previous experience or misconceptions, patients may limit types of treatment. This may be due to fears or reactions that they have had to previous types of treatment.

21. The somatic dysfunction is always reassessed.

22. The patient should be advised that, despite the relative comfort of the treatment, there may be a post-treatment reaction. These reactions can include transient soreness, aches and fatigue. In patients who are prone to bruising, or when there are certain other predisposing factors (e.g. medication), ecchymoses can occur. These may also be found if excessive pressure has been used. Generally, all of these side-effects will resolve in 24–48 hours.

Application

The following two case studies are illustrative of the use of PINS to common myofascial conditions.

Case study 1

The patient was a 25-year-old married female osteopathic medical student who presented with a chief complaint of 'migraine headache'. She had been followed for her musculoskeletal complaints by another osteopathic practitioner who was unavailable on the day of presentation to the clinic. The headache was sharp and focused near the right orbit with radiation to the right frontal and temporal region. The patient had some nausea, blurring of vision, increased lacrimation and neck stiffness. The pain had started a few days beforehand and was unrelieved by the use of non-steroidal anti-inflammatory drugs, sleep or frequent doses of sumatriptan succinate, which she took orally. The patient stated that she takes between 21 and 30 pills of this drug per month. Loud sounds, light and certain food smells appear to worsen the chief complaint. There were no other visual, auditory or olfactory complaints or associations with the presence of headache. The current episode appeared to be unrelated to the patient's menses, since her last menstrual period had been 2 weeks previously.

Past medical history relative to the chief complaint was significant for paraesthesias to the upper extremities secondary to a motor vehicle accident 2 months earlier. She was the driver of a vehicle that was stopped at a traffic light, when it was struck from behind. She did see the other vehicle and had braced herself for impact. She had had a fall at age 12 years, in which she struck the top of her head, and she has had migraines since that time. Family history is significant in that other members of the family have had migraines, a brother has allergies, and her mother has 'colon problems'. The patient has two glasses of wine once per week, during religious observations, and denies use of recreational drugs or tobacco. She has had a tonsillectomy, rhinoplasty and sinus cauterisation. Other medical history was non-contributory.

Other medications included fexofenadine hydrochloride, oral contraceptives, Excedrin® PM (paracetamol (acetaminophen), aspirin and caffeine) and ibuprofen, as well as the sumatriptan. The last three drugs were taken episodically for headaches. At times in the past, she had gone to the emergency room for treatment of unrelieved migraine headaches.

Cranial nerve, sensorimotor and reflex testing were normal. Other neurological and orthopaedic evaluation findings for the patient were essentially normal. Although she had several tender points, there was not a pattern that would suggest fibromyalgia as a component of the patient's condition.

Examination of the head, neck, chest and abdomen were essentially normal, with the exception of photophobia. Vital signs were stable and the patient was alert and oriented for all modalities. Examination resulted in findings of somatic dysfunctions, as described below.

Cranial. Cranial examination revealed restrictive patterns on the right side with relative freedom of left cranial motion.

Cervical. Several single somatic dysfunctions were found in the cervical spine including ones at OA (C0–C1), AA (C1–C2), C2, C3, C6 and C7. There was also hypertonicity of the right trapezius and right sternocleidomastoid muscles.

Thoracic and rib. Hypertonicity of the right levator scapula and of the left scalene muscles; right first rib elevation; myofascial restriction of the hyoid and anterior strap muscles; multiple thoracic type II somatic dysfunctions.

Lumbar. A somatic dysfunction was found at L5 on the right accompanied by thoracolumbar paravertebral muscle spasms.

Sacrum and pelvis. Restrictions of the right sacroiliac joint and the related myofascial structures were noted.

The primary diagnosis for the office visit in question included cephalgia (migraine). Other diagnoses included cervical, thoracic, head, lumbar, sacral and pelvic somatic dysfunctions and strain. Although they were present, the areas other than those related to the patient's head were more chronic in nature and not as crucial to the patient's chief complaint. The patient was clearly anxious regarding her condition.

Much of the treatment that was performed on this single visit was similar to that which had been performed previously for the patient. Many modalities of treatment were utilised to address all related and apparently unrelated strains and dysfunctions. All of these interventions were successful, to some extent, in relieving most of the somatic dysfunctions and complaints, with the exception of the chief one – the cephalgia. The complaints of the 'migraine headache' persisted.

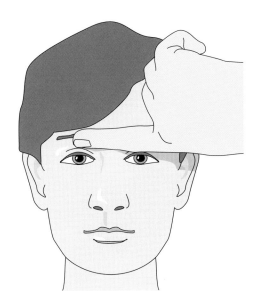

Figure 11.1A   Frontal view.

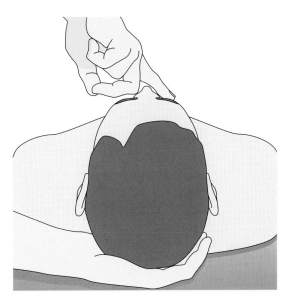

Figure 11.1C   Crown view.

Figure 11.1   Pressure is exerted on the end point at the right suboccipital region and the right supraorbital ridge by using a finger of each hand. Redrawn from Dowling (2000), with permission from The American Osteopathic Association.

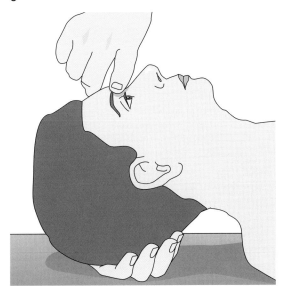

Figure 11.1B   Lateral view.

PINS, as a modality, was added to the other customary treatment. Sensitive points at the right supraorbital ridge at the trochlear notch and in the suboccipital region were identified. Placing his left hand beneath the patient's head and neck, the author inhibited the suboccipital point with his left index finger ('end point'). Simultaneously, the author's right index finger

(Fig. 11.1A,B,C) exerted pressure on the right orbital sensitive point ('primary point').

The patient indicated that the orbital point was the more sensitive of the two. The pressure also seemed to increase her ophthalmic symptoms (nausea, blurring of vision, increased lacrimation). Pressure was maintained for approximately 30 seconds on the anterior, primary point. After this interval, a second point superior to this was simultaneously pressed, with the same amount of pressure as the first, utilising the author's right middle finger (Fig. 11.2A,B). The patient was asked to identify which of the two anterior points was more sensitive. She stated that the second was more so. Pressure was then maintained on this second point and released on the first.

This was then maintained for 30 seconds before a third point was identified approximately 2 cm above the second point. This now was reported as more sensitive than the second point. Pressure was then relieved from the second point and maintained on the third. The same pattern was followed progressively along a parasagittal line

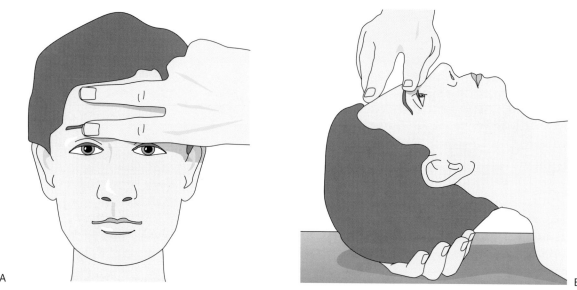

A   B

Figure 11.2A,B   Pressure is typically exerted for 20–30 seconds before searching for a secondary point. The secondary point is usually 2–3 cm from the anterior primary point in the direction of the end point. Pressure is then placed simultaneously on all three locations. If the secondary point is greater or equal in sensitivity to that now experienced at the original primary point, pressure is released from the primary point. The secondary point becomes the new – and temporary – 'primary' point. Each subsequent point between this and the end point is treated similarly. If other 'secondary points' are not found easily in a direct line towards the end point, the practitioner should attempt to press at another location medially or laterally until a point of equal or greater intensity is found. If this is also unsuccessful, a longer period of inhibition on the primary point is performed. Generally, after 1–2 minutes, new secondary points are located more easily. Redrawn from Dowling (2000), with permission from The American Osteopathic Association.

over the frontal, parietal and occipital bones until a final point was identified. This was 1 cm above the end-point location that was being inhibited in the suboccipital region throughout the whole process. The somatic dysfunctions were treated with a combination of other modalities such as cervical strain/counterstrain, facilitated positional release, low-velocity and then high-velocity, low-amplitude techniques to the suboccipital region. These techniques had previously, during this session, either been unsuccessful or could not be performed, because of the patient's symptoms. All the patient's symptoms resolved completely.

Note: Placement and movement of the fingers often requires that the practitioner move the whole hand when selecting subsequent points. This 'finger walking' may mean that the second, third and fourth fingers are primarily used in sequence. Sometimes, the first finger (thumb) can be utilised temporarily to locate a new

secondary point. Once it has been selected, one of the other fingers can be substituted.

Because she understood the process and her own particular patterns, the patient also tried the technique on herself, with positive results. When used early, it could be quite effective in aborting what she felt was the beginning of a migraine headache. When the results were less than optimal, she reported that she could then take a single sumatriptan pill and the symptoms would usually improve to a greater extent. Instead of the 21–30 pills per month, her use of this medication reduced to a more acceptable 2–3 monthly. This remained constant for several months.

Cephalgia or headache is complex, and complicated by overlapping symptoms and findings. The same symptoms can represent multiple aetiologies. A consideration is that all headaches have elements of muscle contraction, regardless of the cause. When initiated during the prodromal phase or during relatively symptom-free intervals, manipulative treatment of migraine headaches appears to be most successful. Migraine headaches, in particular, are vascular with arterial constriction, dilatation and inflammatory phases nearly paralleling the aural, pain and refractory phases. When considering irritation and inflammation of the cranial dura, one must keep in mind that the first branch of the trigeminal nerve innervates the frontal region. The posterior fossa receives a good portion of innervation from the upper cervical region. Generally, treatment during the full-blown sickening headache component of migraine may be more effective in reduction rather than complete elimination of the symptoms.

Other types of headaches, such as muscle tension/contraction headaches, can mimic some of the more typical migraine symptoms. Because all headaches have muscle contraction as a component, there is no reason why migraine and muscle contraction headaches cannot occur in the same person. Patients with chronic headaches of any sort may seek many means of intervention.

It is well documented that pharmacological interventions such as non-steroidal anti-inflammatory drugs and vasoconstrictive medications are frequently the initial and/or most frequently attempted interventions. Caffeine is an ingredient in many other self-treatments, including beverages, foods and pills. Because of their vasoconstrictive effects, they are successful in limiting or eliminating headaches. However, paradoxically, they have also been implicated in recurrences. It is possible to experience a rebound effect once the medication level goes below a critical point. Rather than eliminate headaches as intended, frequent use of anti-inflammatory and/or vasoconstrictive substances may encourage recurrences.

Cephalgia of this type can be approached from a neuromusculoskeletal model by inhibiting discovered sensitive points by using the PINS technique. The location of the initial point, in this particular case, was at the exit of the ophthalmic division of the trigeminal nerve, above the orbit. The same nerve innervates both the dural lining of the brain and the pain-sensitive structures of

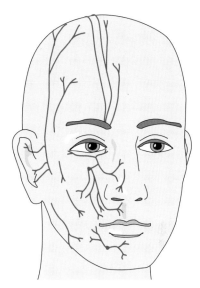

Figure 11.3 Trigeminal innervation of the face and head (frontal view). Redrawn from Dowling (2000), with permission from The American Osteopathic Association.

the forehead. The dura, one of the layers of the meninges, is also a pain-sensitive structure. The attachment of the superior oblique muscle at the trochlear notch of the orbit, as well as sympathetic influences from the upper cervical spine postganglionic fibres, must also be considered.

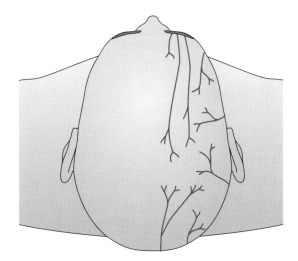

Figure 11.4 Overlapping innervation of the trigeminal nerve and the greater occipital nerves in the watershed region of the scalp (superior view). Redrawn from Dowling (2000), with permission from The American Osteopathic Association.

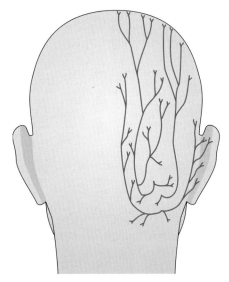

Figure 11.5 Greater occipital nerve innervation of the head (posterior view). Redrawn from Dowling (2000), with permission from The American Osteopathic Association.

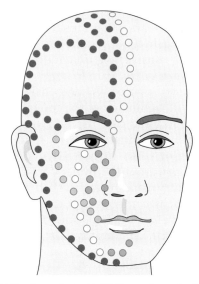

Figure 11.7 Some typical inhibition patterns for the face and head. Redrawn from Dowling (2000), with permission from The American Osteopathic Association.

There are several branchings of the ophthalmic division of the trigeminal nerve (Fig. 11.3), and all project more superiorly along the frontal region. Basically, they track upwards unilaterally into the parietal region and are responsible for sensory

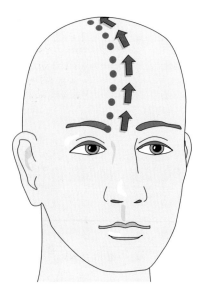

Figure 11.6 Pattern of inhibition points in this case of cephalgia. Redrawn from Dowling (2000), with permission from The American Osteopathic Association.

appreciation from this region. Near their terminations on the top of the head there is a 'watershed' region at the galea aponeurotica (Fig. 11.4). The greater occipital nerve (Fig. 11.5) begins to also innervate the skin and musculature in this region (Moore 1980). This nerve is derived from C2 and C3 nerve roots and perforates the fascia and suboccipital muscles. These nerve roots control the majority of sensory and motor innervation to most of the occipital region. Fibres also travel anteriorly upwards through the foremen magnum to the dura of the posterior fossa. Without inhibition and other treatment of the suboccipital region, resolution of the headache may not occur. With limited treatment, some of the symptoms may abate but the presence of multiple untreated regions may result in fairly rapid recurrence.

The typical direction of treatment of frontal headache utilising PINS (Fig. 11.6) proceeds in a pattern that progresses from orbit to occiput along a typical parasagittal line. The direction may vary in some cases and include other divisions or subdivisions of the trigeminal nerve (Fig. 11.7). The approach may be more anterograde, beginning in the suboccipital region and proceeding to the frontal–orbital region depending on the findings. This depends on the clinical complaints of the patient as well as the experience of the practitioner. Generally, the more sensitive of the points is selected as the beginning location. Sometimes, pressure placed on to the suboccipital region reproduces the symptoms and pain in the region of the eye. Although it is infrequently a terminal point, it is also not unusual to find that one of the intermediate points near the vertex of the head also refers pain towards the initial primary point, either to the eye or to the base of the head.

Finding this point should be taken as a positive sign that the procedure is locating and treating the component factors of the dysfunction. In any case, sometimes a 'search and test' approach determines the location of several involved points. Two or more found points may give an indication of the involved structures by tracing a line and identifying the structures that link them.

Case study 2

The patient was a 72-year-old man with chief complaints of pain in the left lower extremity, specifically in the hip area. He also had a history of Parkinson's disease and osteoarthritis. He described the primary symptom as sharp, almost constant, and with radiation of the pain from the left hip towards the knee and ankle. His Parkinson's disease had progressed slowly and was expressed primarily by stiffness. When added to his arthritis, some activities had become difficult to perform. His posture and gait

were stooped, with head forward and moderate bradykinesia. The recent onset of the hip pain added a limp to his already shuffling gait. Shortly after the examination, radiography revealed apparently symmetrical moderate degenerative joint disease of both hips. The patient denied any changes in bowel or bladder habits.

Range of motion examination revealed equal restriction of motion of both hips. Fabere (Patrick test) and Fadir (Flexion, Adduction and Internal Rotation) ranges of motion, as well as pure flexion, were equally limited and equivalent for both hips. Sacroiliac motion was likewise limited with asymmetry. The left side demonstrated slightly less motion than the right. A left unilateral sacral shear was noted. Equal mobility, or relative lack thereof, of ilia motion was demonstrated. The legs appeared to be of equal length. Moderate somatic dysfunctions were noted throughout the lumbar, thoracic and cervical regions as well. Neurological examination revealed that sensorimotor and deep tendon reflex testing of the lower extremities were equal and normal. Strain/counterstrain tender points were noted in the left gluteal, piriformis, midpole sacral and iliotibial band. Left posterior fibular head somatic dysfunction was also noted.

Manipulative treatment based on these findings was performed on one occasion using techniques such as strain/counterstrain, muscle energy, balanced ligamentous tension, and other means of fascial release. Attempted mobilisation utilising high-velocity, low-amplitude (HVLA)

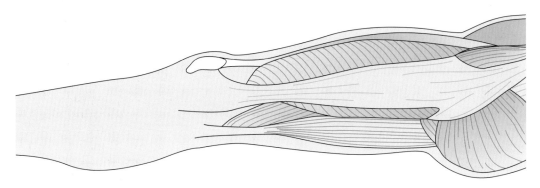

Figure 11.8 Iliotibial band and musculature of the lateral leg. Redrawn from Dowling (2000).

thrust of the posterior fibular head was unsuccessful. Ultrasound modality was utilized along the iliotibial band, both during that office visit and during the twice-a-week physiotherapy sessions, along with other physical medicine modalities. Despite all this, the patient's chief complaint symptoms persisted.

One week later, the same clinical and palpatory findings were noted. PINS technique was then utilised. A sensitive primary point was located at the greater trochanter. The end point was found overlying the fibula head. Location of this point took some trial and error. End points could have been located at the ankle, medial knee, popliteal space, buttock, or even more centrally above the iliac crest. In this case, successive points were also found along the tensor

fascia lata/iliotibial band (Figs 11.8–11.10). Following a process of sequential inhibition of these points, the final 'primary' point that was located close to the end point was approximately 2 cm proximal to the end point. Pressure was maintained for half a minute simultaneously on the two points. Inhibition alone resulted in a reported reduction of at least 50% of the lower extremity pain and radiation. The fibula head was then mobilised successfully with HVLA mobilisation. The patient stated he had only a small amount of residual discomfort after this was performed. Previous attempts at performing HVLA thrust to the fibula head had been unsuccessful.

At the next visit, the patient reported that the improvement had persisted for at least 1 week.

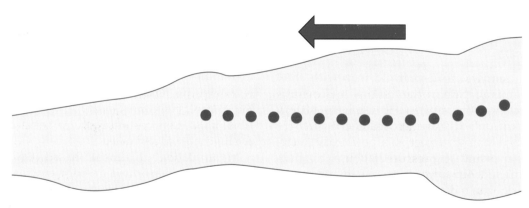

Figure 11.9 Points and direction of treatment of iliotibial band in case study 2. Redrawn from Dowling (2000).

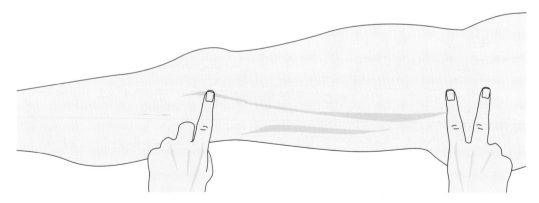

Figure 11.10 Locations of end point (index finger, left hand) and primary point (middle finger, right hand). The index finger of the right hand has located the 'secondary point'. Redrawn from Dowling (2000).

The findings were again present, but to a much lesser degree, and were limited to a single tender point near the left greater trochanter. This was easily treated with only strain/counterstrain technique. PINS was not necessary to the treatment protocol on this visit.

POSSIBLE MECHANISM OF ACTION

The mechanism of action by which the technique of inhibition works can only be postulated. Unfortunately, this is the status with many other modalities of osteopathic manipulative technique: insufficient research has been performed for many manipulative modalities. However, the clinical outcomes have been reported anecdotally many times. Understanding the processes of injury as well as treatment is typically based on the most likely combination of relevant physiological and anatomical components.

One of the important components of inhibition is the use of a low-level (but using a constant amount of force) pressure applied to a dysfunctional tissue.

Accommodation or habituation is a process wherein a stimulus of a constant level, even if initially irritating, becomes less noticeable over time. At first, the subject may be acutely aware of the intrusion or pressure. The patient may state that there is pain, sensitivity, increased pressure or some other sensation. The practitioner may also note that the local tissue reacts by initially increasing in tension. Firm, spasmed muscle may become more so. When the pressure is maintained constantly, these reactions decrease and may disappear altogether as the system adapts (Bailey 1976). The reticular formation as a screen is but one component involved in the process. There are many other occasions where the body accommodates to stimuli. These are evidenced by the relative non-awareness of body contact with eyeglasses, tight belts, stiff clothing, uncomfortable shoes, as well as constant auditory and visual stimuli. It is only when attention is called to them by a new, probably irritating, event that awareness resurfaces. A refrigerator in the kitchen or the sounds from a nearby railway often fail to attract the attention of someone accustomed to them – unless the sounds deviate from the usual. Persons who have worn eyeglasses since infancy may be oblivious to their presence and may even casually adjust the positioning with almost unconscious effort. However, someone who has recently developed the need for visual aids, such as a middle-aged presbyopic adult, may be all too aware of every aspect from the points of contact to the change in appearance of objects. Gradually, this diminishes. This filtering process may also involve lower components, such as the spinal cord, to act as a mediator. Its contribution in this habituation process is to act as a 'brake' when sensory overload occurs (Patterson 1976).

Direct pressure placed upon areas of greatest sensitivity or symptoms may act as a counter-irritant. Rapid, conducting, large nerve afferents gate transmission in the dorsal horn of the spinal cord. Collateral fibres in the substantia gelatinosa or adjacent interneurons then inhibit the transmission of pain to the central nervous system via the spinothalamic tract (Ganong 1995). Pressure acts as a stimulant to the neighbouring tissue, reducing the sensitivity of the original tender point. Scratching in the region of an itch would be an example of this phenomenon. An ischaemia theory concerning the use of a sustained pressure, such as that used in inhibition, describes an effect in the immediate tissue. When a muscle is maintained in prolonged contraction, metabolites are released that were produced from the local tissue damage (Stoddard 1969). Damaged tissue ordinarily demonstrates a decrease in circulation in a progressive fashion. Immediate or acute injury results in hyperaemia and congestion. This is followed by infiltration of vasoactive substances. These appear primarily for the theoretical purpose of dealing with tissue injury. If the injury persists or there is a prolonged reduced function, trophic tissue changes occur. The muscles, ligaments and fascia may develop fibrotic changes. The chronic nature of the dysfunction demonstrates decreased circulation by blanching following any pressure. Normally, the skin shows a brief blanching followed by redness, which also fades. When muscle is maintained in a chronically tightened state, circulation is impaired. The use of further pressure in a therapeutic fashion to cause a relatively increased ischaemia does not initially make sense from the standpoint of nutrient deprivation. One way of appreciating an effect is to postulate that, following pressure, the increased ischaemia reduces the capacity of the nociceptive receptors to process. Once this pressure is removed, the resultant hyperaemia produced after release results in flushing of the waste products from the region. The local vessels are dammed temporarily, there is a build-up of pressure, and then sudden washing away as the compression is released.

Although there may be no visible abnormality, a dysfunctional muscle may appear to be in its neutral position but still be hypertonic. Any further stretch from the shortened attitude increases activity of the muscle spindle mechanisms. Slight increases in length, even if the muscle is halfway between fully shortened and extended, may result in a reflexive and prolonged contraction. Within skeletal muscle, sensory muscle fibres 'monitor' length changes. These specialised muscular fibres lie deep to and occur in parallel with the larger extrafusal fibres. Set in parallel, the sensory nerve fibres to these small muscles track back to the spinal cord. Specific motor nerves (γ motor neurons) modulate muscle spindle contractions. The sensory fibres, the annulospiral and flower-spray afferents, react to either contraction of the nuclear bag and chain fibres or the stretching of these. This is an intrinsic means of protection. A rationale for this is the prevention of tearings of the muscle. Factors that increase the sensitivity and gain of these fibres include stress, anxiety, pain, cold and other general components. Sudden, unexpected stretching, as well as over-stretching of the intrafusal fibres, also increases activity of the special sensory flower-spray and annulospiral fibres. Mediated by the spinal cord segment, this results in a reflex action by activation of the α motor neuron. This causes contraction of the larger extrafusal muscle fibres. When the γ motor neuron gain is set too high, the muscle spindles react earlier in the stretch, to a greater degree than is usually necessary, or are inappro-

priately maintained for longer than is necessary (Becker 1976, Buzzell 1967, Ganong 1995, Korr 1976).

Slow stretching is encouraged, especially before and after exercise, to prevent contractions as a means of 'training' the extrafusal muscles, but also to lower the reactivity of the muscle spindles. Pressure applied during inhibition introduces a gentle stretch while allowing re-setting of the stretch receptors (Korr 1979b). This localised pressure may add a stretch in a region of only a few centimetres without challenging the whole muscle. The component that is initially irritating is at a subcritical level. Once the small, localized component is overwhelmed, any affected adjacent area can subsequently be inhibited, with similar results. The use of digitally applied pressure along the muscle, such as is used in PINS, may be a very effective method as it deals with a series of irritated parts. In this way, the practitioner completes the treatment by progressively treating all of the involved elements.

Myotendinotic changes, which are usually characterised by increased tone, thickening, resistance and decreased plasticity, have been described by some authors (Dvorak & Dvorak 1990). These occur within the muscle. They are particularly tender when the muscle is palpated perpendicular to the direction of the fibres. The tenderness may be elicited when using pressure that should not ordinarily be irritating. Along with the increase in sensitivity, changes in these fibres can be palpated from the origin to the insertion. Other non-pathological fibres that are located in the same or nearby muscles do not evidence the same pattern of irritation. The pathological and physiological fibres can be parallel to one another. However, the pathological aspects of the fibres may occur in relatively isolated bundles from the neighbouring unaffected ones. These tender bands can be found in patterns that are similar to trigger points. The appearance may be related to relatively non-traumatic events. After a variable latency period in which only one site is irritable, the rest of the muscle and attachments become irritable. This phenomenon may explain some of the correlation between locations of Jones' strain/counterstrain tender points and Travell's trigger points (Travell & Simons 1983). Jones' points tend to be related to muscle bands, are sensitive to light pressure, but elicit only tenderness at the site of pressure. The Travell points themselves may be sensitive or not, but the hallmark of their existence is the pain patterns that radiate when they are compressed. The differences in quality between the two types of point may represent a matter of duration and degree of the dysfunction.

A complementary muscular reflex system to the muscle spindle is that of the Golgi tendon system. The Golgi tendon organs are set in series and located in a net-like fashion in the tendon, unlike the muscle spindles, which are set in parallel with the extrafusal muscles. Tendons are the least contractile element of a muscle. The Golgi unit has sensory fibres that become relatively stretched during muscular contraction. This is unlike the activation of the muscle spindles, which occurs during muscular stretch. The Golgi tendon organs can also become activated by passive stretch of the whole unit. Unlike the muscle spindle, increased Golgi tendon organ activity brings about reflex relaxation of the muscle as a whole. The sensory neuron from the Golgi apparatus influences the α motor neuron indirectly through the mediation of an inhibitory interneuron. The reflex is also known as the clasp-knife reflex, and the results can be quite dramatic and sudden. The progressive tightening of muscles recruits more and more Golgi tendon activity. Therefore, the signals bring about greater inhibition of the muscular contraction. When muscles are hypertonic, an intervention whereby initial stretch results in further contraction is then followed by resultant relaxation (Ganong 1995). This reflex system is the one most probably involved in direct active techniques (i.e. muscle energy) and in passive stretch interventions where the region is held at a pathological barrier for a significant amount of time.

A narrow view of compression is that only blood flow is impeded. Impaired flow can be of vascular, lymphatic or neuronal origin. Pressure on the axons can impair the transport of necessary neuropeptides and other substances when considering nerves (Korr 1979c). According to Korr & Appeltauer (1979), the speed with which this flow naturally occurs is quite slow at 40 to several hundred millimetres per day. These rates would therefore not easily explain any immediate effect of inhibitory pressure. The reduction in the soft tissue hypertonicity and the persistence of this effect in response to soft tissue treatments such as PINS may be due in some part to alleviation of the pressure upon nerves (Korr 1979a).

The persistence of somatic dysfunction can occur despite adequate treatment, as has been expressed previously. Sometimes the breakthrough in successful treatment comes with the recognition of the connection of various apparently unrelated elements. Beginning with the postulate that some dysfunctions support others, failure to recognise and initiate improvement of some aspects allows for continuation or recurrence. The more symptomatic elements may receive the attention, while the supportive ones remain relatively silent in the background: the 'noisy' ones are treated while the 'quiet' ones are not. After treatment, the whole problem may resolve, the secondary components may assert themselves, or they may instigate a recurrence of the original problem. Using the analogy of a reverberating circuit, all elements should be 'shut down' to eliminate the process entirely. It is tempting, on first presentation, to focus solely on the region of the patient's chief complaint. If there is good resolution, there may be no need to search further. However, when limited results are obtained, there is a need to search. As a treatment modality, the PINS approach offers an additional means of analysing and treating persistent or difficult dysfunctions.

CONTRAINDICATIONS AND SIDE-EFFECTS

Over the years, repeated use of PINS has demonstrated few contraindications and side-effects. Any condition in which pressure placed on or through the skin might be expected to cause a worsening of the symptoms or signs should preclude the use of PINS. Localised inflammation, abscesses or infection should not be pressed: surgical or other medical interventions may be more appropriate. The aetiology in these instances would preclude the use of PINS or any other technique that may cause more damage. Other manipulative interventions could then possibly include lymphatic or other fluid techniques instead. PINS could be applied to treat any residual sensitive points if sensitive points persist after the resolution of the inflammatory or infectious process. As the pressure applied is just enough to ensure a response of sensitivity, the likelihood of real injury should be minimal. There is always a possibility that the patient may develop some temporary symptoms such as aches or fatigue. These generally begin within 24 hours, are usually vague, and almost always resolve by 48 hours. Preparing the patient for the possibility goes a long way in reassuring and meeting their expectations from treatment. As with all manipulative interventions, the intensity is generally less than the symptoms and disability experienced by the patient before treatment, the localisation varies, and the duration is relatively brief.

CONCLUSION

Inhibition or the use of pressure on dysfunctional areas is one of the oldest forms of treatment. PINS represents a variant of the more traditional approach to using inhibition. Standard methods of palpatory and other techniques of palpatory diagnosis are utilised. PINS offers a theoretical model for searching out the primary and related locations that maintain somatic dysfunction. As a technique, it follows a theoretical framework while allowing for adaptations based on the palpatory findings. As a modality, it can be used solely or in combination with other methods of manipulation. Even though it bears some similarities to previously described methods, PINS is distinctive enough to warrant inclusion as an individual method of osteopathic manipulation. Knowledge of physiology and anatomy is necessary for the determination of primary and end points, as well as of the intervening points. Further adaptations may be necessary for analysis of alterations from the norm, the patient's subjective responses, and the use of appropriate low-level force to inhibit specific connected locations leads to reduction of the underlying aetiology. Rather than being used exclusively, if there are still remnants of the dysfunction, other manipulative techniques should be employed. Previously ineffective treatment modalities may be attempted after PINS, and may then be found to be more effective.

PINS does require an investment of time. The amount of time can be anywhere from 2 to 10 minutes, depending on the process of locating and treating the number of points. Compared with other methods, this may seem excessive: some other point techniques, such as facilitated positional release, take only a few seconds, and strain/counterstrain typically takes 90 seconds. However, when typical interventions are of limited success with recalcitrant dysfunctions, alternative means are required. PINS, by eliminating inappropriately maintained reflexes, restrictions and abnormal function, can be a tool utilised to facilitate the person's intrinsic function. By freeing the restricted elements, this maximises the individual's self-healing and repair functions.

REFERENCES

American Osteopathic Association 1998 Glossary of Osteopathic Terminology 1998 American Osteopathic Association Yearbook and Directory of Osteopathic Practitioners. AOA, Chicago, Illinois

Bailey HW 1976 Some problems in making osteopathic spinal manipulative therapy appropriate and specific. Journal of the American Osteopathic Association 75: 486–499

Becker RF 1976 The gamma system and its relation to the development and maintenance of muscle tone. In: 1976 year book of the American Academy of Osteopathy, pp 26–40. American Academy of Osteopathy, Colorado Springs

Burton Goldberg Group 1994 Alternative medicine: the definitive guide. Future Medicine Publishing, Puyallup, Washington

Buzzell KA 1967 The potential disruptive influence of somatic input. In: The physiological basis of osteopathic medicine, pp 39–51. Postgraduate Institute of Osteopathic Medicine and Surgery, Insight Publishing, New York

Cerney JV 1974 Acupuncture without needles. Parker Publishing, West Nyack, New York

Chaitow L 1980 Neuro-muscular technique. Thorsons, Wellingborough, UK

Chaitow L 1990 Osteopathic self-treatment. Thorsons, Wellingborough, UK

Chaitow L 1996 Modern neuromuscular techniques. Churchill Livingstone, New York

Chila AG 1997 Fascial – ligamentous release: an indirect approach. In: Ward RC, ed. Foundations for osteopathic medicine, pp 819–830. Williams & Wilkins, Baltimore

Cyriax J 1959 Text-book of orthopaedic medicine. vol. II: Treatment by manipulation and message. 6th edn. Harper & Row, New York

Dowling DJ 1997 Myofascial release techniques. In: DiGiovanna EL & Schiowitz S, eds. An osteopathic approach to diagnosis and treatment. 2nd edn, pp 381–383. Lippincott-Raven, Philadelphia

Dowling DJ 1998 S.T.A.R.: a more viable alternative descriptor system of somatic dysfunction. American Academy of Osteopathy Journal 8(2):34–37

Dowling DJ 2000 Progressive inhibition of neuromuscular structures (PINS) technique. Journal of the American Osteopathic Association 100(5):285–297.

Dowling DJ & Scariati PD 1997 Neurophysiology relevant to osteopathic principles and practice. In: DiGiovanna EL & Schiowitz S, eds. An osteopathic approach to diagnosis and treatment. 2nd edn, p 33. Lippincott-Raven, Philadelphia

Dvorak J & Dvorak V 1990 Manual medicine: diagnostics. 2nd edn. Thieme, New York

Ehrenfeuchter WC 1997 Soft tissue techniques. In: Ward RC, ed. Foundations for osteopathic medicine, pp 781–794. Williams & Wilkins, Baltimore

Ganong WF 1995 Review of medical physiology. Lange

Glover JC, Yates HA 1997 Strain and counterstrain techniques. In: Ward RC, ed. Foundations for osteopathic medicine, pp 809–818. Williams & Wilkins, Baltimore

Goetz EW 1905 Manual of osteopathy. 2nd edn. Cincinnati, Ohio

Hazzard C 1905 The practice and applied therapeutics of osteopathy.

Hermann E 1965 The D.O. October: 163–164

Johnston WL 1997 Functional technique: an indirect method. In: Ward RC, ed. Foundations for osteopathic medicine, pp 795–808. Williams & Wilkins, Baltimore

Jones LH 1981 Strain and counterstrain. American Academy of Osteopathy. Newark, Ohio

Jones LH, Kusenose R, Goering E 1995 Jones strain–counterstrain. Jones Strain–Counterstrain Company, Boise, Idaho

Kenyon J 1988 Acupressure techniques: a self help guide. Healing Arts Press, Rochester, Vermont

Korr IM 1976 Proprioceptors and somatic dysfunction. In: 1976 year book of the American Academy of Osteopathy, pp 41–50. American Academy of Osteopathy, Colorado Springs, Colorado

Korr IM 1979a Neurochemical and neurotrophic consequences of nerve deformation: clinical implications in relation to spinal manipulation. Journal of the American Osteopathic Association 75:409–414 (reprinted in: The collected papers of Irvin M Korr, pp 196–199. American Academy of Osteopathy, Colorado Springs)

Korr IM 1979b Proprioceptors and somatic dysfunction. Journal of the American Osteopathic Association 74:638–650 (reprinted in: The collected papers of Irvin M Korr, pp 200–207. American Academy of Osteopathy, Colorado Springs)

Korr IM 1979c The nature and basis of the trophic function of nerves: outline of a research program. Journal of the American Osteopathic Association 66:74–78 (reprinted in: The collected papers of Irvin M Korr, pp 96–99. American Academy of Osteopathy, Colorado Springs)

Korr IM, Appeltauer GS 1979 Continued studies on the axonal transport of nerve proteins to muscle. Journal of the American Osteopathic Association 69:76–78 (reprinted in: The collected papers of Irvin M Korr, pp 100–101. American Academy of Osteopathy, Colorado Springs)

Moore KL 1980 Clinically oriented anatomy. Williams & Wilkins, London

Owens C 1937 An endocrine interpretation of Chapman's reflexes. 2nd edn. Chattanooga Printing and Engraving Company, Chattanooga, Tennessee

Patterson MM 1976 A model mechanism for spinal segmental facilitation. Journal of the American Osteopathic Association 76:62–72

Prudden B 1980 Pain erasure: the Bonnie Prudden way. Ballantine Books, New York

Robbins SL, Cotran RS, Kumar V 1984 Pathologic basis of disease. 3rd edn. WB Saunders, Philadelphia

Schiowitz S 1997 In: DiGiovanna & Schiowitz S, eds. An osteopathic approach to diagnosis and treatment. 2nd edn, p 91. Lippincott-Raven, Philadelphia

Schultz W 1976 Shiatsu: Japanese finger pressure therapy. Bell Publishing, New York

Still AT 1902 The philosophy and mechanical principles of osteopathy. Hudson-Kimberly, Kansas City, Missouri

Still AT 1908 Autobiography of AT Still. Revised edn. Self-published, Kirksville, Missouri

Stoddard A 1969 Manual of osteopathic practice. Hutchinson Medical, London

Tasker DD 1916 Principles of osteopathy. 4th edn. Bireley & Elson, Los Angeles

Travell JG, Simmons DG 1983 Myofascial pain and dysfunction: the trigger point manual. Vol. I: The upper extremities. Williams & Wilkins, Baltimore

Typaldos S 1994 Introducing the fascial distortion model. American Academy of Osteopathy Journal 4(2)

van Buskirk VL 1996 A manipulative technique of Andrew Taylor Still as reported by Charles Hazzard, DO, in 1905. Journal of the American Osteopathic Association 96(10):597–602

Ward RC 1997 Integrated neuromusculoskeletal release and myofascial release: an introduction to diagnosis and treatment. In: Ward RC, ed. Foundations for osteopathic medicine, pp 846–849. Williams & Wilkins, Baltimore

Weil A 1995 Spontaneous healing. Ballantine Books, New York

Index

Numbers in **bold** refer to figures and tables

Multimedia CD-ROM
Single User License Agreement

1. NOTICE. WE ARE WILLING TO LICENSE THE MULTI-MEDIA PROGRAM PRODUCT TITLED *Modern Neuromuscular Techniques 2e* ("MULTIMEDIA PROGRAM") TO YOU ONLY ON THE CONDITION THAT YOU ACCEPT ALL OF THE TERMS CONTAINED IN THIS LICENSE AGREEMENT. PLEASE READ THIS LICENSE AGREEMENT CAREFULLY BEFORE OPENING THE SEALED DISK PACKAGE. BY OPENING THAT PACKAGE YOU AGREE TO BE BOUND BY THE TERMS OF THIS AGREEMENT. IF YOU DO NOT AGREE TO THESE TERMS WE ARE UNWILLING TO LICENSE THE MULTIMEDIA PROGRAME TO YOU, AND YOU SHOULD NOT OPEN THE DISK PACKAGE. IN SUCH CASE, PROMPTLY RETURN THE UNOPENED DISK PACKAGE AND ALL OTHER MATERIAL IN THIS PACKAGE, ALONG WITH PROOF OF PAYMENT, TO THE AUTHORISED DEALER FROM WHOM YOU OBTAINED IT FOR A FULL REFUND OF THE PRICE YOU PAID.

2. **Ownership and License**. This is a license agreement and NOT an agreement for sale. It permits you to use one copy of the MULTIMEDIA PROGRAM on a single computer. The MULTIMEDIA PROGRAM and its contents are owned by us or our licensors, and are protected by U.S. and international copyright laws. Your rights to use the MULTIMEDIA PROGRAM are specified in this Agreement, and we retain all rights not expressly granted to you in this Agreement.

- You may use one copy of the MULTIMEDIA PROGRAM on a single computer
- After you have installed the MULTIMEDIA PROGRAM on your computer, you may use the MULTIMEDIA PROGRAM on a different computer only if you first delete the files installed by the installation program from the first computer.
- You may not copy any portion of the MULTIMEDIA PROGRAM to your computer hard disk or any other media other than printing out or downloading non-substantial portions of the text and images in the MULTIMEDIA PROGRAM for your own internal informational use.
- Your may not copy any of the documentation or other printed materials accompanying the MULTIMEDIA PROGRAM.

Neither concurrent use on two or more computers nor use in a local area network or other network is permitted without separate authorisation and the payment of additional license fees.

3. **Transfer and Other Restrictions**. You may not rent, lend, or lease this MULTIMEDIA PROGRAM. Save as permitted by law, you may not and you may not permit others to (a) disassemble, decompile, or otherwise derive source code from the software included in the MULTIMEDIA PROGRAM (the "Software"), (b) reverse engineer the Software, (c) modify or prepare derivative works of the MULTIMEDIA PROGRAM (d) use the Software in an on-line system, or (e) use the MULTIMEDIA PROGRAM in any manner that infringes on the intellectual property or other rights of another party.

However, you may transfer this license to use the MULTI-MEDIA PROGRAM to another party on a permanent basis by transferring this copy of the License Agreement, the MULTIMEDIA PROGRAM, and all documentation. Such transfer of possession terminates your license from us. Such other party shall be licensed under the terms of this Agreement upon its acceptance of this Agreement by its initial use of the MULTIMEDIA PROGRAM. If you transfer the MULTIMEDIA PROGRAM, you must remove the installation files from your hard disk and you may not retain any copies of those files for your own use.

4. **Limited Warranty and Limitation of Liability**. For a period of sixty (60) days from the date you acquired the MULTIMEDIA PROGRAM from us or our authorised dealer, we warrant that the media containing the MULTIMEDIA PROGRAM will be free from defects that prevent you from installing the MULTIMEDIA PROGRAM on your computer. If the disk fails to conform to this warranty you may as your sole and exclusive remedy, obtain a replacement free of charge if you return the defective disk to us with a dated proof of purchase. Otherwise the MULTIMEDIA PROGRAM is licensed to you on an "AS IS" basis without any warranty of any nature.

WE DO NOT WARRANT THAT THE MULTIMEDIA PROGRAM WILL MEET YOUR REQUIREMENTS OR THAT ITS OPERATION WILL BE UNINTERRUPTED OR ERROR-FREE. THE EXPRESS TERMS OF THIS AGREEMENT ARE IN LIEU OF ALL WARRANTIES, CONDITIONS, UNDERTAKINGS, TERMS AND OBLIGATIONS IMPLIED BY STATUTE, COMMON LAW, TRADE USAGE, COURSE OF DEALING OR OTHERWISE ALL OF WHICH ARE HEREBY EXCLUDED TO THE FULLEST EXTENT PERMITTED BY LAW, INCLUDING THE IMPLIED WARRANTIES OF SATISFACTORY QUALITY AND FITNESS FOR A PARTICULAR PURPOSE.

WE SHALL NOT BE LIABLE FOR ANY DAMAGE OR LOSS OF ANY KIND (EXCEPT PERSONAL INJURY OR DEATH RESULTING FROM OUR NEGLIGENCE) ARISING OUT OF OR RESULTING FROM YOUR POSSESSION OR USE OF THE MULTIMEDIA PROGRAM (INCLUDING DATA LOSS OR CORRUPTION), REGARDLESS OF WHETHER SUCH LIABILITY IS BASED IN TORT, CONTRACT OR OTHERWISE AND INCLUDING, BUT NOT LIMITED TO, ACTUAL, SPECIAL, INDIRECT, INCIDENTAL OR CONSEQUENTIAL DAMAGES. IF THE FOREGOING LIMITATION IS HELD TO BE UNENFORCEABLE OUR MAXIMUM LIABILITY TO YOU SHALL NOT EXCEED THE AMOUNT OF THE LICENSE FEE PAID BY YOU FOR THE MULTIMEDIA PROGRAM. THE REMEDIES AVAILABLE TO YOU AGAINST US AND THE LICENSORS OF MATERIALS INCLUDED IN THE MULTIMEDIA PROGRAM ARE EXCLUSIVE.

5. **Termination.** This license and your right to use this MULTIMEDIA PROGRAM automatically terminate if you fail to comply with any provisions of this Agreement, destroy the copy of the MULTIMEDIA PROGRAM in your possession, or voluntarily return the MULTIMEDIA PROGRAM to us. Upon termination you will destroy all copies of the MULTIMEDIA PROGRAM and documentation.

6. **Miscellaneous Provisions.** This Agreement will be governed by and construed in accordance with English law and you hereby submit to the non-exclusive jurisdiction of the English Courts. This is the entire agreement between us relating to the MULTIMEDIA PROGRAM, and supersedes any prior purchase order, communications, advertising or representations concerning the contents of this package, No change or modification of this Agreement will be valid unless it is in writing and is signed by us.